Advancements in Artificial Intelligence for Dentomaxillofacial Radiology

Advancements in Artificial Intelligence for Dentomaxillofacial Radiology

Guest Editors

Andre Luiz Ferreira Costa
Kaan Orhan
Sérgio Lúcio Pereira de Castro Lopes

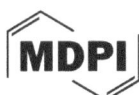

Basel • Beijing • Wuhan • Barcelona • Belgrade • Novi Sad • Cluj • Manchester

Guest Editors

Andre Luiz Ferreira Costa
Postgraduate Program in
Dentistry
Cruzeiro do Sul University
(UNICSUL)
São Paulo
Brazil

Kaan Orhan
Department of
Dentomaxillofacial Radiology
Ankara University
Ankara
Turkey

Sérgio Lúcio Pereira de
Castro Lopes
Department of Diagnosis and
Surgery
São Paulo State University
(UNESP)
São José dos Campos
Brazil

Editorial Office
MDPI AG
Grosspeteranlage 5
4052 Basel, Switzerland

This is a reprint of the Special Issue, published open access by the journal *Diagnostics* (ISSN 2075-4418), freely accessible at: https://www.mdpi.com/journal/diagnostics/special_issues/W73BWEI0B6.

For citation purposes, cite each article independently as indicated on the article page online and as indicated below:

Lastname, A.A.; Lastname, B.B. Article Title. *Journal Name* **Year**, *Volume Number*, Page Range.

ISBN 978-3-7258-4269-8 (Hbk)
ISBN 978-3-7258-4270-4 (PDF)
https://doi.org/10.3390/books978-3-7258-4270-4

© 2025 by the authors. Articles in this book are Open Access and distributed under the Creative Commons Attribution (CC BY) license. The book as a whole is distributed by MDPI under the terms and conditions of the Creative Commons Attribution-NonCommercial-NoDerivs (CC BY-NC-ND) license (https://creativecommons.org/licenses/by-nc-nd/4.0/).

Contents

Preface . . . . **vii**

Kaan Orhan, Andre Luiz Ferreira Costa and Sérgio Lúcio Pereira de Castro Lopes
Closing Editorial: Advancements in Artificial Intelligence for Dentomaxillofacial Radiology—Current Trends and Future Directions
Reprinted from: *Diagnostics* **2025**, *15*, 1222, https://doi.org/10.3390/diagnostics15101222 . . . . **1**

Kader Azlağ Pekince, Adem Pekince and Buse Yaren Kazangirler
Improving TMJ Diagnosis: A Deep Learning Approach for Detecting Mandibular Condyle Bone Changes
Reprinted from: *Diagnostics* **2025**, *15*, 1022, https://doi.org/10.3390/diagnostics15081022 . . . . **4**

Serap Akdoğan, Muhammet Üsame Öziç and Melek Tassoker
Development of an AI-Supported Clinical Tool for Assessing Mandibular Third Molar Tooth Extraction Difficulty Using Panoramic Radiographs and YOLO11 Sub-Models
Reprinted from: *Diagnostics* **2025**, *15*, 462, https://doi.org/10.3390/diagnostics15040462 . . . . . **22**

Gulfem Ozlu Ucan, Omar Abboosh Hussein Gwassi, Burak Kerem Apaydin and Bahadir Ucan
Automated Age Estimation from OPG Images and Patient Records Using Deep Feature Extraction and Modified Genetic–Random Forest
Reprinted from: *Diagnostics* **2025**, *15*, 314, https://doi.org/10.3390/diagnostics15030314 . . . . . **45**

Can Arslan, Nesli Ozum Yucel, Kaan Kahya, Ezgi Sunal Akturk and Derya Germec Cakan
Artificial Intelligence for Tooth Detection in Cleft Lip and Palate Patients
Reprinted from: *Diagnostics* **2024**, *14*, 2849, https://doi.org/10.3390/diagnostics14242849 . . . . **72**

Wojciech Kazimierczak, Róża Wajer, Oskar Komisarek, Marta Dyszkiewicz-Konwińska, Adrian Wajer, Natalia Kazimierczak, et al.
Evaluation of a Vendor-Agnostic Deep Learning Model for Noise Reduction and Image Quality Improvement in Dental CBCT
Reprinted from: *Diagnostics* **2024**, *14*, 2410, https://doi.org/10.3390/diagnostics14212410 . . . . **84**

Hakan Amasya, Mustafa Alkhader, Gözde Serindere, Karolina Futyma-Gąbka, Ceren Aktuna Belgin, Maxim Gusarev, et al.
Evaluation of a Decision Support System Developed with Deep Learning Approach for Detecting Dental Caries with Cone-Beam Computed Tomography Imaging
Reprinted from: *Diagnostics* **2023**, *13*, 3471, https://doi.org/10.3390/diagnostics13223471 . . . . **99**

Wael I. Ibraheem
Accuracy of Artificial Intelligence Models in Dental Implant Fixture Identification and Classification from Radiographs: A Systematic Review
Reprinted from: *Diagnostics* **2024**, *14*, 806, https://doi.org/10.3390/diagnostics14080806 . . . . . **114**

Bogdan Constantin Costăchel, Anamaria Bechir, Mihail Târcolea, Lelia Laurenţa Mihai, Alexandru Burcea and Edwin Sever Bechir
The Stresses and Deformations in the Abfraction Lesions of the Lower Premolars Studied by the Finite Element Analyses: Case Report and Review of Literature
Reprinted from: *Diagnostics* **2024**, *14*, 788, https://doi.org/10.3390/diagnostics14080788 . . . . . **135**

Preface

This Special Issue Reprint of *Diagnostics*, titled "Advancements in Artificial Intelligence for Dentomaxillofacial Radiology", brings together a curated selection of original research articles and reviews that highlight current trends, novel methodologies, and emerging technologies in the field of oral and maxillofacial imaging. The contributions focus particularly on the integration of artificial intelligence (AI), radiomics, and advanced imaging techniques, which are increasingly shaping the future of diagnostics in dentistry and maxillofacial care.

This Special Issue aimed to provide a platform for interdisciplinary dialogue between clinicians, radiologists, computer scientists, and researchers involved in the development and clinical application of AI-driven tools. As oral health care enters the era of precision diagnostics, it becomes critical to explore how imaging modalities such as cone-beam computed tomography (CBCT), magnetic resonance imaging (MRI), and digital radiography can be enhanced through machine learning and texture analysis to improve diagnostic accuracy, treatment planning, and patient outcomes.

This reprint is addressed to a diverse audience, including dental practitioners, oral and maxillofacial radiologists, researchers in dental imaging, as well as data scientists interested in biomedical image analysis. By compiling these innovative contributions, we hope to support ongoing research and stimulate new approaches to diagnostic challenges in oral health.

We extend our sincere thanks to all the authors who contributed their work, to the reviewers for their critical insights, and to the editorial team of *Diagnostics* for their continuous support throughout the peer-review and publication process. Their dedication ensured the scientific rigour and high quality of the articles featured in this issue.

Andre Luiz Ferreira Costa, Kaan Orhan, and Sérgio Lúcio Pereira de Castro Lopes
Guest Editors

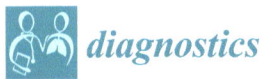

Editorial

Closing Editorial: Advancements in Artificial Intelligence for Dentomaxillofacial Radiology—Current Trends and Future Directions

Kaan Orhan [1,2,3,*], Andre Luiz Ferreira Costa [4] and Sérgio Lúcio Pereira de Castro Lopes [5]

[1] Department of Dentomaxillofacial Radiology, Faculty of Dentistry, Ankara University, Ankara 06560, Turkey
[2] Department of Dental and Maxillofacial Radiodiagnostics, Medical University of Lublin, 20-059 Lublin, Poland
[3] Medical Design Application and Research Center (MEDITAM), Ankara University, Ankara 06000, Turkey
[4] Postgraduate Program in Dentistry, Cruzeiro do Sul University (UNICSUL), São Paulo 08060-070, SP, Brazil; alfcosta@gmail.com
[5] Department of Diagnosis and Surgery, São José dos Campos School of Dentistry, São Paulo State University (UNESP), São José dos Campos 12245-000, SP, Brazil; sergio.lopes@unesp.br
* Correspondence: knorhan@dentistry.ankara.edu.tr; Tel.: +90-(312)-296-5504

Artificial intelligence (AI) continues to redefine diagnostic approaches across medical disciplines, and its impact on dentomaxillofacial radiology has increased exponentially in recent years. With advances in deep learning (DL), large annotated datasets, and computational power, AI has become a powerful tool in analyzing complex craniofacial imaging data, offering precision, speed, and reproducibility beyond human capacity in many contexts.

This Special Issue of *Diagnostics*, entitled "Advancements in Artificial Intelligence for Dentomaxillofacial Radiology", sought to capture this dynamic shift by curating original research and reviews that span the spectrum of AI applications in dental imaging—from traditional 2D panoramic radiography to 3D CBCT and emerging dental MRI technologies.

A key focus of this Issue was on algorithmic performance in real-world diagnostic scenarios. Contributions employing YOLOv8 and similar architectures demonstrated the near-perfect detection of critical anatomical structures, including the mandibular canal, condyles, and dental implants, across variable image qualities and devices. These studies reflect a crucial trend toward the development of device-agnostic AI models with clinically reliable precision. For instance, George et al. (2023) analyzed panoramic dental radiographs using the YOLOv8 model and examined its effectiveness for diagnosis [1].

Segmentation-based models also featured prominently. U-Net, nnU-Net, and U^2-Net-based frameworks were used to delineate pulp chambers, periapical lesions, and maxillofacial bones, yielding Dice Similarity Coefficients (DSCs) above 0.90 in most cases. These models not only enhance reproducibility but also facilitate downstream applications such as volumetric assessment, AI-assisted treatment planning, and augmented surgical navigation. For example, Baydar et al. (2023) utilized a U-Net architecture to evaluate dental bite-wing radiographs, achieving high accuracy in detecting various dental conditions [2].

Of particular interest are the articles examining explainability—a growing imperative in AI-driven diagnostics. Black-box models, while powerful, face resistance in clinical implementation, being without interpretability. Research using Grad-CAM, SHAP, and attention maps demonstrated how AI can transparently highlight diagnostic cues, thereby improving clinician trust and legal defensibility. A scoping review by Ghosh et al. (2023)

emphasized the importance of interpretability and explainability in medical AI applications, highlighting the need for transparent models in clinical settings [3].

Despite these strides, several barriers remain. First, model generalizability is often limited by dataset homogeneity. Even the most promising models can falter when applied to imaging protocols or populations not represented in the training data. Second, integration into clinical workflow requires alignment with standards like DICOM, PACS systems, and regulatory approval pathways (e.g., CE/FDA clearances). Third, few studies have addressed longitudinal AI model performance or outcomes-based validation in dental radiology—critical aspects for widespread adoption [4–11].

Future research should aim to achieve the following objectives:

- Multimodal fusion—combining radiographic, intraoral, and clinical data for holistic AI-based diagnostics [8].
- Real-time integration—deploying AI tools at the point of care, especially in underserved areas or during tele-dentistry sessions [9].
- Texture analysis as a valuable technique in dentomaxillofacial diagnosis, providing an advanced method for quantification and characterization of different image modalities [10].
- Ethical AI frameworks—ensuring bias mitigation, privacy preservation, and transparent model auditing across global dental populations [11].

This Special Issue was enriched by contributions from researchers across multiple continents, reflecting the global relevance of AI in oral and maxillofacial imaging. The breadth of work underscores both the maturity and future potential of this interdisciplinary field. We thank all authors, reviewers, and editorial staff for their efforts and encourage readers to build on the strong foundation laid by this collection.

We hope the studies here serve as a catalyst for translational research and encourage the deeper integration of AI into dental radiology education, clinical care, and policymaking [4–11].

Author Contributions: Conceptualization, K.O., A.L.F.C. and S.L.P.d.C.L.; writing—original draft preparation, K.O.; writing—review and editing, A.L.F.C. and S.L.P.d.C.L.; supervision, K.O.; project administration, K.O. All authors have read and agreed to the published version of the manuscript.

Funding: This research received no external funding.

Conflicts of Interest: The authors declare no conflicts of interest.

References

1. George, A.; Hemanth, D.J. Dental Radiography Analysis and Diagnosis Using YOLOv8. ResearchGate. 2023. Available online: https://www.researchgate.net/publication/376283755_Dental_Radiography_Analysis_and_Diagnosis_using_YOLOv8 (accessed on 1 May 2025).
2. Baydar, O.; Różyło-Kalinowska, I.; Futyma-Gąbka, K.; Sağlam, H. The U-Net Approaches to Evaluation of Dental Bite-Wing Radiographs: An Artificial Intelligence Study. *Diagnostics* **2023**, *13*, 453. [CrossRef] [PubMed]
3. Champendal, M.; Müller, H.; Prior, J.O.; Dos Reis, C.S. A scoping review of interpretability and explainability concerning artificial intelligence methods in medical imaging. *Eur. J. Radiol.* **2023**, *169*, 111159. [CrossRef] [PubMed]
4. Altındağ, A.; Bahrilli, S.; Çelik, Ö.; Bayrakdar, İ.Ş.; Orhan, K. The Detection of Pulp Stones with Automatic Deep Learning in Panoramic Radiographies: An AI Pilot Study. *Diagnostics* **2024**, *14*, 890. [CrossRef] [PubMed]
5. Bayati, M.; Savareh, B.A.; Ahmadinejad, H.; Mosavat, F. Advanced AI-driven detection of interproximal caries in bitewing radiographs using YOLOv8. *Sci. Rep.* **2025**, *15*, 4641. [CrossRef] [PubMed]
6. Wang, Y.C.C.; Chen, T.L.; Vinayahalingam, S.; Wu, T.H.; Chang, C.W.; Chang, H.H.; Wei, H.J.; Chen, M.H.; Ko, C.C.; Moin, D.A.; et al. Artificial Intelligence to Assess Dental Findings from Panoramic Radiographs—A Multinational Study. *arXiv* **2025**, arXiv:2502.10277. [CrossRef]
7. Budagam, D.; Kumar, A.; Ghosh, S.; Shrivastav, A.; Imanbayev, A.Z.; Akhmetov, I.R.; Kaplun, D.; Antonov, S.; Rychenkov, A.; Cyganov, G.; et al. Instance Segmentation and Teeth Classification in Panoramic X-rays. *arXiv* **2024**, arXiv:2406.03747. [CrossRef]

8. Xu, X.; Li, J.; Zhu, Z.; Zhao, L.; Wang, H.; Song, C.; Chen, Y.; Zhao, Q.; Yang, J.; Pei, Y. A Comprehensive Review on Synergy of Multi-Modal Data and AI Technologies in Medical Diagnosis. *Bioengineering* **2024**, *11*, 219. [CrossRef] [PubMed]
9. Abdat, M.; Herwanda Jannah, M.; Soraya, C. Detection of caries and determination of treatment needs using DentMA teledentistry: A deep learning approach. *Dent. J.* **2024**, *57*, 62–67. [CrossRef]
10. Barioni, E.D.; Lopes, S.L.P.C.; Silvestre, P.R.; Yasuda, C.L.; Costa, A.L.F. Texture Analysis in Volumetric Imaging for Dentomaxillofacial Radiology: Transforming Diagnostic Approaches and Future Directions. *J. Imaging* **2024**, *10*, 263. [CrossRef] [PubMed]
11. Topol, E.J. High-performance medicine: The convergence of human and artificial intelligence. *Nat. Med.* **2019**, *25*, 44–56. [CrossRef] [PubMed]

Disclaimer/Publisher's Note: The statements, opinions and data contained in all publications are solely those of the individual author(s) and contributor(s) and not of MDPI and/or the editor(s). MDPI and/or the editor(s) disclaim responsibility for any injury to people or property resulting from any ideas, methods, instructions or products referred to in the content.

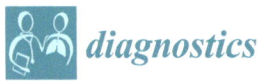

Article

Improving TMJ Diagnosis: A Deep Learning Approach for Detecting Mandibular Condyle Bone Changes

Kader Azlağ Pekince [1], Adem Pekince [1,*] and Buse Yaren Kazangirler [2,3]

[1] Department of Oral and Maxillofacial Radiology, Karabuk University, Karabuk 78600, Turkey; azlagkader@karabuk.edu.tr
[2] Department of Computer Engineering, Karabuk University, Karabuk 78600, Turkey; buseyaren@uky.edu or byarenkazangirler@gmail.com
[3] Department of Internal Medicine, University of Kentucky, Lexington, KY 40506, USA
* Correspondence: adempekince@karabuk.edu.tr; Tel.: +90-4440478-1201; Fax: +90-370-4187880

Abstract: Objectives: This paper evaluates the potential of using deep learning approaches for the detection of degenerative bone changes in the mandibular condyle. The aim of this study is to enable the detection and diagnosis of mandibular condyle degenerations, which are difficult to observe and diagnose on panoramic radiographs, using deep learning methods. **Methods**: A total of 3875 condylar images were obtained from panoramic radiographs. Condylar bone changes were represented by flattening, osteophyte, and erosion, and images in which two or more of these changes were observed were labeled as "other". Due to the limited number of images containing osteophytes and erosion, two approaches were used. In the first approach, images containing osteophytes and erosion were combined into the "other" group, resulting in three groups: normal, flattening, and deformation ("deformation" encompasses the "other" group, together with osteophyte and erosion). In the second approach, images containing osteophytes and erosion were completely excluded, resulting in three groups: normal, flattening, and other. The study utilizes a range of advanced deep learning algorithms, including Dense Networks, Residual Networks, VGG Networks, and Google Networks, which are pre-trained with transfer learning techniques. Model performance was evaluated using datasets with different distributions, specifically 70:30 and 80:20 training-test splits. **Results**: The GoogleNet architecture achieved the highest accuracy. Specifically, with the 80:20 split of the normal-flattening-deformation dataset and the Adamax optimizer, an accuracy of 95.23% was achieved. The results demonstrate that CNN-based methods are highly successful in determining mandibular condyle bone changes. **Conclusions**: This study demonstrates the potential of deep learning, particularly CNNs, for the accurate and efficient detection of TMJ-related condylar bone changes from panoramic radiographs. This approach could assist clinicians in identifying patients requiring further intervention. Future research may involve using cross-sectional imaging methods and training the right and left condyles together to potentially increase the success rate. This approach has the potential to improve the early detection of TMJ-related condylar bone changes, enabling timely referrals and potentially preventing disease progression.

Keywords: temporomandibular joint; mandibular condyle; degenerative bone changes; deep learning; convolutional neural networks; panoramic radiography

1. Introduction

The temporomandibular joint (TMJ) is a pair of joints formed by the articulation of the mandibular bone with the temporal bones, located symmetrically on both sides of the head.

The space between the condylar process of the mandibular bone and the articular fossa of the temporal bone is divided into upper and lower joint compartments by the articular disc. This joint is supported by ligaments.

Due to its anatomical structure, the temporomandibular joint can move in three planes. This allows the physiological movements of speaking, chewing and swallowing to be easily performed. These physiological movements are made possible by the combination of the elevation–depression, protrusion–retraction and lateral translation movements [1,2] of the TMJ. The TMJs are connected via the mandible, which adds to the complexity of these movements. Although each TMJ is an independent joint [3,4], they move together and affect each other's direction and range of motion.

Exceeding the physiological limits of joint movements, infections, trauma, or biological factors can cause pain and dysfunction in the chewing muscles and TMJ. This condition is called temporomandibular disorder (TMD). TMD can progress from disc dysfunction to osteoarthritis, but this outcome is not always certain. In cases where osteoarthritis does develop, radiographic findings are often seen in the mandibular condyle and articular eminence [5].

TMD is a common health problem that significantly reduces quality of life, affecting an average of 34% (Asia—33%, South America—47%, North America—26%, Europe—29%) of the world's population according to a meta-analysis study [6]. Okeson has classified TMDs into muscle-related disorders, disc displacements, inflammatory joint diseases, and genetic and acquired anatomical abnormalities. This classification demonstrates that TMD encompasses a broad spectrum of diverse pathologies and can manifest with a variety of symptoms.

Temporomandibular joint osteoarthritis, an inflammatory joint disease and a subtype of TMD, is one of the most frequently observed degenerative joint disorders. Osteoarthritis is a painful inflammatory condition. Osteoarthritis is defined by clinical symptoms and radiological signs [7]. It causes changes in the joint surfaces and arises as a consequence of disc displacement, trauma, functional overload, and developmental anomalies [8]. These factors contribute to the joint components being loaded beyond their adaptive capacity, and in some instances, to their exposure to prolonged and destructive loads [9]. This scenario initiates a physiological process characterized by degenerative changes in the bones, aimed at accommodating the joint surfaces to the functional demands [10]. As these processes persist and advance, morphological alterations manifest in the bones. Such alterations are more prevalent in the mandibular condyle than in the glenoid fossa or articular eminence [11]. Degenerative bone changes occurring in the TMJ can be observed as erosion, osteophyte formation, sclerosis and subcortical cyst formation in the mandibular condyle [8,12].

Often the arthritic condition can become adaptive once the load is reduced, but the bony morphology remains altered. The adaptive stage is known as osteoarthrosis.

Osteoarthritis and osteoarthrosis are classified as degenerative joint diseases (DJD) of the temporomandibular joint [5].

Meta-analysis findings revealed that TMJ DJD is observed in 10% of the general adult population and ranges from 18% to 85% among patients with TMD [13]. Furthermore, a study of elderly people with TMD found that 70% of elderly people had bone changes in their temporomandibular joints, and 69.93% of these changes were seen in the condyles [14].

The multifactorial etiology of TMD leads to a diversity of treatment approaches. In some cases, TMD treatment requires an interdisciplinary approach involving collaboration among specialists. Correct and early diagnosis of this condition, which affects a large segment of society, is critical for determining appropriate treatment strategies and managing the disease.

In some studies conducted to measure the level of knowledge of general dentists about TMD, it was concluded that the level of knowledge of general dentists was inadequate and would be insufficient to provide effective care to patients with TMD [15,16].

Artificial Intelligence (AI) is now widely used in every field, bringing convenience and practicality to every area where it is applied. With the increase in workload and time requirements, AI has become very useful. Today, the application of AI and especially computer vision techniques in the medical field is becoming much more widespread [17]. For this reason, a decision support mechanism that will receive support from AI rather than a determination based on human power is often a preferred solution [18].

Artificial Intelligence (AI), including the development of machine learning tools and neural networks, has developed rapidly over the last decade. Various medical applications have been developed with the support of AI to save clinicians' time during examinations and to demonstrate the ability to make more objective diagnoses [19,20]. Neural network cells used for AI are a type of network that makes up artificial neural networks. In particular, Convolutional Neural Networks (CNN), a type of artificial neural network, are used in detection and image classification studies for image data. Medical imaging technology plays a vital role in several critical applications, from early detection of diseases to surgical planning. Innovative approaches in this field include medical image classification and detection, allowing for faster and more accurate detection of diseases. While traditional classification methods are often inadequate for this complex task, deep learning techniques, especially CNN, have revolutionized this field. These algorithms used by AI can analyze large amounts of clinical data on different diseases and consequently aim to minimize diagnostic and treatment errors that are common in standard clinical settings [21]. CNN are deep learning algorithms for 2D data that take input images and perform convolution with filters or kernels to extract features. Moreover, CNN networks have been proven to outperform experts in many image detection studies and tasks [22]. In particular, CNN algorithms have been chosen for image classification and interpretation, considering that CNN algorithms are a powerful and effective choice in common literature studies of researchers. Thus, in this study, deep learning techniques were developed to make decisions about the clinical condition of patients. As a result, CNNs offer an innovative approach to medical image classification, providing healthcare professionals with powerful applications for more accurate diagnosis and treatment planning. This paper will explore the potential of CNN-based approaches in detecting different condyle degenerative bone changes in TMJ.

Transfer Learning with Convolutional Neural Networks

One of the main reasons why CNNs are especially preferred in medical image classification is the ability to emphasize local features and extract hierarchical features thanks to convolutional layers [9,23]. Transfer learning is a strategy that allows knowledge learned in one task to be used more quickly and effectively in another task. CNN-based transfer learning can improve the model's performance when working with limited datasets in image classification [24]. Moreover, by transferring knowledge from a general dataset to a specialized dataset, transfer learning allows for more specific results in a specific medical application area. Therefore, using transfer learning for CNN networks saves time by avoiding the need to re-learn attributes and weights. Thus, it offers the potential to overcome dataset limitations during the model's training and learning phase and increase its generalization capability [25]. Farook et al. [26], who presented a comprehensive review study for the clinical classification of degenerative disorders in TMJ, presented many approaches to traditional diagnostics obtained from radiographs while addressing the causes of deformations and included studies in the literature in detail. According to the study's results, neural network models learned through deep learning were found to diagnose the detection in 2D or 3D radiographs as accurately as clinicians. According to the research mentioned in the study (depending on the dataset used, types of deformation, etc.), the top-performing deep learning algorithms are usually pretrained algorithms such as Random Forest (RF), Multi-Layer Perceptron (MLP), AlexNet, Support Vector Machine (SVM), Extreme Gradient Boost (XGBoost), LightGBM, Residual Network (ResNet), Visual Geometry Group Network (VGGNet), etc. However, algorithms such as SVM, RF, XGBoost, LightGBM, etc., are frequently used in machine learning and leave feature extraction to the user [27].

Deep learning has revolutionized medical image analysis by enabling more precise and efficient diagnostic processes. This study aims to leverage deep learning techniques, particularly CNNs to enhance the accuracy and efficiency of medical image classification in detecting degenerative bone changes in the TMJ. The selection of pre-trained CNN architectures was guided by their proven effectiveness in medical image classification tasks and their architectural diversity. The purpose of this was to facilitate a comprehensive performance comparison of the models. The models selected for the study were AlexNet, VGG16, VGG19, ResNeXt (18, 101), DenseNet (121, 169, 201), ResNeXt and GoogleNet. It is important to note that these models represent different network depths, connectivity models and parameter efficiencies. The prevailing trend in the field of healthcare towards a greater reliance on AI-driven decision support systems is the focus of this research. The potential of CNN-based models, including pretrained architectures such as AlexNet, VGGNet, ResNet, and DenseNet, to improve diagnostic precision will be explored. Furthermore, transfer learning strategies will be employed to optimize model performance on limited medical imaging data. The integration of cutting-edge deep learning methodologies is a key aspect of this study, with the aim of contributing to the advancement of automated diagnostic tools. These tools are expected to reduce human error and provide clinicians with more objective and reliable assessments. This study uses various proposed CNN architectures to improve the corresponding system performance while keeping the underlying learning topologies constant. In this study, the most widely used pretrained CNN algorithms are AlexNet, VGG16 and VGG19, DenseNet121, DenseNet169, DenseNet201, ResNet18, ResNet101, ResNeXt, and GoogleNet. These algorithms are famous CNN architectures introduced for object recognition and classification tasks [25,28,29].

Several studies have used different radiological methods and classification systems to evaluate temporomandibular joint osteoarthritis. One study [30] examined 3514 cone-beam computed tomography (CBCT) images from 314 patients and classified changes in condylar structure were divided into three groups: no evidence of TMJOA, indeterminate for TMJOA, and evidence of TMJOA. Another study [31] using panoramic radiographs used the same classification system. A separate study [32] of 858 panoramic radiographs classified the presence of osteoarthritis as "osteoarthritis" or "normal".

Bony changes observed in the mandibular condyle may show different variations, ranging from erosion to deformation of the condyle morphology. A detailed classification of these findings provides the clinician with information about the status of the disease.

Given the progressive nature of TMD, early detection of osseous alterations in the mandibular condyle, irrespective of etiology, is important.

Because patients frequently present to general dental practitioners as their initial point of contact, and given the constraints faced by these practitioners in accessing and interpreting CBCT, the significance of panoramic imaging in detecting bone changes is increasing.

Panoramic radiography, which is widely used in routine clinical practice, has the potential to contribute to the early diagnosis of TMD by allowing the evaluation of the temporomandibular joint. Based on previous research, this study aims to comprehensively evaluate the potential of deep learning in detecting and classifying degenerative bone changes of the mandibular condyle on panoramic radiographs through comparative analysis of multiple CNN architectures on a large dataset.

2. Materials and Methods

2.1. Selection, Preparation and Evaluation of Images

For the evaluation of mandibular condyle bone changes, 2300 randomly selected panoramic radiographic images in DICOM format taken between January 2023 and September 2023 from the X-ray archive of Karabük Oral and Dental Health Training and Research Hospital were examined. These images were obtained using the same panoramic radiography device (I-Max touch, Owandy Radiology, Croissy-Beaubourg, France) in accordance with the manufacturer's instructions (80 kV tube voltage, 9 mA and 14.4 s).

2.2. Dataset and Preprocessing Steps

Of the panoramic radiographic images examined by the oromaxillofacial radiology specialist, a total of 725 condylar images were excluded from the study, including 248 with superposition that impaired the observation of condylar borders, 189 with artifacts, and 288 images from 144 individuals under the age of 18. Given that age and sex are not matched in the condyle, all models and results presented in this study could be sex and gender biased. Further research is required to address this limitation in future studies with balanced data. Furthermore, all experiments were performed in a subject-independent manner in the study, meaning that images from the same subject were not used in the training and testing phases. A total of 3875 condylar images from individuals over the age of 18, in which the mandibular condyles could be clearly observed, without artifacts, were included in the study. The study included a total of 3875 subjects with 1 image per subject.

The borders of the mandibular condyle are normally straight, continuous, and convex. Therefore, it is assumed that the outlines of normal condyles should have a convex configuration everywhere and that there should be symmetry between both condyles in the same individual [33]. However, anatomical variations such as slight flattening or pronounced convexity on the upper surface of the condylar head may be seen. In this case, the size and shape of the right and left condylar heads should be compared and the symmetry of both sides should be evaluated [34].

Another preprocessing step is to make the data compatible with CNN algorithms. CNN algorithms typically work in 224 × 224 dimensions. These dimensions may increase and decrease depending on the working structure of CNNs and the feature mapping technique. The images were automatically cropped for the CNN architectures used, and the input data were subjected to specific preprocessing steps to normalize them [21]. This will help the network improve learning performance because transfer learning will be provided with previously learned weights. For the standardization process, normalization was performed using mean values [0.485, 0.456, 0.406] and standard deviation values [0.229, 0.224, 0.225] [22].

In our study, condyles with regular convex and continuous borders were evaluated together with their symmetry and labeled as normal. Condyles that did not meet these criteria, with interrupted borders, straight but not symmetrical or concave borders, were included in the other class. Condyles with mild flattening or significant convexity were included in the normal class when they were symmetrical and were included in the other class when they were unilateral. All condyles with osteoarthritic changes such as erosion and osteophyte formation, other than significant flattening, were labeled as other. Images in which the convexity at the outer borders of the mandibular condyles was disrupted in favor of flattening were labeled as flattening. Images in which the continuity of the outer borders of the condyle was disrupted were labeled as erosion.

In addition, while evaluating condylar bone changes in our study, flattening, osteophyte, erosion and images in which two or more of these changes were observed together were classified as the other group. Images in which condyles with pseudocysts were observed were not evaluated as a separate class because they did not affect the outer borders of the mandibular condyle observed on the panoramic images.

Classifications were made for the study. Since each group did not contain enough images for computer learning, two separate approaches were made for the images belonging to the condyles with erosion and osteophyte formation. In the first approach, osteophyte formation and erosion groups were included in the other group and the images were collected in three groups: normal, flattening and deformation. In the second approach, osteophyte and erosion groups were removed from the study and grouped as normal, flattening and other. The deformation group became a more comprehensive group compared to the other group.

The mandibular condyles were resized to 224×224 (width and height) dimensions to be compatible as input to CNN models. Nonetheless, there was an absence of coordinate labeling of the condyle images. Instead, the mandibular condyles were categorized into clusters by an oromaxillofacial radiologist. This approach is informed by the nature of the study, which is an image classification task. To ensure optimal feature extraction and to focus on clinically relevant areas, a preprocessing step was implemented before feeding images into CNN architectures. Since CNN models require a fixed input size, the following methodology was applied:

Region of Interest (ROI) Selection: Rather than employing full panoramic radiographs, which comprise a large amount of extraneous background information, radiologists manually identified the mandibular condyle regions in the images. The ROIs were then cropped so as to isolate the condylar region. This was performed in order to ensure that the CNN models focus on the most relevant anatomical structures.

Automated Resizing to Proper Sizes: Following the cropping of the ROI, the images were resized to 224×224 pixels by means of bilinear interpolation. This step is of paramount importance as it ensures compatibility with pretrained CNN models while preserving critical features necessary for classification. This approach has been demonstrated to minimize irrelevant variations in input images, thereby improving the data of model focus on clinically significant patterns and optimizing the learning process. A randomly selected 25% of the labelled images were re-examined by the same clinician at a different time to assess intra-observer agreement. The agreement of the results was assessed using Cohen's kappa analysis. SPSS (Statistical Package for Social Sciences) for Windows 20.0 was used for the Kappa test. When the obtained κ value ($\kappa = 0.8$) was interpreted according to Landis and Koch, it was found that there was sufficient agreement.

Mandibular condyle changes: mandibular condyle regions in panoramic radiographs were cropped and labeled by the oromaxillofacial radiology specialist. Mandibular condyle changes and regions in panoramic radiographs were cropped and labeled. Classifications were made for the study. Since each group did not contain enough images for computer learning, two separate approaches were made for condyles with erosion and osteophyte formation images. In the first approach, osteophyte formation and erosion groups were included in the other group, and the images were collected in three groups: normal, flattening, and deformation (N,F,D). The second approach removed osteophytes and erosion groups from the study and grouped them into normal, flattening, and other (N,F,O) groups. The deformation group became a more comprehensive group compared to the other group. A deep learning-based algorithm approach was applied for high-performance detection and classification of condyle bone changes in cropped images as normal, flattening, and other (N,F,O) and normal, flattening, and deformation (N,F,D). The study applied two different datasets to CNN architecture, and their successes were discussed. To develop the Artificial Intelligence (AI) approach, two different sets will be separated into different sets for the training and testing process. In AI applications, randomness should be used as a basis for applying the data to the training and testing process. The set is divided into 70:30 and 80:20 training tests, respectively, as shown in Figure 1. In the experimental findings section of the study, this separated set will reveal the differences in the success of CNN algorithms. Different dataset separations are applied to solve the balance problem.

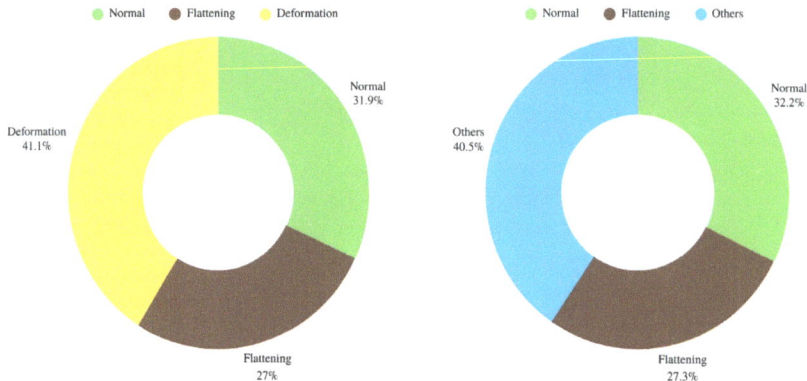

Figure 1. Weighted scatter plot of prepared data classes including normal-flattening-deformation and normal-flattening-others classes.

In AI applications, randomness should be taken as a basis for applying the data to the training and testing process. The set was split into 70:30 and 80:20 training–testing, respectively, as shown in Figure 1. The experimental findings section of the study will reveal the differences in the success of the CNN algorithms. The different separations of the data were applied to solve the balance problem.

The processing step was applied separately for training and testing steps Figure 2 is an architectural visualization representing the working structure of the different CNN architectures proposed for detecting degenerative bone changes in the temporomandibular joints in panoramic images. First, the size of the input images from the TMJ region should be standardized for all instances. The figure shows that this standard form is set to 224 × 224 for the example CNNs. For this reason, the TMJ regions cropped by the oromaxillofacial radiology specialist are scaled to 224 × 224 by a preprocessing step before being fed to the model. Many different architectures were used in this study to access the experimental findings for the pretrained CNN algorithms with version 1.13.1 of the PyTorch library. Therefore, each architecture contains different layers, such as convolution, pooling, etc., in its internal structure. For this reason, a typical internal architecture structure is depicted in Figure 2.

In the present study, a range of pretrained architectures was utilized to assess the efficacy of models. The input data are constituted by an image, upon which sequential mathematical operations are applied in the context of pretrained CNN algorithms. In CNN models, these parameters comprise convolution kernels (filters), weights, and biases of the fully connected layers. For fully connected layers within CNNs, refer to the following sources: the linear transformation is modeled as W weight matrix, b bias term, and X input vector in Equation (1).

$$Y = WX + b \qquad (1)$$

The image X matrix as an input vector denotes the value of each pixel and typically assumes the form of a 3D tensor (height, width, number of channels. In this context, the prediction function of the model is denoted by $\hat{y} = f(X, \theta)$. According to the specified equation, X denotes the input data received by the model. The class prediction function is usually expressed as $\hat{y}$ is the class or probability distribution predicted by the model. In the context of an image-based AI model, X corresponds to an image matrix. Conversely, θ encompasses the weights and bias values that the model must learn. Furthermore, the Rectified Linear Unit (ReLU) function, a widely utilized activation function, is formulated in Equation (2).

$$ReLU(x) = \max(0, x) \qquad (2)$$

Accordingly, x represents the weighted sum, and the output of the neuron is calculated by inserting x into the ReLU activation function. As the model undergoes training, the optimization algorithm updates these parameters to ensure the most accurate prediction. During the training process, the categorical cross entropy loss function is employed to minimize the classification error. The optimization process involved the update of model weights using the SGD and Adamax algorithms. In addition, the Adamax algorithm has been shown to outperform the SGD algorithm in other models. The formulas for mean moment estimation, infinite norm estimation, and parameter update are given in Equations (3), (4), and (5), respectively. It is noteworthy that this algorithm utilizes infinite-norm estimation; consequently, it provides more balanced updates when the weights are substantial. According to these equations, β_1 is the momentum term for the first-moment estimate, g_t is gradient time step t, and also m_t is the first-moment vector. On the other hand, β_2 refers to the decay rate for the exponentially weighted infinity norm, u_t is an infinity norm (maximum absolute value of past gradients), Θ_t model parameter at time step t, and also α is a learning rate.

$$m_t = \beta_1 \times m_t - 1 + (1 - \beta_1) \times g_t \qquad (3)$$

$$u_t = \max(\beta_2 \times u_t - 1, |g_t|) \qquad (4)$$

$$\Theta_{t+1} = \Theta_t - ((\alpha/u_t) \times m_t) \qquad (5)$$

Figure 2 shows a typical internal architecture. The automatically cropped data are organized into folders according to the selected study. For example, for approach 1, normal, flattening, deformation; for approach 2, normal, flattening, others. Both datasets were subjected to the standardization above and normalization for preprocessing. The convolution layers, especially the first convolution layer from which the input is taken, use multiple filters to capture various edge and texture information. Then, the activation function is appropriate for the chosen CNN algorithm. The pooling layer follows to reduce the dimensionality and preserve important features. Multiple convolutions and pooling layers are added to increase the depth. This enables capturing more complex features (e.g., detailed characteristics of degenerative changes). After the convolution and pooling layers, the resulting feature map is smoothed and fed into multiple fully connected layers to reach the output layer. In the output layer, the appropriate activation function is designed to classify different condyle bone changes, and the classification process is completed depending on the number of classes. Furthermore, CNNs were trained using the Adam optimizer with a learning rate of 0.001 to provide adaptive learning adjustments to enhance convergence. To enhance stability during the training process, a step learning rate scheduler was employed, which reduced the learning rate by a factor of 0.1 every 10 epochs.

This approach prevented overshooting and ensured gradual refinement of the model's parameters. The training process was conducted for 200 epochs, enabling the model to acquire robust feature representations. The loss function employed was categorical cross-entropy, a well-suited choice for multiclass classification problems. The hyperparameter choices were made to balance training efficiency and classification accuracy while ensuring optimal model performance.

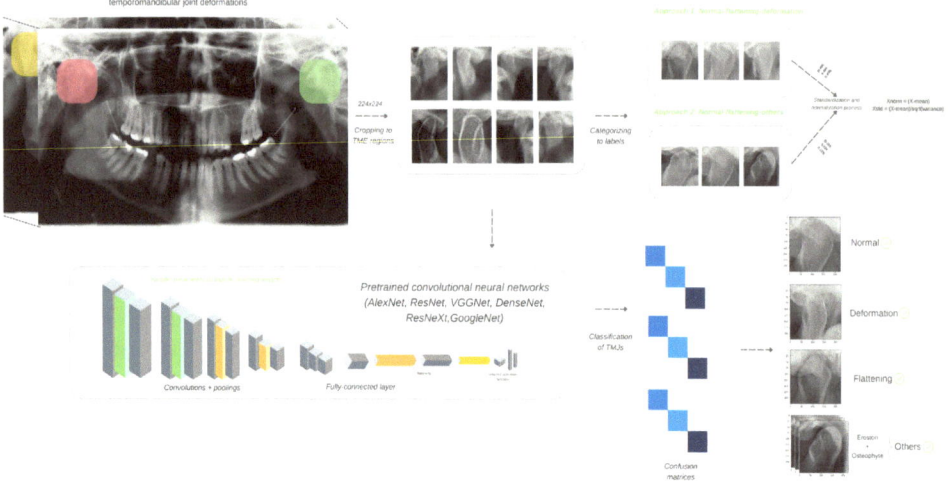

Figure 2. Different CNN architectures are proposed for the detection of morphologies caused by degenerative bone changes in temporomandibular joints in panoramic images.

3. Results

In this study, the mandibular condyle regions are cropped on panoramic radiographs, and the approach of artificial intelligence-based algorithms is applied to classify the condyle bone changes into normal, flattening, deformation, and variants belonging to the normal, flattening, and other categories for high-performance detection. To achieve the main objective of the study, which is to detect different condyle degenerative bone changes in the temporomandibular joint most successfully, various datasets belonging to different distributions were used and evaluated with different learning techniques. Many different pretrained CNN algorithms were applied in the study, and their experimental findings are given in Tables 1 and 2. For the experimental findings in the tables, the accuracy, precision, recall, and F1-score metrics in Equations (6)–(9), which are frequently used in object detection and classification studies, were used. These metrics capture not only the accuracy performance of the model but also the miss rates and successes of negative and positive classes. In particular, the F1-score metric provides an overall view by obtaining the harmonic mean of the precision and recall metrics [35]. Thus, it proved why CNN algorithms are preferred for convolutional filtering and classification of health images.

$$Accuracy = \frac{TP + TN}{TP + FP + TN + FN} \quad (6)$$

$$Precision = \frac{TP}{TP + FP} \quad (7)$$

$$Recall = \frac{TP}{TP + FN} \quad (8)$$

$$F1 - Score = 2 \times \frac{Precision \times Recall}{Precision + Recall} \qquad (9)$$

Table 1. Performance results for normal, flattening, and other data classes with a certain distribution range.

Model	Distribution	Learning Rate	Optimizer	Accuracy	Precision	Recall	F1-Score
DenseNet121	70:30	0.001	Adamax	64.85%	64.45%	64.22%	63.88%
ResNet18	70:30	0.0001	Adamax	69.23%	65.52%	66.41%	65.65%
AlexNet	70:30	0.0001	Adamax	70.71%	68.74%	68.55%	68.47%
DenseNet169	70:30	0.0001	Adamax	73.43%	71.05%	71.04%	70.66%
GoogleNet	70:30	0.0001	Adamax	86.61%	85.92%	85.60%	85.73%

Table 2. Comparative performance results for normal, flattening, others and normal, flattening, deformation data classes with different distribution ranges (N: Normal, F: Flattening, O: Others, D: Deformation).

Model	Distribution	Dataset	Optimizer	Accuracy	Precision	Recall	F1-Score
DenseNet169	70:30	N-F-O	Adamax	73.43%	73.29%	73.12%	73.20%
GoogleNet	70:30	N-F-O	Adamax	86.61%	85.92%	85.60%	85.73%
GoogleNet	80:20	N-F-D	SGD	92.65%	92.29%	92.36%	92.33%
ResNeXt	80:20	N-F-D	Adamax	94.32%	94.15%	94.07%	94.08%
GoogleNet	80:20	N-F-D	Adamax	95.23%	94.89%	95.08%	94.98%

Table 1 presents simple statistical analyses for a single dataset (N, F, O) with different CNN algorithms. Experiments were performed on equal terms at this stage when using multiple pretrained neural networks. At the beginning of the experiments, the learning rate was chosen as 0.001, but it was found that the results were more successful with a learning rate of 0.0001. For this reason, in the experimental findings, only the best results (lr = 0.001) for DenseNet121 are included, while the results for the other algorithms (lr = 0.0001) are compared in the table. Since the analysis sets were divided into 70:30 and 80:20 in the study, their ratios are given in the table as a distribution. Table 2 shows the results for N-F-O and N-F-D by applying multiple experimental tests. In addition, Adamax and Stochastic Gradient Descent (SGD) algorithms, commonly used for CNN architectures, were also applied for the optimization algorithm.

Considering the many architectures proposed in the study, the GoogleNet algorithm gave the best results even when different data classes and datasets were considered. It should be noted that the algorithm performance is high, and the test data are prepared separately from the training data. Since the GoogleNet algorithm provides high performance on the datasets, the results of Adamax and SGD optimizers are given in Table 2. Accordingly, for the dataset belonging to the 80:20 distribution of N-F-D classes, the accuracy value of 95.23% with the Adamax optimizer was the highest compared to other data classes. For N-F-O with 70:30 data distribution, the GoogleNet algorithm gave the highest result, 86.61%.

By combining the benefits of the repeated blocks in the GoogleNet algorithm with transfer learning using pre-trained weights, we improve the model's test performance. Based on the Inception architecture, GoogleNet overcomes a major challenge for a neural network with 22 layers by avoiding feature loss. The performance difference between the Inception-v3 and the GoogleNet classifier is assumed to be due to Inception modules allowing the choice between multiple convolutional filter sizes in each block [26]. The network includes a 1 × 1 convolutional layer with 128 filters and a 70% dropout of the neural network cells to prevent over-memorization [36].

Figure 3 shows the performance graphs of the best and worst-performing models of DenseNet and GoogleNet architectures. Accordingly, following the performance findings in Tables 1 and 2, the 121-layer model of DenseNet shows the worst result with 64.85% accuracy for the 70:30 distribution. In comparison, GoogleNet shows the best result with 95.23% accuracy for the 80:20 distribution. Graphs (a) and (c) show the change in total training time per iteration, while (b) and (d) represent the error (loss) rate of the model per iteration. When graph (b) is analyzed, we see that the loss value has difficulty approaching 0 and shows a very variable structure.

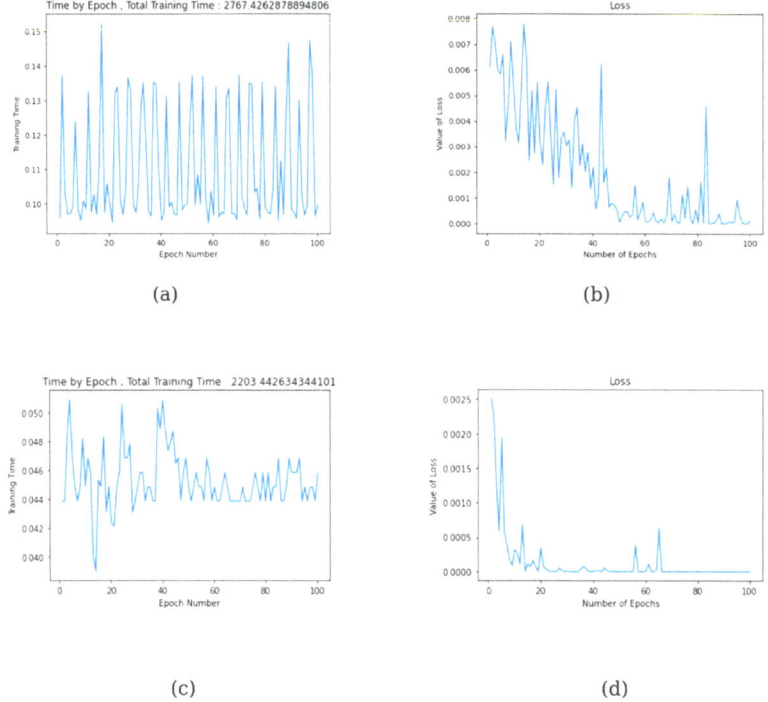

Figure 3. (**a**) DenseNet121 graph of worst total training time-epoch, (**b**) DenseNet121 graph of worst loss-epoch, (**c**) GoogleNet graph of best total training time-epoch, (**d**) GoogleNet graph of best loss-epoch.

Figure 4 indicates the training, and validation results up to a certain number of epochs. The blue line (training accuracy) shows a steady rise, reaching about 90%, indicating the model is learning from the data. The orange line (validation accuracy) is more unstable, with frequent ups and downs. While it does generally rise, the possible over-fitting is concerning. The model's poor generalization capabilities to unseen data are indicated by the widening gap between the training and validation accuracies. Consequently, it can be posited that GoogleNet, as opposed to DenseNet, yields optimal outcomes in this study.

This proves that the model cannot learn enough and is not a very desirable situation. However, in graph (d), the graph starts with a relatively high loss value and gradually tends to approach 0. This is a very common and desirable situation in classification studies. If the training is continued with many iterations, the model becomes over-memorized.

For this reason, it was also concluded that further training is inappropriate using enough anti-over-memorization probability.

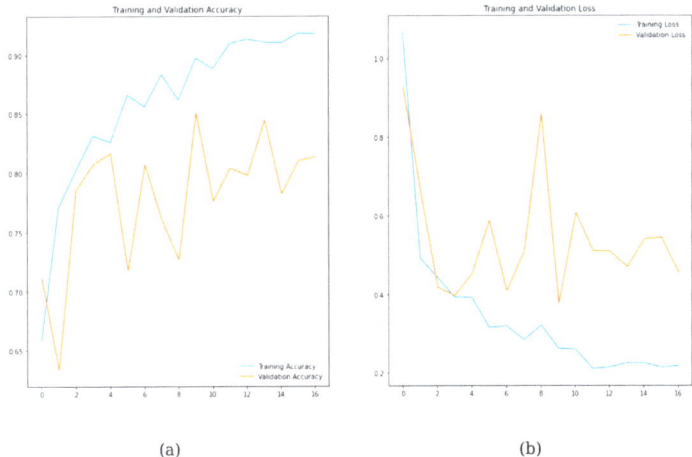

Figure 4. DenseNet121 graph of training and validation results for the epoch. (**a**) DenseNet121 training and validation accuracy values, (**b**) DenseNet121 training and validation loss values.

The results of the confusion matrices in Figure 5 are visual evidence for inferring the performance metrics calculated in the equations. When the matrix is examined in detail, the values on the diagonal represent the TP values. TP values indicate that the class to be detected is detected correctly. For this reason, the TP values of each class are expected to be as high as possible. In this case, the relevant TP, TN, FP, and FN values for the performance metrics in the equations are obtained from this matrix and calculated. For the confusion matrix, the horizontal axis shows the predicted labels while the vertical axis contains the actual labels, i.e., oromaxillofacial radiology specialist knowledge. Figure 5 shows the results of the 70:30 dataset distribution for the flattening-normal-others dataset. Here, three confusion matrices are expressed as a percentage ratio. Accordingly, when the first left image is analyzed for the GoogleNet model in the confusion matrix, 76% of correct predictions were made for the "Flattening" class in total. However, 11% of "Normal" and 13% of "Others" were incorrectly predicted. As the highest TP value, 94% correct prediction was made for the "Others" class, but 1% "Normal" and 5% "Flattening" predictions were made.

Figure 6 numerically expresses the results of the 70:30 dataset distribution for the normal-flattening-deformation dataset. Considering the measurement results in Tables 1 and 2, the complexity matrix error values in the figures are appropriate. Accordingly, for the GoogleNet-Adamax optimizer model in the complexity matrix, the "Deformation" class made 310 correct predictions in total. Seven were obtained as "Flattening" and six as "Normal". When we examine the "Normal" class, while 227 "Normal" predictions were made, 7 "Flattening" and 3 "Deformation" results were obtained. Again, when the matrix is analyzed here, the deformation group was detected with higher success and the flattening and normal groups were detected with relatively lower success.

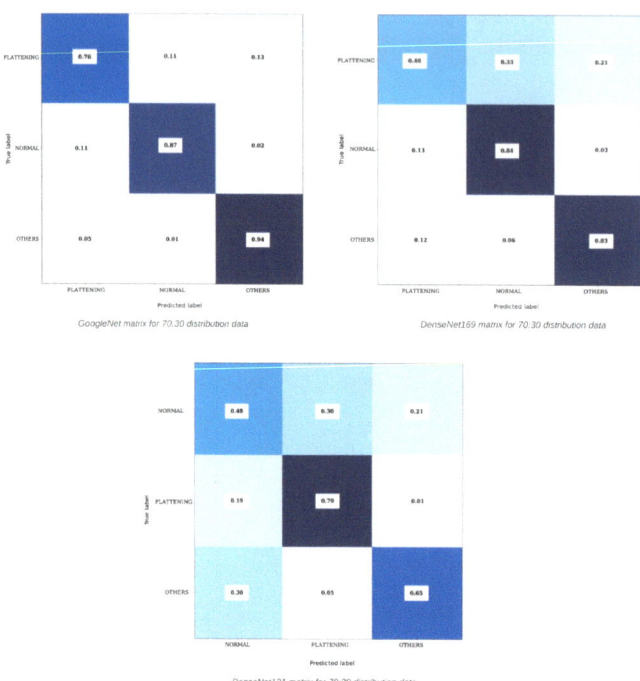

Figure 5. Confusion matrix results obtained with different algorithms for normal-flattening-others classes.

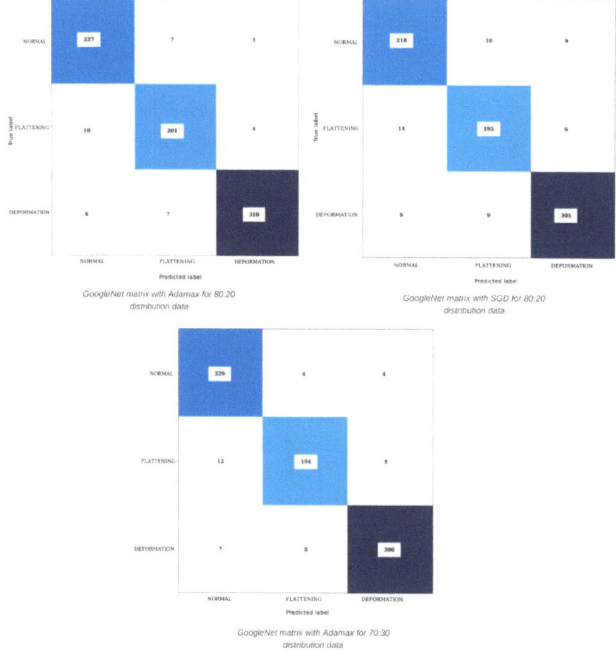

Figure 6. Confusion matrix results were obtained with different algorithms for normal-flattening-deformation classes.

4. Discussion

Mandibular condyle bony changes manifest in a spectrum of variations, ranging from subtle erosions to gross deformities of condylar morphology. A granular classification of these findings furnishes clinicians with valuable insights into disease status. Discordance may exist between clinical symptomatology and radiographic evidence, and inflammatory changes within the temporomandibular joint (TMJ) may, at times, follow a subclinical course.

While ultrasonography and magnetic resonance imaging are the modalities of choice for evaluating the soft tissues of the temporomandibular joint [37,38], conventional radiography and CBCT remain frequently employed for assessing osseous structures.

Panoramic radiography, a conventional radiographic technique utilized for imaging the hard tissues of the temporomandibular joint, offers ready accessibility and cost-effectiveness for general dental practitioners, coupled with a relatively low radiation dose compared to CBCT. However, inherent limitations constrain its utility in TMJ imaging. Panoramic films, acquired with the mandible in a slightly open and protruded position, fail to accurately depict the condyle's natural position within the glenoid fossa. Furthermore, the superimposition of cranial structures onto the osseous components of the TMJ impedes the detection of subtle alterations [39]. As a result of these shortcomings, panoramic radiographs may prove insufficient for comprehensive condylar and TMJ assessment.

Despite its limitations in accurately evaluating mandibular condyle morphology [40], panoramic radiography possesses the potential to facilitate early diagnosis of TMD due to its low cost, low radiation dose, and routine application [41].

CBCT offers tomographic imaging in all planes, eliminating superimposition and enabling unobstructed visualization of the TMJ region. CBCT demonstrates superior reliability compared to conventional methods in the evaluation of condylar erosions. Consequently, the application of CBCT is advocated as an effective tool for identifying TMJ osteoarthritis [39,42–44]. However, CBCT is associated with increased radiation exposure and cost compared to panoramic imaging. Given these considerations, CBCT should be reserved as an advanced imaging modality, with panoramic imaging serving as the preferred initial evaluation to mitigate unnecessary exposure.

These factors impose practical constraints on the widespread adoption of CBCT in clinical settings, thereby impeding researchers' ability to attain adequate sample sizes for robust investigations.

Accordingly, the present study employed panoramic images to assess the concordance between AI-driven diagnostic outcomes and oromaxillofacial radiology specialist assessments. Achieving alignment between AI diagnostic capabilities and those of an oromaxillofacial radiology specialist would streamline clinical workflows for general dental practitioners.

This study evaluated the agreement between diagnoses rendered by an oromaxillofacial radiology specialist via panoramic images and those derived from AI analysis. Future investigations could explore training AI models using diagnoses informed by both CBCT and panoramic images, enabling a more comprehensive assessment of AI diagnostic accuracy.

Moreover, the implementation of CBCT, an imaging technique that mitigates limitations inherent to panoramic films, may further reduce the likelihood of diagnostic errors by oromaxillofacial radiology specialists, potentially enhancing study outcomes.

Prior literature has predominantly focused on patients with osteoarthritis [31,32,45] and has utilized CBCT imaging [30,45]. The present study sought to classify condylar alterations resulting from both active symptomatic disease (osteoarthritis) and chronic degenerative processes (osteoarthrosis), often used interchangeably, according to features such as flattening, osteophyte formation, erosion, and deformation.

Within this framework, mandibular condyles were categorized into five groups—normal, flattening, osteophyte, erosion, and other—and presented to a CNN for evaluation. The resulting performance was deemed satisfactory.

Notably, the oromaxillofacial radiology specialist incorporated right–left symmetry considerations into condyle classification, particularly in the presence of subtle flattening or pronounced convexity. However, in the context of CNN analysis, condyles were cropped from panoramic images and were not explicitly labeled as right or left. This resulted in a unilateral evaluation of data otherwise interpreted with symmetry, leading the CNN to analyze each condyle independently, disregarding this symmetry.

This study focused on evaluating the performance of CNN models in detecting and classifying mandibular condyle bone changes in panoramic radiographs. As a result of the necessary research and application of the methods, the study showed that CNN-based methods were CNN-based methods demonstrated a high success rate in determining the mandibular condyle bone changes. However, it was concluded that the condyles should be taught dependently with the prediction that the success rate could be further increased. İt is posited that CNN performance could be augmented by segmenting condyles within a single panoramic image and incorporating right–left labeling during training.

Given the limited number of images within the osteophyte and erosion categories, discrete analysis of these conditions was precluded. We anticipate that augmenting the sample size for these groups, while ensuring balanced representation within the overall dataset, would contribute to more robust and accurate findings.

In the present study, a range of deep learning architectures were utilized for the purpose of detecting TMJ-related condylar bone changes using panoramic radiographs. These architectures included AlexNet, VGG16, VGG19, DenseNet121, DenseNet169, DenseNet201, ResNet18, ResNet101, ResNeXt, and GoogleNet. The objective of this research is to illustrate the potential of AI-driven diagnostic support in dentistry and maxillofacial radiology specialists. A distinguishing feature of this study is its rigorous classification strategy. The mandibular condyles were grouped into different categories based on their morphological characteristics, using a novel classification scheme that considers symmetry for images with slight flattening or pronounced convexity. Addressing the challenge of imbalanced datasets is a central tenet of this study, which explores the impact of erosion and osteophyte formation under varied grouping strategies. This exploration aims to enhance the model's generalizability. Furthermore, model performance was systematically examined using different splits (70:30 and 80:20) to reduce the effects of class imbalance and assess the robustness of the models across different distributions. This methodological approach ensures the reliability and generalizability of the findings. The results show that CNN-based methods achieve a remarkable level of accuracy in detecting mandibular condyle bone changes. These results underscore the effectiveness of deep learning models in providing automated diagnostic assistance that can help clinicians identify patients requiring further intervention. To further validate our labeling methodology, we performed an intra-observer agreement analysis using Cohen's kappa coefficient, which indicates significant agreement. This step serves to strengthen the reliability of our dataset and classification framework.

Notwithstanding the encouraging outcomes of this study, it is imperative to acknowledge its limitations. First, in our study, panoramic images of individuals over 18 years of age were used to eliminate morphological changes in the condyle during growth and development. However, the AI was trained using panoramic images of individuals over 18 years of age, regardless of age and gender. Future studies can investigate the effects of age and gender differences on AI training. In this way, it will reveal whether age and gender factors have a significant effect on the learning process of AI.

Furthermore, the data utilized in this research are modest in size, which may impede the model's generalizability. The incorporation of more extensive and varied data could enhance the robustness and precision of the proposed AI models. Notably, the inclusion of erosion and osteophyte classes as other classes and training was necessitated by the limited number of patients. However, the labeling process for annotations and categorization information, a fundamental component of the supervised learning technique, is subject to inter-observer variability and potential bias in ground truth annotations due to the reliance on expert judgment. Ultimately, it is imperative to emphasize that real-world clinical validation remains a crucial step in the development of AI-assisted diagnostic systems. Addressing these limitations in future research will contribute to the development of more robust and clinically applicable AI-assisted diagnostic systems.

5. Conclusions

Early and accurate diagnosis of individuals with TMD and referral to specialists for appropriate treatment approaches are critical to the prognosis of the disease. Considering the limited knowledge of general dentists about TMD, the development and integration of AI-supported neural networks into clinical practice could increase the effectiveness of panoramic radiographs in TMJ assessment. It is believed that this approach could provide significant advantages to both general dentists and patients by providing AI-based support in the diagnosis and treatment processes.

As a result, this study achieved a high success rate by using CNNs to determine the mandibular condyle bone changes. We think that identifying the changes in this region, which are difficult to evaluate on panoramic images, with CNN will make it easier for clinicians to refer patients to physicians who are experts in this field.

Author Contributions: Conceptualization, A.P. and K.A.P.; Methodology: A.P.; Formal Analysis: A.P. and K.A.P.; Resources: A.P., K.A.P. and B.Y.K.; Data Curation: K.A.P. and B.Y.K.; Writing—Original Draft Preparation: K.A.P. and B.Y.K.; Writing—Review and Editing: A.P., K.A.P. and B.Y.K.; Supervision: A.P. All authors have read and agreed to the published version of the manuscript.

Funding: This research received no external funding.

Institutional Review Board Statement: This study was conducted in accordance with the Declaration of Helsinki, and approved by the Karabuk University Non-Interventional Clinical Research Ethics Committee (Date: 8 February 2024, Decision No: 1680).

Informed Consent Statement: Informed consent was obtained from all subjects involved in the study.

Data Availability Statement: The original contributions presented in this study are included in this article, and further inquiries can be directed to the corresponding author.

Conflicts of Interest: The authors declare no conflicts of interest.

References

1. Sritara, S.; Tsutsumi, M.; Fukino, K.; Matsumoto, Y.; Ono, T.; Akita, K. Evaluating the morphological features of the lateral pterygoid insertion into the medial surface of the condylar process. *Clin. Exp. Dent. Res.* **2021**, *7*, 219–225. [CrossRef] [PubMed]
2. Suh, M.; Park, S.; Kim, Y.-K.; Yun, P.-Y.; Lee, W. 18F-NaF PET/CT for the evaluation of temporomandibular joint disorder. *Clin. Radiol.* **2018**, *73*, 414.e7–414.e13. [CrossRef] [PubMed]
3. Minervini, G.; D'Amico, C.; Cicciù, M.; Fiorillo, L. Temporomandibular joint disk displacement: Etiology, diagnosis, imaging, and therapeutic approaches. *J. Craniofacial Surg.* **2023**, *34*, 1115–1121. [CrossRef] [PubMed]
4. Crincoli, V.; Anelli, M.G.; Quercia, E.; Piancino, M.G.; Di Comite, M. Temporomandibular disorders and oral features in early rheumatoid arthritis patients: An observational study. *Int. J. Med. Sci.* **2019**, *16*, 253. [CrossRef]

5. Schiffman, E.; Ohrbach, R.; Truelove, E.; Look, J.; Anderson, G.; Goulet, J.-P.; List, T.; Svensson, P.; Gonzalez, Y.; Lobbezoo, F. Diagnostic criteria for temporomandibular disorders (DC/TMD) for clinical and research applications: Recommendations of the International RDC/TMD Consortium Network and Orofacial Pain Special Interest Group. *J. Oral Facial Pain Headache* **2014**, *28*, 6. [CrossRef]
6. Zieliński, G.; Pająk-Zielińska, B.; Ginszt, M. A meta-analysis of the global prevalence of temporomandibular disorders. *J. Clin. Med.* **2024**, *13*, 1365. [CrossRef]
7. Bliddal, H. Definition, pathology and pathogenesis of osteoarthritis. *Ugeskr. Laeger* **2020**, *182*, V06200477.
8. Cardoneanu, A.; Macovei, L.A.; Burlui, A.M.; Mihai, I.R.; Bratoiu, I.; Rezus, I.I.; Richter, P.; Tamba, B.-I.; Rezus, E. Temporomandibular joint osteoarthritis: Pathogenic mechanisms involving the cartilage and subchondral bone, and potential therapeutic strategies for joint regeneration. *Int. J. Mol. Sci.* **2022**, *24*, 171. [CrossRef]
9. Mureșanu, S.; Hedeșiu, M.; Iacob, L.; Eftimie, R.; Olariu, E.; Dinu, C.; Jacobs, R.; Team Project Group. Automating Dental Condition Detection on Panoramic Radiographs: Challenges, Pitfalls, and Opportunities. *Diagnostics* **2024**, *14*, 2336. [CrossRef]
10. ArunKumar, G. Bone changes in condyles of asymptomatic temperomandibular joints & its correlation with age, gender and occlusal condition; a digital panoramic study. *J. Dent. Health Oral Disord. Ther.* **2021**, *12*, 111–115.
11. Görürgöz, C.; İçen, M.; Kurt, M.; Aksoy, S.; Bakırarar, B.; Rozylo-Kalinowska, I.; Orhan, K. Degenerative changes of the mandibular condyle in relation to the temporomandibular joint space, gender and age: A multicenter CBCT study. *Dent. Med. Probl.* **2023**, *60*, 127–135. [CrossRef] [PubMed]
12. Schroder, Â.G.D.; Gonçalves, F.M.; Germiniani, J.d.S.; Schroder, L.D.; Porporatti, A.L.; Zeigelboim, B.S.; de Araujo, C.M.; Santos, R.S.; Stechman-Neto, J. Diagnosis of TMJ degenerative diseases by panoramic radiography: Is it possible? A systematic review and meta-analysis. *Clin. Oral Investig.* **2023**, *27*, 6395–6412. [CrossRef] [PubMed]
13. Valesan, L.F.; Da-Cas, C.D.; Réus, J.C.; Denardin, A.C.S.; Garanhani, R.R.; Bonotto, D.; Januzzi, E.; de Souza, B.D.M. Prevalence of temporomandibular joint disorders: A systematic review and meta-analysis. *Clin. Oral Investig.* **2021**, *25*, 441–453. [CrossRef]
14. Mani, F.M.; Sivasubramanian, S.S. A study of temporomandibular joint osteoarthritis using computed tomographic imaging. *Biomed. J.* **2016**, *39*, 201–206. [CrossRef]
15. Osiewicz, M.; Kojat, P.; Gut, M.; Kazibudzka, Z.; Pytko-Polończyk, J. Self-Perceived Dentists' Knowledge of Temporomandibular Disorders in Krakow: A Pilot Study. *Pain Res. Manag.* **2020**, *2020*, 9531806. [CrossRef]
16. Mozhdeh, M.; Caroccia, F.; Moscagiuri, F.; Festa, F.; D'Attilio, M. Evaluation of knowledge among dentists on symptoms and treatments of temporomandibular disorders in Italy. *Int. J. Environ. Res. Public Health* **2020**, *17*, 8760. [CrossRef]
17. Schwendicke, F.; Golla, T.; Dreher, M.; Krois, J. Convolutional neural networks for dental image diagnostics: A scoping review. *J. Dent.* **2019**, *91*, 103226. [CrossRef]
18. Shafi, I.; Fatima, A.; Afzal, H.; Díez, I.D.L.T.; Lipari, V.; Breñosa, J.; Ashraf, I. A Comprehensive Review of Recent Advances in Artificial Intelligence for Dentistry E-Health. *Diagnostics* **2023**, *13*, 2196. [CrossRef]
19. Özbay, Y.; Kazangirler, B.Y.; Özcan, C.; Pekince, A. Detection of the separated endodontic instrument on periapical radiographs using a deep learning-based convolutional neural network algorithm. *Aust. Endod. J.* **2024**, *50*, 131–139. [CrossRef]
20. Bayrakdar, I.S.; Orhan, K.; Akarsu, S.; Çelik, Ö.; Atasoy, S.; Pekince, A.; Yasa, Y.; Bilgir, E.; Sağlam, H.; Aslan, A.F. Deep-learning approach for caries detection and segmentation on dental bitewing radiographs. *Oral Radiol.* **2022**, *38*, 468–479. [CrossRef]
21. Kreiner, M.; Viloria, J. A novel artificial neural network for the diagnosis of orofacial pain and temporomandibular disorders. *J. Oral Rehabil.* **2022**, *49*, 884–889. [CrossRef] [PubMed]
22. Chauhan, R.; Ghanshala, K.K.; Joshi, R. Convolutional neural network (CNN) for image detection and recognition. In Proceedings of the 2018 First International Conference on Secure Cyber Computing and Communication (ICSCCC), Jalandhar, India, 15–17 December 2018; IEEE: Piscataway, NJ, USA, 2018; pp. 278–282.
23. Ozsari, S.; Güzel, M.S.; Yılmaz, D.; Kamburoğlu, K. A Comprehensive Review of Artificial Intelligence Based Algorithms Regarding Temporomandibular Joint Related Diseases. *Diagnostics* **2023**, *13*, 2700. [CrossRef] [PubMed]
24. Zhu, Z.; Lin, K.; Jain, A.K.; Zhou, J. Transfer learning in deep reinforcement learning: A survey. *IEEE Trans. Pattern Anal. Mach. Intell.* **2023**, *45*, 13344–13362. [CrossRef]
25. Shaha, M.; Pawar, M. Transfer learning for image classification. In Proceedings of the 2018 Second International Conference on Electronics, Communication and Aerospace Technology (ICECA), Coimbatore, India, 29–31 March 2018; IEEE: Piscataway, NJ, USA, 2018; pp. 656–660.
26. Farook, T.H.; Dudley, J. Automation and deep (machine) learning in temporomandibular joint disorder radiomics: A systematic review. *J. Oral Rehabil.* **2023**, *50*, 501–521. [CrossRef]
27. Yazici, İ.; Shayea, I.; Din, J. A survey of applications of artificial intelligence and machine learning in future mobile networks-enabled systems. *Eng. Sci. Technol. Int. J.* **2023**, *44*, 101455. [CrossRef]
28. Nishiyama, M.; Ishibashi, K.; Ariji, Y.; Fukuda, M.; Nishiyama, W.; Umemura, M.; Katsumata, A.; Fujita, H.; Ariji, E. Performance of deep learning models constructed using panoramic radiographs from two hospitals to diagnose fractures of the mandibular condyle. *Dentomaxillofacial Radiol.* **2021**, *50*, 20200611. [CrossRef]

29. Ahn, Y.; Hwang, J.J.; Jung, Y.-H.; Jeong, T.; Shin, J. Automated mesiodens classification system using deep learning on panoramic radiographs of children. *Diagnostics* **2021**, *11*, 1477. [CrossRef]
30. Lee, K.; Kwak, H.; Oh, J.; Jha, N.; Kim, Y.; Kim, W.; Baik, U.; Ryu, J. Automated detection of TMJ osteoarthritis based on artificial intelligence. *J. Dent. Res.* **2020**, *99*, 1363–1367. [CrossRef]
31. Choi, E.; Kim, D.; Lee, J.-Y.; Park, H.-K. Artificial intelligence in detecting temporomandibular joint osteoarthritis on orthopantomogram. *Sci. Rep.* **2021**, *11*, 10246. [CrossRef]
32. Jung, W.; Lee, K.; Suh, B.; Seok, H.; Lee, D. Deep learning for osteoarthritis classification in temporomandibular joint. *Oral Dis.* **2023**, *29*, 1050–1059. [CrossRef]
33. Hegde, S.; Praveen, B.; Shetty, S.R. Morphological and radiological variations of mandibular condyles in health and diseases: A systematic review. *Dentistry* **2013**, *3*, 154.
34. Mallya, S.; Lam, E. *White and Pharoah's Oral Radiology: Principles and Interpretation*; Elsevier Health Sciences: Chennai, India, 2018.
35. Tekin, B.Y.; Ozcan, C.; Pekince, A.; Yasa, Y. An enhanced tooth segmentation and numbering according to FDI notation in bitewing radiographs. *Comput. Biol. Med.* **2022**, *146*, 105547.
36. Szegedy, C.; Liu, W.; Jia, Y.; Sermanet, P.; Reed, S.; Anguelov, D.; Erhan, D.; Vanhoucke, V.; Rabinovich, A. Going deeper with convolutions. In Proceedings of the IEEE Conference on Computer Vision and Pattern Recognition, Boston, MA, USA, 1–12 June 2015; pp. 1–9.
37. Pekince, K.A.; Caglayan, F.; Pekince, A. Imaging of masseter muscle spasms by ultrasonography: A preliminary study. *Oral Radiol.* **2020**, *36*, 85–88. [CrossRef] [PubMed]
38. Pekince, K.A.; Çağlayan, F.; Pekince, A. The efficacy and limitations of USI for diagnosing TMJ internal derangements. *Oral Radiol.* **2020**, *36*, 32–39. [CrossRef]
39. Walewski, L.Â.; de Souza Tolentino, E.; Yamashita, F.C.; Iwaki, L.C.V.; da Silva, M.C. Cone beam computed tomography study of osteoarthritic alterations in the osseous components of temporomandibular joints in asymptomatic patients according to skeletal pattern, gender, and age. *Oral Surg. Oral Med. Oral Pathol. Oral Radiol.* **2019**, *128*, 70–77. [CrossRef]
40. Schmitter, M.; Gabbert, O.; Ohlmann, B.; Hassel, A.; Wolff, D.; Rammelsberg, P.; Kress, B. Assessment of the reliability and validity of panoramic imaging for assessment of mandibular condyle morphology using both MRI and clinical examination as the gold standard. *Oral Surg. Oral Med. Oral Pathol. Oral Radiol. Endodontology* **2006**, *102*, 220–224. [CrossRef]
41. Singh, B.; Kumar, N.R.; Balan, A.; Nishan, M.; Haris, P.S.; Jinisha, M.; Denny, C.D. Evaluation of normal morphology of mandibular condyle: A radiographic survey. *J. Clin. Imaging Sci.* **2020**, *10*, 51. [CrossRef]
42. Abrahamsson, A.-K.; Kristensen, M.; Arvidsson, L.Z.; Kvien, T.K.; Larheim, T.A.; Haugen, I.K. Frequency of temporomandibular joint osteoarthritis and related symptoms in a hand osteoarthritis cohort. *Osteoarthr. Cartil.* **2017**, *25*, 654–657. [CrossRef]
43. Sonnesen, L.; Petersson, A.; Wiese, M.; Jensen, K.E.; Svanholt, P.; Bakke, M. Osseous osteoarthritic-like changes and joint mobility of the temporomandibular joints and upper cervical spine: Is there a relation? *Oral Surg. Oral Med. Oral Pathol. Oral Radiol.* **2017**, *123*, 273–279. [CrossRef]
44. Dumbuya, A.; Gomes, A.F.; Marchini, L.; Zeng, E.; Comnick, C.L.; Melo, S.L.S. Bone changes in the temporomandibular joints of older adults: A cone-beam computed tomography study. *Spec. Care Dent.* **2020**, *40*, 84–89. [CrossRef]
45. de Dumast, P.; Mirabel, C.; Cevidanes, L.; Ruellas, A.; Yatabe, M.; Ioshida, M.; Ribera, N.T.; Michoud, L.; Gomes, L.; Huang, C.; et al. A web-based system for neural network based classification in temporomandibular joint osteoarthritis. *Comput. Med. Imaging Graph.* **2018**, *67*, 45–54. [CrossRef]

Disclaimer/Publisher's Note: The statements, opinions and data contained in all publications are solely those of the individual author(s) and contributor(s) and not of MDPI and/or the editor(s). MDPI and/or the editor(s) disclaim responsibility for any injury to people or property resulting from any ideas, methods, instructions or products referred to in the content.

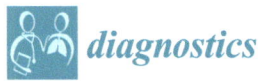

Article

Development of an AI-Supported Clinical Tool for Assessing Mandibular Third Molar Tooth Extraction Difficulty Using Panoramic Radiographs and YOLO11 Sub-Models

Serap Akdoğan [1], Muhammet Üsame Öziç [1,*] and Melek Tassoker [2]

[1] Department of Biomedical Engineering, Faculty of Technology, Pamukkale University, Denizli 20160, Türkiye; sakdogan18@posta.pau.edu.tr
[2] Department of Oral and Maxillofacial Radiology, Faculty of Dentistry, Necmettin Erbakan University, Konya 42090, Türkiye; dishekmelek@gmail.com
* Correspondence: muozic@pau.edu.tr

Abstract: Background/Objective: This study aimed to develop an AI-supported clinical tool to evaluate the difficulty of mandibular third molar extractions based on panoramic radiographs. **Methods:** A dataset of 2000 panoramic radiographs collected between 2023 and 2024 was annotated by an oral radiologist using bounding boxes. YOLO11 sub-models were trained and tested for three basic scenarios according to the Pederson Index criteria, taking into account Winter (angulation) and Pell and Gregory (ramus relationship and depth). For each scenario, the YOLO11 sub-models were trained using 80% of the data for training, 10% for validation, and 10% for testing. Model performance was assessed using precision, recall, F1 score, and mean Average Precision (mAP) metrics, and different graphs. **Results:** YOLO11 sub-models (nano, small, medium, large, extra-large) showed high accuracy and similar behavior in all scenarios. For the calculation of the Pederson index, nano for Winter (average training mAP@0.50 = 0.963; testing mAP@0.50 = 0.975), nano for class (average training mAP@0.50 = 0.979; testing mAP@0.50 = 0.965), and medium for level (average training mAP@0.50 = 0.977; testing mAP@0.50 = 0.989) from the Pell and Gregory categories were selected as optimal sub-models. Three scenarios were run consecutively on panoramic images, and slightly difficult, moderately difficult, and very difficult Pederson indexes were obtained according to the scores. The results were evaluated by an oral radiologist, and the AI system performed successfully in terms of Pederson index determination with 97.00% precision, 94.55% recall, and 95.76% F1 score. **Conclusions:** The YOLO11-supported clinical tool demonstrated high accuracy and reliability in assessing mandibular third molar extraction difficulty on panoramic radiographs. These models were integrated into a GUI for clinical use, offering dentists a simple tool for estimating extraction difficulty, and improving decision-making and patient management.

Keywords: mandibular third molar extraction; oral surgery; panoramic radiography; Pederson difficulty index; YOLO11

1. Introduction

The frequency of impacted mandibular molars is reported in the literature to be between 16.7% and 68.6% [1]. The surgical extraction of impacted mandibular third molars is one of the most frequently performed and challenging procedures in oral and maxillofacial surgery. Proper evaluation of the procedure's difficulty before surgery is crucial to estimating postoperative risks, such as swelling, pain, limited mouth opening, dry socket, and inferior alveolar nerve injury. Additionally, it is essential to predict the operation's duration and determine the time the patient should allocate for the appointment [1,2]. The difficulty of extracting impacted third molars varies significantly between cases. In some instances, the procedure can be relatively straightforward, involving the removal of alveolar bone and tooth separation. However, extraction may require general anesthesia in more complex cases where the molar is deeply embedded [2]. Therefore, the operating oral surgeon needs scientific evidence regarding each case's estimated surgical difficulty level [1,3]. This way, the patient will be better informed and mentally prepared before surgery, and the physician can obtain appropriate informed consent regarding the clinical scenario [4]. Several indices have been suggested in the literature to evaluate the extraction difficulty of impacted mandibular third molars preoperatively [4]. The most widely used of these, the Pederson index [5], is derived from the Winter and Pell and Gregory classifications [2,6,7]. This evaluates and scores third molar extractions based on radiographic factors, including the tooth's position, depth, and its relationship to the mandibular ramus [1]. An important limitation of the Pederson index is that it does not include clinical judgment. However, due to its high specificity, the index is reported to be effective in efficiently planning surgeries by eliminating cases that are unlikely to present significant difficulties [4]. Panoramic radiographs (PRs), which are routinely taken in the clinic and provide a single view of the entire jaw structure, provide a clear view for positioning the mandibular third molars. However, for detailed analysis of the molars, such as their relationship with the inferior alveolar canal, cone beam computed tomography (CBCT) images may provide higher diagnostic accuracy [8].

Over the last decade, advancements in artificial intelligence (AI) and its integration into medicine and dentistry have led to a rapid increase in research on deep learning-based models for AI-assisted medical diagnosis [9–11]. Studies that were carried out with conventional machine learning for a long time have been replaced by deep learning models because deep learning models automatically extract and select features across layers. Many feature extraction and selection methods had to be tried in traditional machine learning methods, and the best methodology was determined after many trials. Due to these advantages, many deep learning models have been proposed in recent years [12,13]. Deep learning studies focused on mandibular third molars in PRs have included the determination of the eruption potential of mandibular third molars [14], wisdom tooth detection [9,15,16], segmentation [17,18], age estimation [19], estimation of the time required for mandibular third molar extraction [20], classification of the developmental stages of third molars in a fully automated way [21], determination of the anatomical relationship of mandibular third molars to the mandibular canal [16,22–28], classification of mandibular third molars with different approaches [24], prediction of Pell and Gregory classes [29–31], determination of Winter angulation [9,15,29–32], and prediction of extraction difficulty according to indexes [33–37]. The variety of studies conducted on mandibular third molars clearly demonstrates the clinical importance of these teeth. AI-based studies have provided significant advances in many areas such as the detection, classification, segmentation, determination of anatomical relationships, and prediction of the extraction difficulty of these teeth. However, despite all these developments, manual evaluation of extraction difficulty is still a common practice [38,39]. These traditional approaches are time-consuming and prone to human error. Conversely, studies evaluating extraction difficulty with AI-based methods in PRs are quite limited and their current accuracy rates are still insufficient. This study aimed to automatically detect, classify, and score the extraction difficulty of impacted mandibular third molars based on the Pederson index on panoramic radiographs using YOLO11 state-of-the-art models. YOLO11, the latest version of the YOLO (You Only Look Once) family, which is popularly used in the literature for object detection, segmentation, pose estimation, object tracking, and classification, was introduced in October 2024. This model has increased feature extraction capabilities with improved spine and neck architectures and provides higher efficiency, speed, and accuracy values compared to previous versions and competing models. YOLO11, which can adapt to the environment in difficult tasks, offers a practical use to researchers with its user-friendly interface and framework provided by the Ultralytics library (https://github.com/ultralytics accessed on 1 December 2024). Because of its efficiency and ease of integration into different systems, YOLO11 is expected to have many future applications across various industrial sectors, including healthcare [40]. Many applications to be performed with this algorithm will take their place in medicine to reduce complications that inexperienced general practitioners may encounter, increase the patient's postoperative comfort, and eliminate the need for a jaw surgeon's expertise when necessary. At the end of this study, the tooth extraction difficulties obtained with YOLO11 are automatically printed on the images, a graphical user interface (GUI) is designed for clinical use, and the results are discussed.

2. Materials and Methods

2.1. Data Collection and Image Preprocessing

This study was performed in accordance with the Declaration of Helsinki and protocol number 2024/424 obtained from the Ethics Committee of Necmettin Erbakan University Faculty of Dentistry, Department of Oral and Maxillofacial Radiology, on 25 April 2024. A total of 2000 PRs of mandibular third molars were collected from patients who visited the Faculty of Dentistry for dental check-ups between 2023 and 2024. The dataset was obtained from two different devices: NewTom GiANO HR (Verona, Italy) and 2D Veraviewpocs (J MORITA MFG corp, Kyoto, Japan). Clear visualizations of the root structure, tooth positioning, and bone level of the third molars were established as the inclusion criteria, while cases involving complete extractions, surgical interventions, trauma, cystic lesions, tumors, or severe maxillofacial deformities were designated as exclusion criteria. All images were converted to Portable Network Graphics (PNG) format with 8-bit depth and resized to 1024×532 using the bilinear interpolation method.

2.2. Radiological Assessment and Image Annotation

Radiologic evaluations were performed according to the Pederson index [5], which is widely used in the literature to predict the difficulty of extraction of mandibular third molars. This index divides the spatial position and depth of the third molars into 3 subcategories according to the Pell and Gregory system [6] and the angulation into 4 subcategories according to the Winter classification system [7]. Thus, 36 different possibilities were calculated (Table 1) and extraction difficulty was slightly difficult, moderately difficult, and very difficult. According to the Pell and Gregory and Winter classification systems, the following criteria were used for the radiologic evaluation of PRs. Table 1 shows the scores for each subcategory and total score values.

Table 1. Criteria and scores of the Pederson index [5,41–43].

	Criterion	Values
Winter	Mesioangular	1
	Horizontal/Transverse	2
	Vertical	3
	Distoangular	4
Depth	Level A	1
	Level B	2
	Level C	3

Table 1. Cont.

	Criterion	Values
Ramus	Class 1	1
	Class 2	2
	Class 3	3
Score	Slightly difficult	3–4
	Moderately difficult	5–6
	Very difficult	7–10

* Pederson's original index classified 5–7 scores as 'Moderately Difficult' [43].

Angulation (Winter) [7]:

Vertical: There is an angle between $10°$ and $-10°$ between the long axis of the mandibular third molar and the long axis of the second molar, and the tooth is in a vertical position.

Mesioangular: There is an angle between $11°$ and $79°$ between the long axis of the mandibular third molar and the long axis of the second molar, and the crown of the tooth is inclined towards the second molar.

Horizontal: There is an angle between $80°$ and $100°$ between the long axis of the mandibular third molar and the long axis of the second molar, and the tooth is in a horizontal position.

Distoangular: There is an angle between $-11°$ and $-79°$ between the long axis of the mandibular third molar and the long axis of the second molar and the crown of the tooth is inclined towards the back of the jaw.

Ramus Relation (Pell and Gregory): Position of the third molar relative to the mandibular ramus [6].

Class I: The space between the mandibular ramus and the distal root of the second molar is sufficient for the mesiodistal diameter of the third molar to be located.

Class II: The space between the mandibular ramus and the distal root of the second molar is insufficient for the mesiodistal diameter of the third molar to be located.

Class III: The third molar tooth is completely located in the mandibular ramus.

Depth (Pell and Gregory): Depth level according to the occlusal plane [6].

Level A: The uppermost part of the third molar (occlusal surface) is at or above the occlusal plane of the adjacent second molar.

Level B: The uppermost part of the third molar is between the cementoenamel junction of the second molar and the occlusal plane.

Level C: The uppermost part of the third molar is located apical to the cementoenamel junction of the adjacent second molar.

Considering these criteria, all PRs were examined by an oral radiologist (MT) with 13 years of experience and prepared for this study. Figure 1 shows the image patches prepared according to the relevant criteria from the dataset and the class information is specified. As seen in Figure 1, since the dental anatomical structures of individuals are different, each patch shows a unique pattern. From the 2000 collected PRs, 1400 datasets were created separately for class, level, and angulation. Since each scenario needs to be evaluated independently, a separate AI model should be created for each. The PRs were doubled by horizontally flipping them. Therefore, a total of 8400 PRs were created from 2800 data for each scenario. PRs were annotated using the bounding box with the browser-based labeling tool makesense (https://www.makesense.ai/ accessed on 1 December 2024). In the annotation performed by MT, the inclusion of the third and second molar teeth with their roots in the bounding box was taken into account as the labeling criterion, and a total of 8400 PR images were annotated. Figure 2 shows how an original and a horizontally flipped image were annotated.

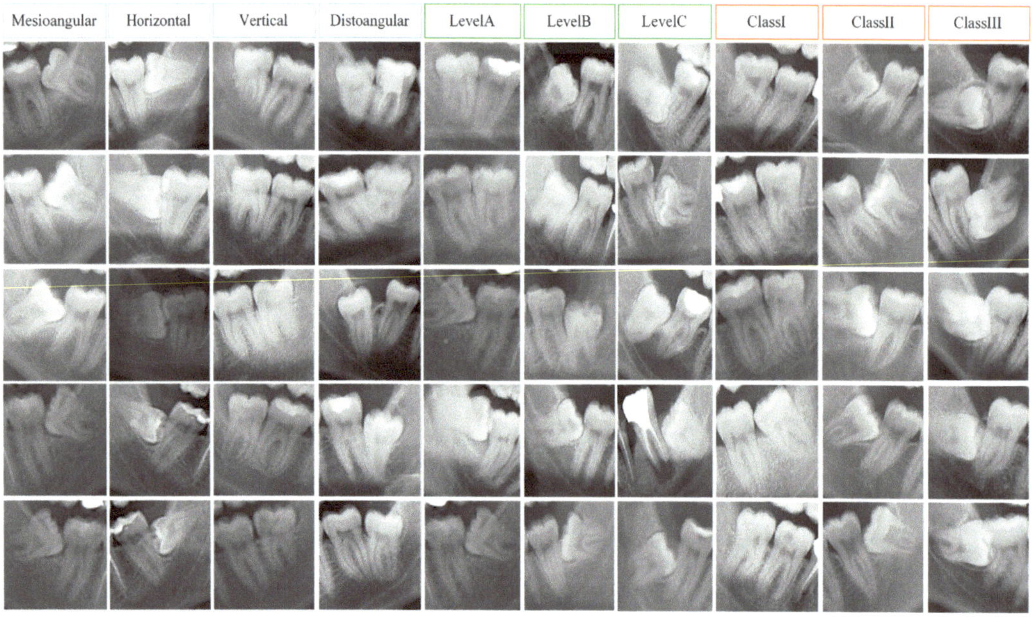

Figure 1. Radiological evaluation of mandibular third molar PR patches based on Pell and Gregory classification and Winter's angulation.

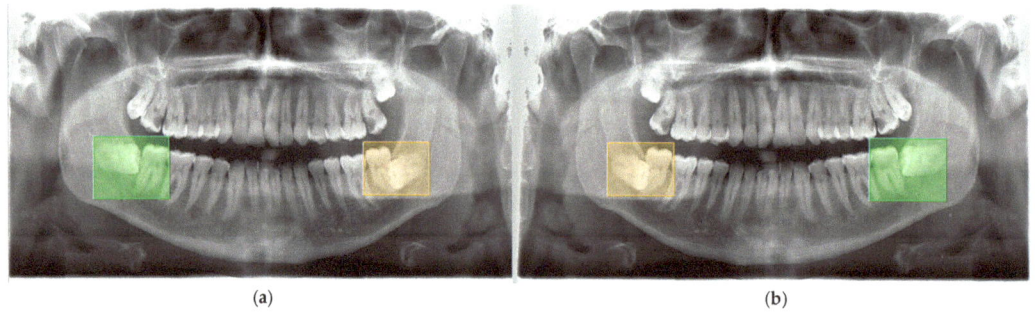

Figure 2. (a) Original annotated PR. (b) Horizontally flipped and annotated PR.

2.3. YOLO11 Sub-Models, Transfer Learning and Fine-Tuning

In this study, the n (nano), s (small), m (medium), l (large), and x (extra-large) sub-models of the YOLO11 algorithm were trained and tested for three different scenarios. The library released by Ultralytics was preferred because it offers user-friendly Python scripts and cloud-based training support. Training and testing operations were performed on TESLA A100 GPUs using Google COLAB Pro+. Data were divided into 80% training, 10% validation, and 10% test sets for each scenario. Data augmentation was performed after the data were separated to ensure that horizontally flipped versions of the original images were not present in other files. Since the current YOLO models were trained with the COCO dataset, they can recognize 80 objects. However, to train with specialized datasets, the capabilities of existing networks can be transferred to the new model using transfer learning operations. Among the hyperparameters of these models, the epoch count was set to 600 and the mini-batch size was set to 8, while the other parameters were left at their default values (optimizer: SGD (lr = 0.01, momentum = 0.9), patience: 100). Due to the structure of the model, the following mosaic data augmentation operations were applied before the images entered the network (Blur (p = 0.01, blur_limit = (3, 7)), MedianBlur (p = 0.01, blur_limit = (3, 7)), ToGray (p = 0.01, num_output_channels = 3, method = 'weighted_average'), and CLAHE (p = 0.01, clip_limit = (1.0, 4.0), tile_grid_size = (8, 8)). So, the generalization ability of the model was increased by using the mosaic data augmentation technique. As a result of the training, artificial intelligence files with the .pt extension were produced by the framework. Test data that the system had not seen before were passed through these models, and the test performance was evaluated separately for three scenarios.

2.4. Performance Evaluation Metrics

The performance of the training and testing processes was evaluated separately for each scenario. The Ultralytics framework automatically calculates the performance metrics. The system first calculates TP (True Positive), which indicates instances that the model predicts as positive, FP (False Positive), which indicates instances that the model predicts incorrectly, and FN (False Negative), which indicates instances that the model fails to predict or does not find an essentially positive instance. Based on these values, precision (P), which indicates the ratio of TP predictions to total positive predictions (Equation (1)), and recall (R), which demonstrates the ratio of TP predictions to total TPs and FNs (Equation (2)), are calculated, and the F1 score (F1-S) is acquired with the harmonic average of these two metrics (Equation (3)). Average Precision (AP) is used to measure the overall performance of the model at different threshold values (Equation (4)) (k: number of classes). The mean Average Precision (mAP) value is then calculated by taking the average AP across all classes (Equation (5)). In particular, mAP@0.5 and mAP@0.5:0.95 metrics are calculated by taking the average of the 50% IoU (Intersection over Union) threshold and IoU thresholds ranging from 50% to 95%, respectively. These metrics provide a detailed analysis of the performance of an object detection model. The results of this study are supported with graphs showing the performances according to the number of epochs, confusion matrices, and precision–recall graphs.

$$precision = \frac{TP}{TP + FP} \tag{1}$$

$$recall = \frac{TP}{TP + FN} \tag{2}$$

$$F1 - score = 2 \times \frac{Precision \times Recall}{Precision + Recall} \tag{3}$$

$$AP_k = \int_0^1 P_k(R_k)dR_k \tag{4}$$

$$mAP = \frac{1}{k}\sum_{i=1}^{k} AP_i \tag{5}$$

3. Results

3.1. Training and Testing Performance Results

Evaluating the performance of the models in both the training and testing phases provides important information about the generalization ability and correct detection ability regarding the detection and classification of third molars under three different scenarios. In this section, the performances will be examined according to the basic performance measurement metrics of precision, recall, F1 score, mAP, precision–recall, confusion matrix (CM), and loss graphs obtained during the training and testing processes. Table 2 shows the training and testing results for Winter angulation (Img: images; Ins: instances). As shown in Table 2, the performance values of the YOLO11 models are close to each other, but they appear to maintain a good balance between precision and recall, particularly in the Distoangular class. In the "Mesioangular" and "Horizontal" classes, all models show strong results, while in the "Distoangular" and "Vertical" classes, the accuracies are relatively lower. The nano model, with its lightweight structure, provides a balanced performance with high generalization capability, and has more stable results than other models, especially in the "Distoangular" class. Due to these advantages, the YOLO11n model (average testing mAP@0.5 = 0.975, mAP@0.5:0.95 = 0.849) was selected for Winter classification in extraction difficulty index calculations.

Table 2. Training and testing results for YOLO11 sub-models on Winter angulation.

Model				Training						Testing				
YOLO11	Prediction	Img	Inst	P	R	F1-S	mAP@.5	mAP@.5:.95	Img	Inst	P	R	F1-S	mAP@.5	mAP@.5:.95
nano	Mesioangular	118	160	0.939	0.975	0.957	0.984	0.900	136	174	0.970	0.989	0.979	0.983	0.875
	Distoangular	56	62	0.962	0.809	0.879	0.946	0.812	20	26	0.851	0.876	0.863	0.933	0.791
	Horizontal	68	88	0.935	0.977	0.956	0.965	0.853	76	92	0.99	0.989	0.989	0.994	0.874
	Vertical	124	184	0.811	0.973	0.885	0.956	0.815	148	200	0.949	0.965	0.957	0.988	0.858
	All	280	494	0.912	0.934	0.923	0.963	0.845	280	492	0.940	0.955	0.947	0.975	0.849
small	Mesioangular	118	160	0.951	1.00	0.975	0.989	0.899	136	174	0.962	0.977	0.969	0.983	0.872
	Distoangular	56	62	0.946	0.742	0.832	0.946	0.836	20	26	0.682	0.769	0.723	0.810	0.685
	Horizontal	68	88	0.967	0.977	0.972	0.964	0.86	76	92	0.962	0.989	0.975	0.994	0.884
	Vertical	124	184	0.876	0.963	0.917	0.958	0.829	148	200	0.941	0.970	0.955	0.980	0.860
	All	280	494	0.935	0.921	0.928	0.964	0.856	280	492	0.887	0.926	0.906	0.942	0.825
medium	Mesioangular	118	160	0.924	0.994	0.958	0.991	0.896	136	174	0.959	0.994	0.976	0.991	0.885
	Distoangular	56	62	0.963	0.842	0.898	0.958	0.842	20	26	0.675	0.88	0.764	0.869	0.715
	Horizontal	68	88	0.965	0.941	0.953	0.956	0.854	76	92	0.989	0.978	0.983	0.990	0.876
	Vertical	124	184	0.893	0.962	0.926	0.949	0.812	148	200	0.950	0.955	0.952	0.986	0.870
	All	280	494	0.936	0.935	0.935	0.964	0.851	280	492	0.893	0.952	0.922	0.959	0.837
large	Mesioangular	118	160	0.939	0.981	0.960	0.987	0.89	136	174	0.969	1.00	0.984	0.990	0.869
	Distoangular	56	62	0.954	0.666	0.784	0.921	0.804	20	26	0.984	0.769	0.863	0.942	0.769
	Horizontal	68	88	0.927	0.977	0.951	0.972	0.868	76	92	0.951	1.00	0.975	0.995	0.880
	Vertical	124	184	0.822	0.954	0.883	0.944	0.803	148	200	0.941	0.985	0.962	0.989	0.860
	All	280	494	0.910	0.895	0.902	0.956	0.842	280	492	0.961	0.939	0.950	0.979	0.845
extra large	Mesioangular	118	160	0.949	1.00	0.974	0.993	0.916	136	174	0.967	0.983	0.975	0.990	0.880
	Distoangular	56	62	0.914	0.790	0.847	0.917	0.808	20	26	0.749	0.917	0.825	0.905	0.770
	Horizontal	68	88	0.935	0.976	0.955	0.971	0.861	76	92	0.979	0.996	0.987	0.995	0.884
	Vertical	124	184	0.834	0.973	0.898	0.947	0.809	148	200	0.934	0.984	0.958	0.990	0.870
	All	280	494	0.908	0.935	0.921	0.957	0.848	280	492	0.907	0.97	0.937	0.970	0.851

Table 3 shows that Class I and Class II models achieve high precision and recall values, with their performance outputs exhibiting similar behavior. In Class III, strong performance is observed despite the relatively low data volume, but its performance is relatively low compared to the other classes. The YOLO11n model provides similar accuracy metrics compared to larger models while offering the advantage of lower computational cost and faster processing. The YOLO11n model (average testing mAP@0.5 = 0.965; mAP@0.5:0.95 = 0.886) was used to determine the extraction difficulty index because of its lightweight structure and its effectiveness, especially in dense sample groups such as Class I and II. In general, all models demonstrated consistency at Levels A, B, and C, achieving high precision and recall values. In particular, the larger models (large and extra-large) achieved high accuracy values at all levels, while the smaller models (nano and small) achieved sufficient accuracy with low computational cost. The YOLO11 medium model stands out with a balanced performance at all levels and reaches a high value of 0.949 mAP@0.5:0.95 on average, especially on the test data. The YOLO11m model was preferred for the determination of extraction difficulty because it is advantageous in terms of computational cost compared to larger models and has the highest test mAP@0.5:0.95. When all the results were evaluated, it was decided to use YOLO11n for Winter angulation (average testing mAP@0.5 = 0.975; mAP@0.5:0.95 = 0.849), YOLO11n for class (average testing mAP@0.5 = 0.965; mAP@0.5:0.95 = 0.886), and YOLO11m for level (average testing mAP@0.5 = 0.989; mAP@0.5:0.95 = 0.949) in GUI design and determination of the tooth extraction difficulty index. Figure 3 graphically shows the performance of these three selected models at the time of training and validation. The fact that the training and validation losses (box_loss, cls_loss, and dfl_loss) decreased rapidly in all tasks and stabilized before the completion of 600 epochs with the early stopping operation reveals that the model performs strong learning in both location estimation and classification. Precision and recall values above 0.9 indicate that the model performs with high accuracy and low error rate, while mAP@0.5 values above 0.9 and mAP@0.5:0.95 values above 0.8 in Winter, class, and level tasks prove that the models perform consistently and successfully at IoU thresholds. Moreover, the validation losses are in line with the training losses, indicating that there are no signs of overlearning and that the model has a high generalization capacity across different datasets. For the nano model, training in the class scenario lasted 1 h and 57 min, with early stopping applied at the 262nd epoch, while in the Winter scenario, training lasted 1 h and 31 min, with early stopping occurring at the 204th epoch; for the medium model in the level scenario, training lasted 3 h and 25 min, with early stopping applied at the 363th epoch. While 5.5 MB AI files with the *.pt extension were obtained for nano models, 40.5 MB AI files were obtained for the medium model. For the selected models, training and testing confusion matrices for level, class, and Winter are given in Figure 4, and precision-recall plots are shown in Figure 5.

Table 3. Training and testing results for YOLO11 sub-models on Pell and Gregory.

Model YOLO11	Prediction	Training							Testing						
		Img	Inst	P	R	F1-S	mAP@.5	mAP@.5:.95	Img	Inst	P	R	F1-S	mAP@.5	mAP@.5:.95
nano	Class I	96	120	0.973	0.983	0.978	0.990	0.913	100	124	0.936	0.950	0.943	0.979	0.901
	Class II	226	360	0.954	0.980	0.967	0.991	0.937	200	308	0.899	0.981	0.938	0.976	0.919
	Class III	54	60	0.876	0.883	0.879	0.956	0.885	76	96	0.931	0.844	0.885	0.940	0.838
	All	280	540	0.934	0.949	0.941	0.979	0.911	280	528	0.922	0.925	0.923	0.965	0.886
small	Class I	96	120	0.959	0.992	0.975	0.995	0.917	100	124	0.910	0.977	0.942	0.974	0.895
	Class II	226	360	0.918	0.992	0.954	0.991	0.938	200	308	0.888	0.990	0.936	0.964	0.902
	Class III	54	60	0.884	0.892	0.888	0.925	0.872	76	96	0.963	0.808	0.879	0.908	0.831
	All	280	540	0.921	0.958	0.939	0.970	0.909	280	528	0.920	0.925	0.922	0.949	0.876
medium	Class I	96	120	0.973	0.992	0.982	0.995	0.927	100	124	0.871	0.984	0.924	0.983	0.913
	Class II	226	360	0.929	0.997	0.962	0.982	0.932	200	308	0.804	1.000	0.891	0.968	0.912
	Class III	54	60	0.922	0.817	0.866	0.926	0.878	76	96	0.847	0.865	0.856	0.908	0.834
	All	280	540	0.941	0.935	0.938	0.968	0.912	280	528	0.841	0.949	0.892	0.953	0.886
large	Class I	96	120	1.00	0.979	0.989	0.994	0.911	100	124	0.931	0.986	0.958	0.982	0.899
	Class II	226	360	0.938	1.00	0.968	0.993	0.936	200	308	0.861	0.990	0.921	0.979	0.919
	Class III	54	60	0.961	0.816	0.883	0.961	0.870	76	96	0.863	0.771	0.814	0.921	0.817
	All	280	540	0.966	0.932	0.949	0.983	0.906	280	528	0.885	0.916	0.900	0.961	0.878
extra large	Class I	96	120	0.957	0.983	0.970	0.992	0.907	100	124	0.886	0.992	0.936	0.956	0.882
	Class II	226	360	0.903	0.994	0.946	0.985	0.927	200	308	0.861	0.974	0.914	0.956	0.901
	Class III	54	60	0.866	0.860	0.863	0.935	0.886	76	96	0.920	0.721	0.808	0.888	0.791
	All	280	540	0.909	0.946	0.927	0.971	0.907	280	528	0.889	0.896	0.892	0.933	0.858
nano	LevelA	106	146	0.966	0.945	0.955	0.99	0.923	96	134	0.947	0.955	0.951	0.985	0.924
	LevelB	130	162	0.818	0.969	0.955	0.973	0.925	106	134	0.967	0.865	0.913	0.976	0.927
	LevelC	146	206	0.935	0.990	0.887	0.991	0.923	136	190	0.950	0.958	0.954	0.988	0.931
	All	280	514	0.906	0.968	0.936	0.985	0.923	280	458	0.955	0.926	0.940	0.983	0.928
small	LevelA	106	146	0.958	0.930	0.944	0.981	0.924	96	134	0.970	0.963	0.966	0.989	0.933
	LevelB	130	162	0.851	0.969	0.906	0.966	0.928	106	134	0.948	0.952	0.950	0.984	0.946
	LevelC	146	206	0.959	0.966	0.962	0.992	0.946	136	190	0.959	0.987	0.973	0.990	0.940
	All	280	514	0.922	0.955	0.938	0.980	0.933	280	458	0.959	0.967	0.963	0.988	0.940
medium	LevelA	106	146	0.942	0.925	0.933	0.982	0.93	96	134	0.970	0.967	0.968	0.990	0.946
	LevelB	130	162	0.833	0.956	0.890	0.96	0.925	106	134	0.955	0.940	0.947	0.985	0.953
	LevelC	146	206	0.948	0.969	0.958	0.987	0.939	136	190	0.954	0.992	0.973	0.992	0.947
	All	280	514	0.908	0.950	0.929	0.977	0.931	280	458	0.960	0.966	0.963	0.989	0.949
large	LevelA	106	146	0.934	0.971	0.952	0.98	0.923	96	134	0.963	0.975	0.969	0.991	0.951
	LevelB	130	162	0.827	0.944	0.882	0.965	0.931	106	134	0.942	0.963	0.952	0.983	0.951
	LevelC	146	206	0.944	0.981	0.962	0.981	0.937	136	190	0.974	0.970	0.972	0.985	0.937
	All	280	514	0.902	0.965	0.932	0.975	0.93	280	458	0.96	0.969	0.964	0.986	0.946
extra large	LevelA	106	146	0.934	0.963	0.948	0.976	0.915	96	134	0.93	0.970	0.950	0.977	0.931
	LevelB	130	162	0.858	0.935	0.895	0.951	0.916	106	134	0.966	0.925	0.945	0.982	0.949
	LevelC	146	206	0.939	0.961	0.950	0.984	0.938	136	190	0.984	0.983	0.983	0.987	0.937
	All	280	514	0.910	0.953	0.931	0.970	0.923	280	458	0.960	0.960	0.960	0.982	0.939

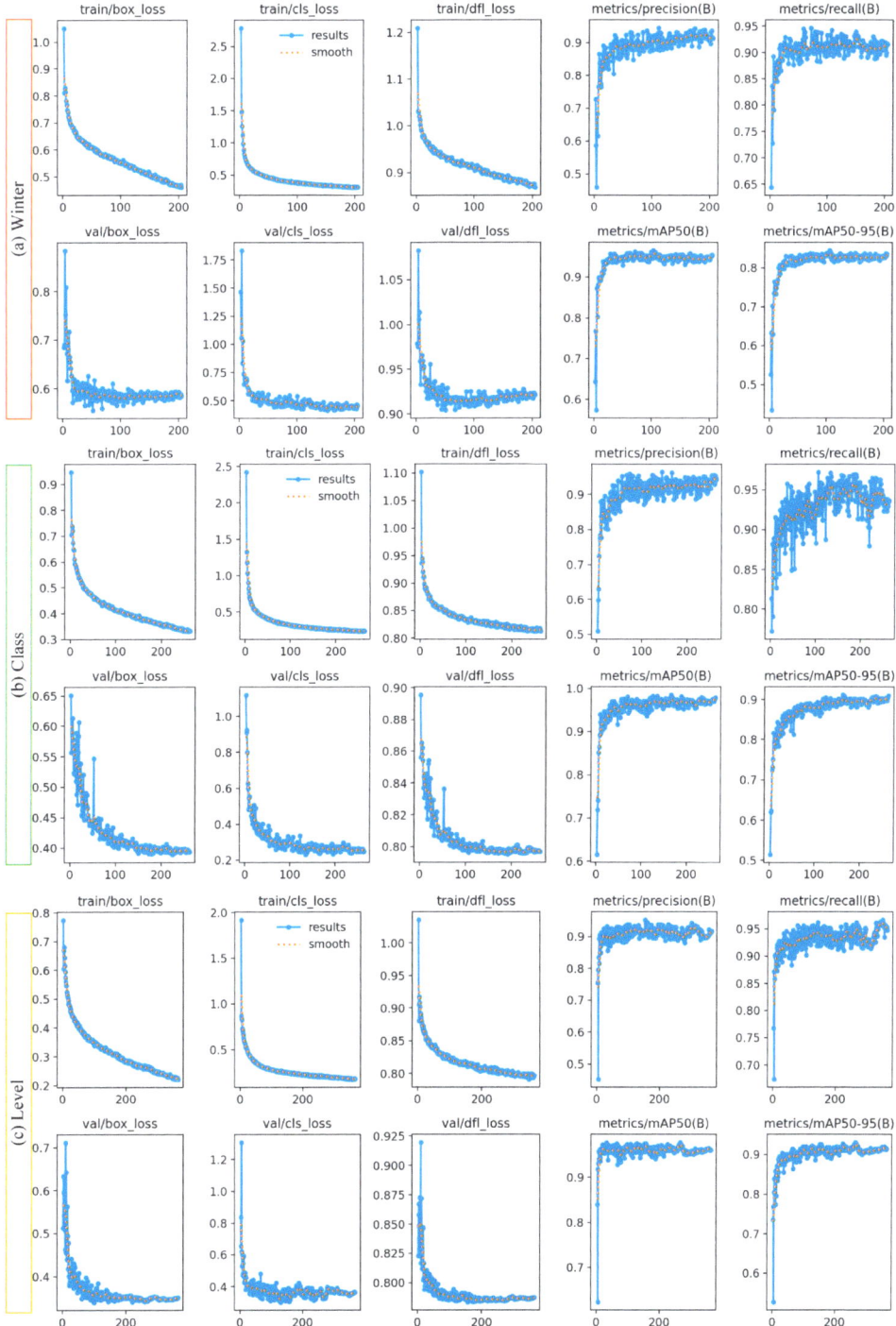

Figure 3. Graphs showing the loss values (box_loss, cls_loss, dfl_loss) and performance metrics (precision, recall, mAP50, mAP50–95) of the model during the training and validation processes across epochs: (**a**) Winter for YOLO11n, (**b**) class for YOLO11n, (**c**) level for YOLO11m.

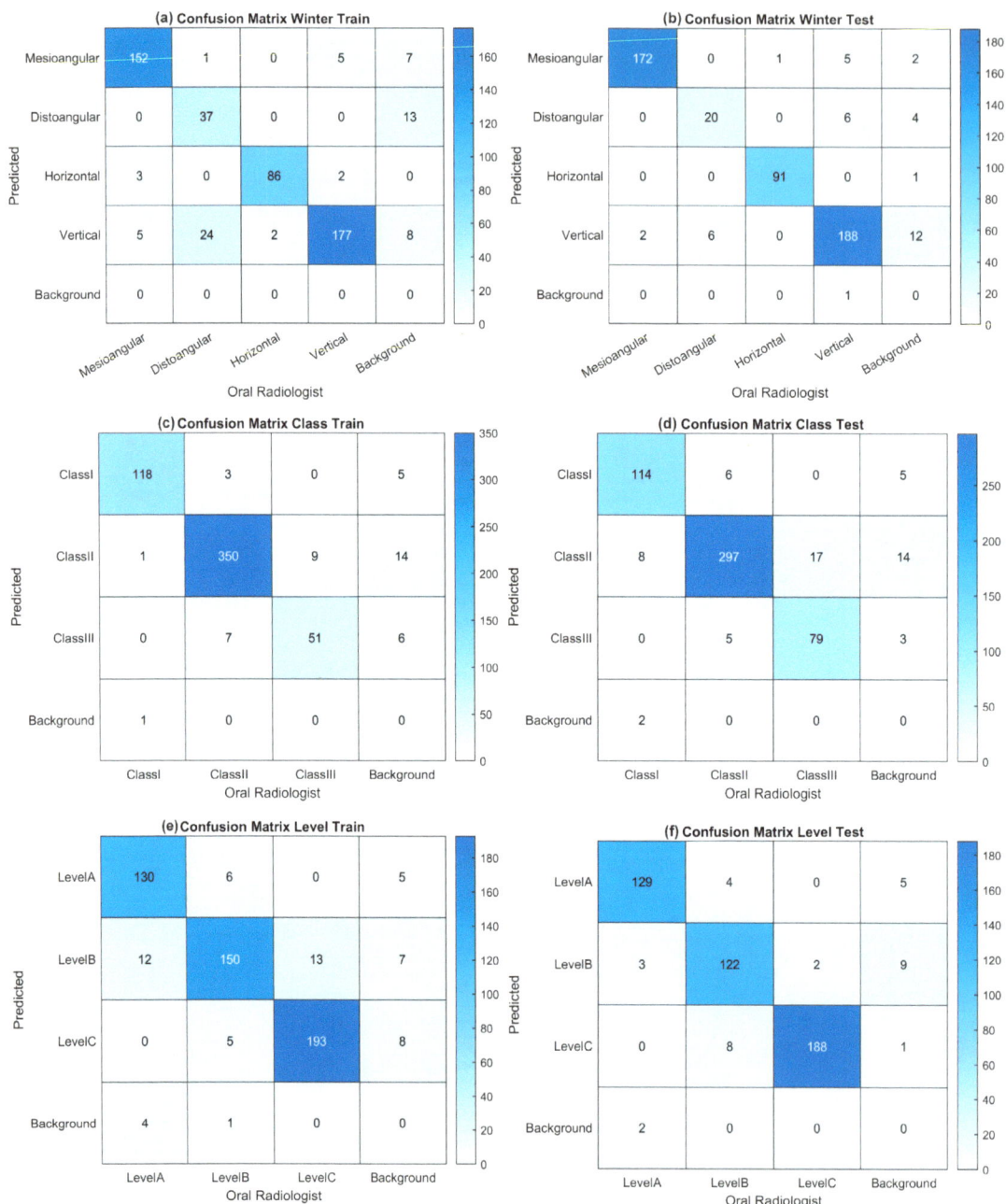

Figure 4. (**a**) Training CM for Winter angulation. (**b**) Testing CM for Winter angulation. (**c**) Training CM for class. (**d**) Testing CM for class. (**e**) Training CM for level. (**f**) Testing CM for level.

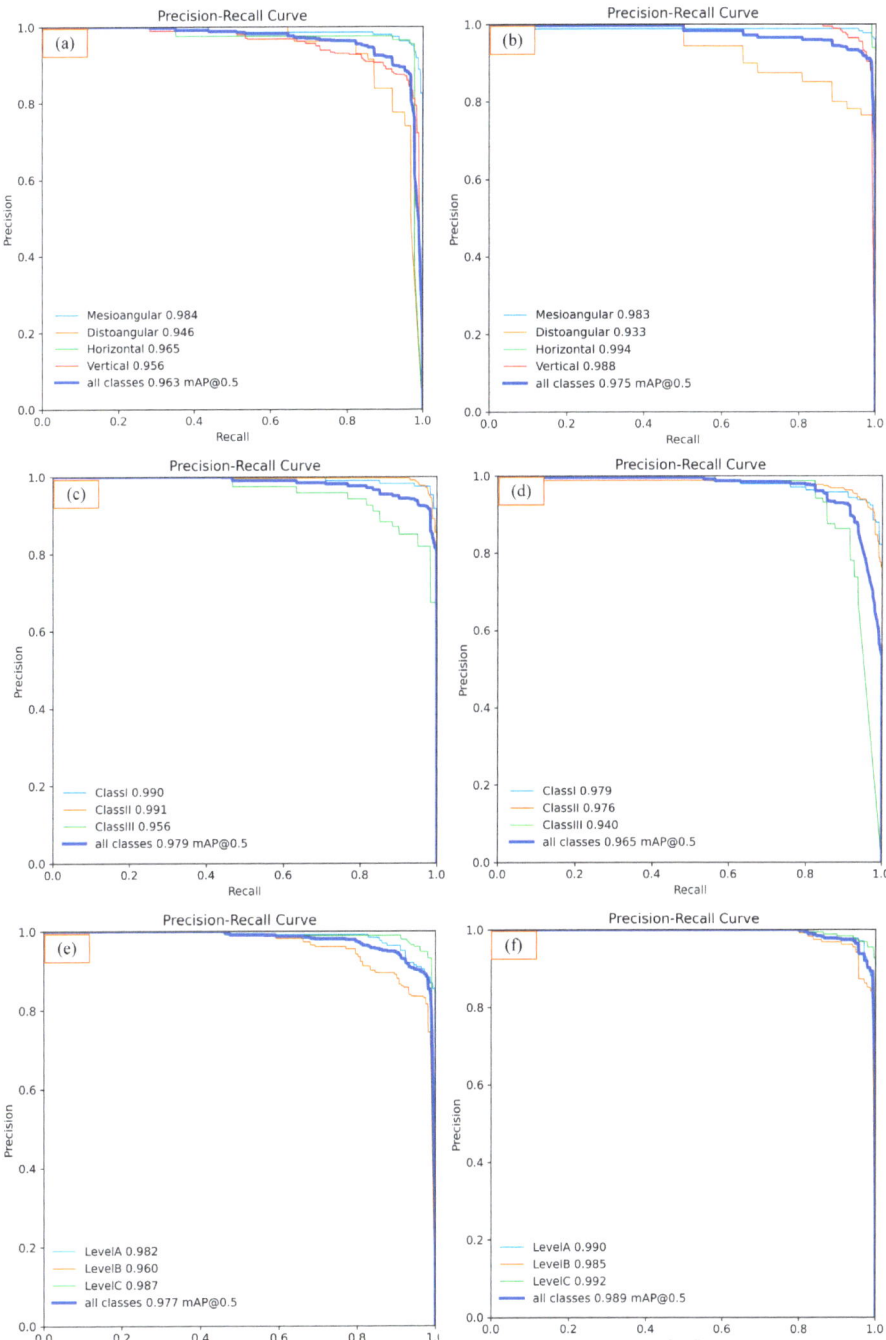

Figure 5. (**a**) Training precision–recall curve for Winter angulation, (**b**) testing precision–recall curve for Winter angulation, (**c**) training precision–recall curve for class, (**d**) testing precision–recall curve for class, (**e**) training precision–recall curve for level, (**f**) testing precision–recall curve for level.

3.2. Visual Results

The prediction results in the test images created for Winter angulation, class, and level were examined by an oral radiologist. It was observed that the second and third molars were correctly boxed in all images, accurately detecting the corresponding localizations. Only some class information was occasionally mispredicted in relation to each other. Since each PR image is personalized and has different anatomical structures, it was observed that the YOLO11 model gave a high success rate in localizing the relevant region. Figure 6 shows six test images with automatic localization and class prediction.

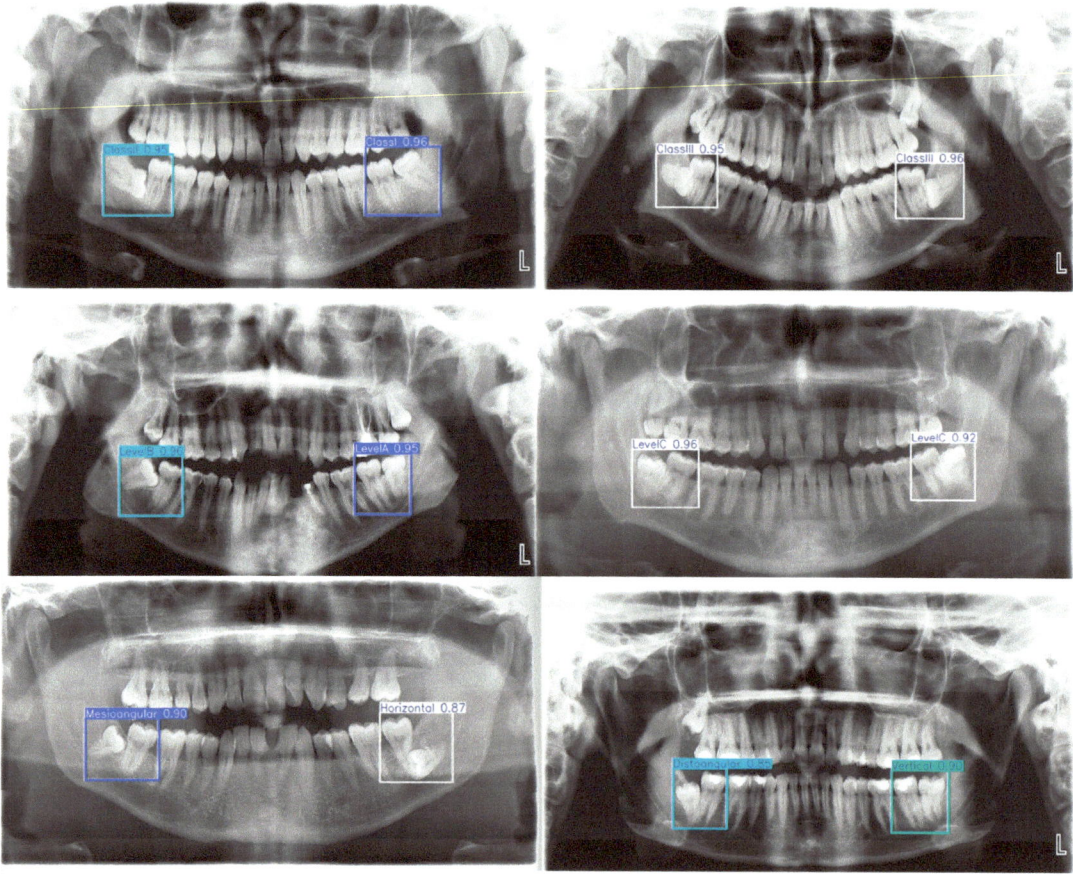

Figure 6. Winter angulation and Pell and Gregory class prediction on six test images using YOLO11 weights. 'L' is the left side of the patient.

3.3. Calculation of Pederson Index and Assistant GUI Tool

The Pederson index, a scoring system used to assess the difficulty level of third molar extractions, is calculated based on the tooth's position relative to the occlusal plane, angulation, and the relationship of the tooth to the mandibular ramus. Angulation is scored as mesioangular (1), vertical (3), horizontal (2), and distoangular (4), with the relationship to the ramus denoted as Class I (1) Class II (2), and Class III (3), and depth denoted as Level A (1), Level B (2), and Level C (3). According to the combination of conditions in the tooth, the values obtained as a result of the total are 3–4 points: slightly difficult; 5–6 points: moderately difficult; 7–10 points: very difficult. Table 4 shows all possible combinations (36 different combinations) and total scores based on angulation, ramus relationship, and depth.

Table 4. All possible combinations and scores for the Pederson index.

Angulation	Ramus	Depth	Score	Difficulty	Angulation	Ramus	Depth	Score	Difficulty
Mesioangular (1)	Class I (1)	Level A (1)	3	Slightly	Vertical (3)	Class I (1)	Level A (1)	5	Moderately
Mesioangular (1)	Class I (1)	Level B (2)	4	Slightly	Vertical (3)	Class I (1)	Level B (2)	6	Moderately
Mesioangular (1)	Class I (1)	Level C (3)	5	Moderately	Vertical (3)	Class I (1)	Level C (3)	7	Very
Mesioangular (1)	Class II (2)	Level A (1)	4	Slightly	Vertical (3)	Class II (2)	Level A (1)	6	Moderately
Mesioangular (1)	Class II (2)	Level B (2)	5	Moderately	Vertical (3)	Class II (2)	Level B (2)	7	Very
Mesioangular (1)	Class II (2)	Level C (3)	6	Moderately	Vertical (3)	Class II (2)	Level C (3)	8	Very
Mesioangular (1)	Class III (3)	Level A (1)	5	Moderately	Vertical (3)	Class III (3)	Level A (1)	7	Very
Mesioangular (1)	Class III (3)	Level B (2)	6	Moderately	Vertical (3)	Class III (3)	Level B (2)	8	Very
Mesioangular (1)	Class III (3)	Level C (3)	7	Very	Vertical (3)	Class III (3)	Level C (3)	9	Very
Horizontal (2)	Class I (1)	Level A (1)	4	Slightly	Distoangular (4)	Class I (1)	Level A (1)	6	Moderately
Horizontal (2)	Class I (1)	Level B (2)	5	Moderately	Distoangular (4)	Class I (1)	Level B (2)	7	Very
Horizontal (2)	Class I (1)	Level C (3)	6	Moderately	Distoangular (4)	Class I (1)	Level C (3)	8	Very
Horizontal (2)	Class II (2)	Level A (1)	5	Moderately	Distoangular (4)	Class II (2)	Level A (1)	7	Very
Horizontal (2)	Class II (2)	Level B (2)	6	Moderately	Distoangular (4)	Class II (2)	Level B (2)	8	Very
Horizontal (2)	Class II (2)	Level C (3)	7	Very	Distoangular (4)	Class II (2)	Level C (3)	9	Very
Horizontal (2)	Class III (3)	Level A (1)	6	Moderately	Distoangular (4)	Class III (3)	Level A (1)	8	Very
Horizontal (2)	Class III (3)	Level B (2)	7	Very	Distoangular (4)	Class III (3)	Level B (2)	9	Very
Horizontal (2)	Class III (3)	Level C (3)	8	Very	Distoangular (4)	Class III (3)	Level C (3)	10	Very

Figure 7 shows the pipeline designed in this study to calculate the extraction difficulty for a single tooth. The system takes an image and first converts it to 8-bit depth and then rescales it to 1024×532. The image is sent to a YOLO11n model trained for angulation prediction, a YOLO11n model trained for class prediction, and a YOLO11m model trained for level prediction, respectively. Each model stores both the prediction results and class localization in a variable and can provide visualization outputs. This process is performed separately for the left and right third molars to determine the extraction difficulty score and grade.

Using the pipeline developed in Figure 7, the prediction and scoring images of three test images are given in Figure 8. The pipeline designed in Figure 7 was developed as a Python script and embedded in a GUI, as seen in Figure 9. In the GUI designed using the PyQT library, all analysis can be performed with a single button. Thus, dentists will be able to calculate the third molar extraction difficulty score without being exposed to complex coding processes.

In the experiments conducted to calculate the Pederson index of a total of 514 mandibular third molars on 300 test images performed using the GUI, the model detected 507 bounding boxes. Of these detected boxes, 12 were evaluated as FP, and 7 were not detected at all and were included in the FN category. However, out of the 24 boxes for which the Pederson index could not be calculated (N/A), 3 were added to FP due to over-detection, and 21 were added to FN due to under-detection. As a result of these adjustments, the total number of FPs was determined as 15, the total number of FNs was 28, and the total number of TPs was determined as 486. When the model's performance was examined, precision was calculated as 97.00%, recall as 94.55%, and F1 score as 95.76%. These results demonstrate that the proposed method based on YOLO11 offers high accuracy and reliability in the detection of mandibular third molars and the calculating of the Pederson index.

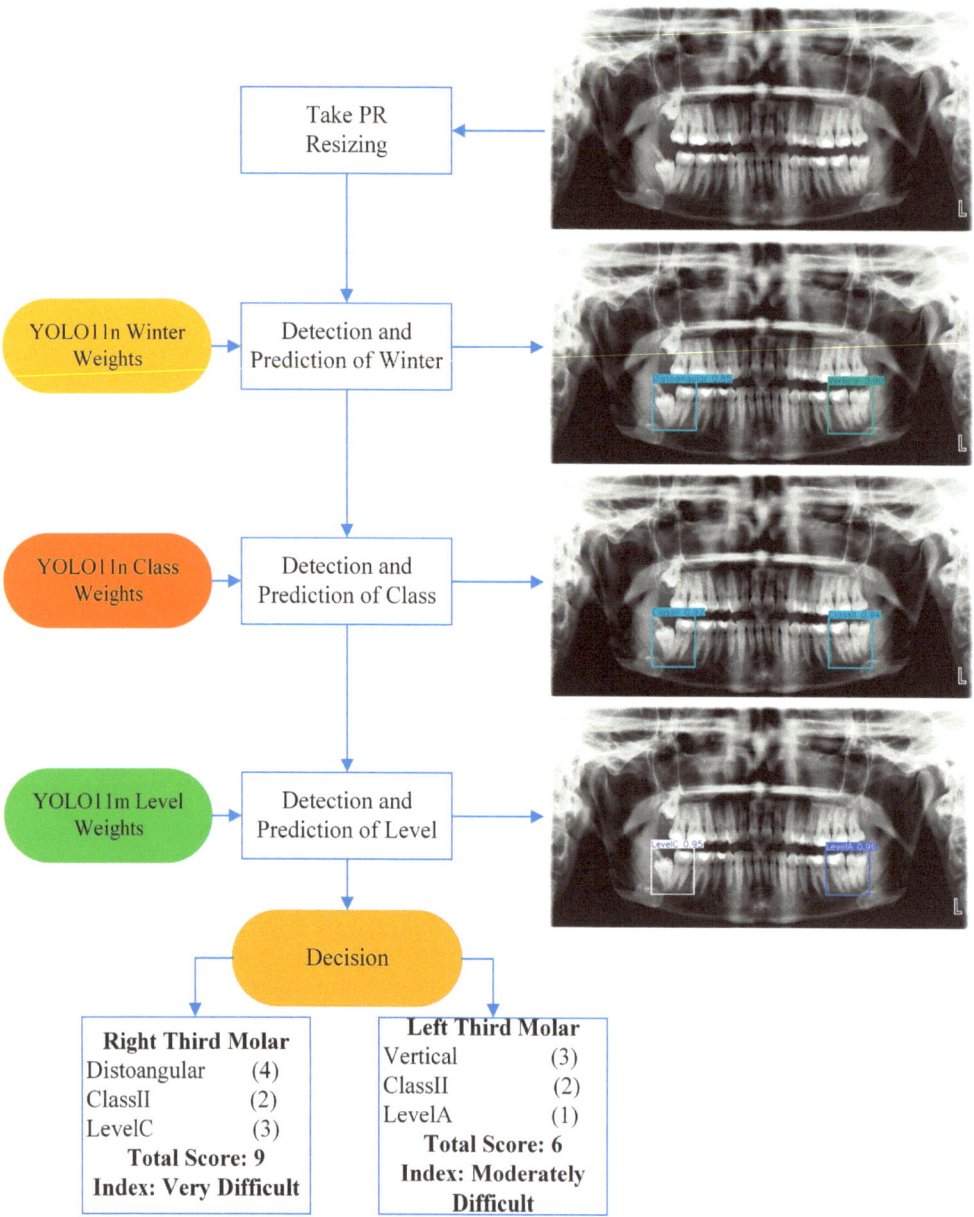

Figure 7. Flow diagram of the system designed for the automatic determination of the mandibular third molar extraction difficulty index.

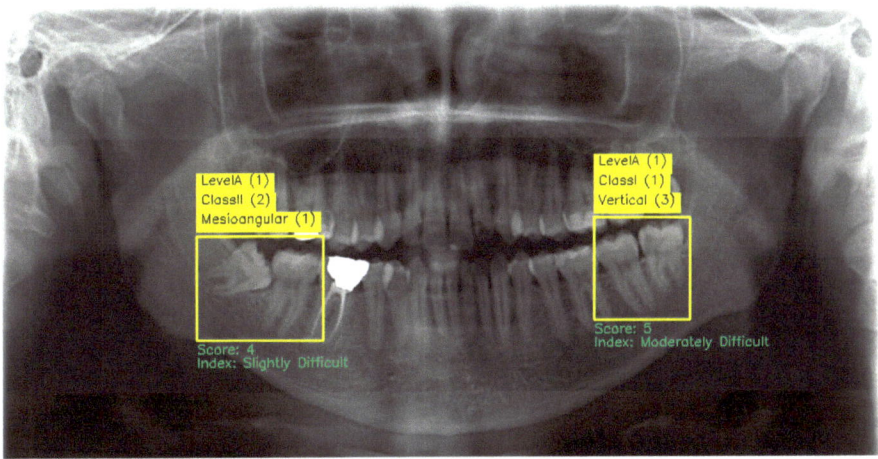
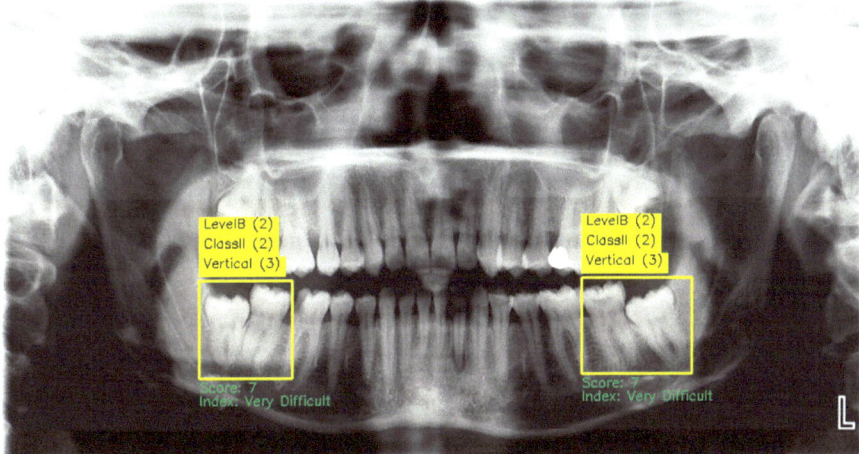
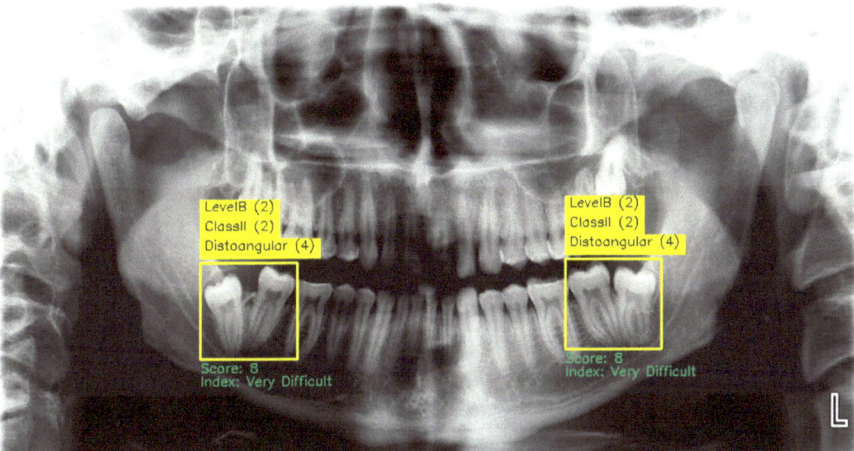

Figure 8. Analysis of 3 test images in terms of the Pederson index using the pipeline developed in Figure 7.

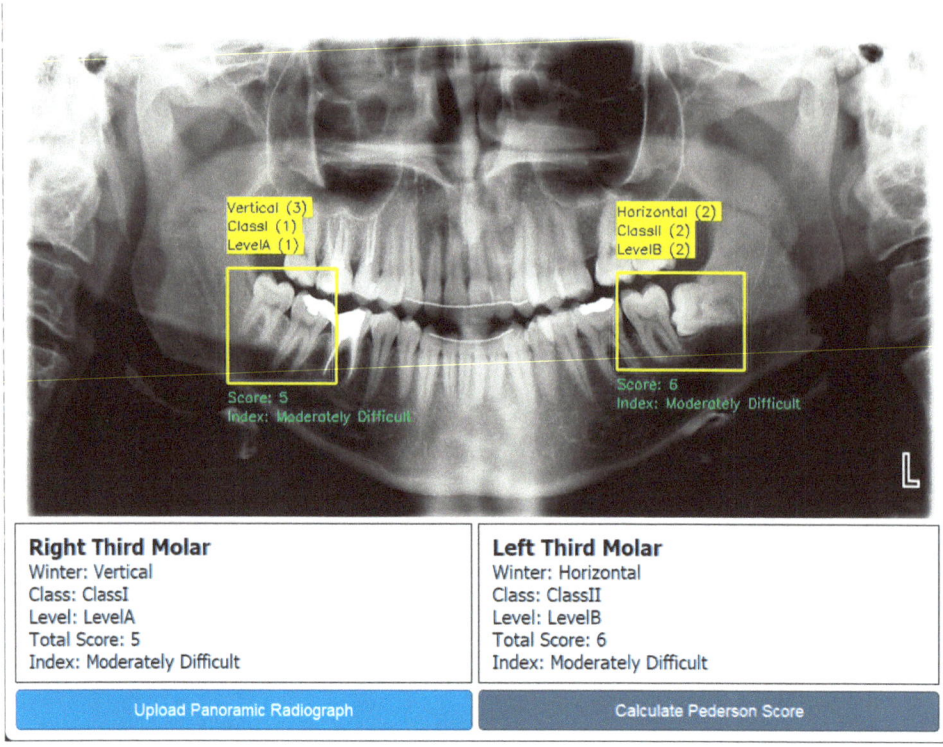

Figure 9. GUI developed for automatic calculation of Pederson index.

4. Discussion

This study developed an AI-assisted clinical tool employing YOLO11 models to predict the difficulty of mandibular third molar extractions, utilizing the widely accepted and validated [44] Pederson difficulty index criteria. As a result of the comparison of YOLO11 sub-models, the nano model for class, the medium model for level in the Pell and Gregory category, and the nano model in the Winter category were preferred for index calculation. It became evident that the sub-models generally yielded similar results to each other, and high results were obtained especially in terms of mAP@50 (mean Average Precision at IoU threshold 0.5) values. High values of mAP@50 indicate that the model performs well, detects the correct objects in positive predictions in the Pell and Gregory and Winter categories, and matches them with a high confidence score. YOLO11 weights were applied sequentially for class, level, and Winter on a PR image and Pederson difficulty index scores were automatically determined. In the evaluation performed by an oral radiologist on 150 test images, the proposed pipeline performed well, achieving 97.00% precision, 94.55% recall, and 95.76% F1 score. The developed Python script was integrated into a GUI, making it a minimal program that dentists can use in the clinic without having to deal with complex coding processes.

The degree of difficulty associated with tooth extractions can range from minimally invasive procedures to complex surgical interventions needing general anesthesia. Categorizing the difficulty of tooth extractions and calculating the time required are important for oral and maxillofacial surgeons [20]. It may also be important for some insurance systems in Asian countries [4]. According to Parant [45], easy extractions are classified as Grade I (requiring only forceps) or Grade II (requiring the osteotomy), while difficult extractions are classified as Grade III (requiring both osteotomy and coronal section) or Grade IV (involving complex procedures such as root resection). Kwon et al. [20] introduced a hybrid model that integrates a convolutional neural network (CNN) utilizing panoramic X-ray images with a multilayer perceptron (MLP) leveraging patient clinical data to estimate the extraction time for mandibular third molars. The combined CNN+MLP model achieved a strong correlation (R = 0.8315) with the test data, predicting extraction times with a mean error of 2.95 min.

In the literature, some studies detect only Pell and Gregory [29–31] and Winter [9,15,29–32] categories based on AI; however, articles on determining the extraction difficulty of mandibular third molars are extremely limited [33–37]. Yoo et al. (2021) [33] proposed a CNN-based model to predict the extraction difficulty of mandibular third molars using PRs. A total of 1053 mandibular third molars from 600 panoramic images were used and labeled according to the Pederson difficulty index by three experts. Zero-padding was applied to the images for preprocessing. The proposed method utilized a two-stage process of region-of-interest (ROI) detection and classification. For ROI detection, a Single-Shot Multibox detector-based object detection model was used and VGG16 acted as a pre-trained backbone. The detected regions were then sent to the ResNet-34-based model for the classification of Pederson difficulty scores. Accuracies of 78.91%, 82.03%, and 90.23% were achieved for C1 (depth), C2 (ramal relationship), and C3 (angulation), respectively. The RMSE value was calculated as 0.6738 when the model predicted the PDS scores. The use of only PRs was mentioned in the study as a limitation that may affect the accuracy of the model. It was emphasized that although PRs extend the range of anatomical structures in 2D, the possibility of unavoidable distortions in both vertical and horizontal dimensions, as well as transverse angulation and dilacerations were extremely difficult to assess. Lee et al. [34] (2022) developed a deep learning approach to predict the extraction difficulty of mandibular third molars from PRs and the probability of inferior alveolar nerve (IAN) injury. A total of 8720 mandibular third molars in 4903 PRs were evaluated by seven dentists. The Retinanet (ResNet-152) model was used for detection, and the Vision Transformer (R50+ViT-L/32) was used for classification. Preprocessing of images involved size adjustment, Contrast-Limited Adaptive Histogram Equalization (CLAHE), and data augmentation. In addition, the ROI was cropped to 700 × 700 pixels to contain the mandibular third molar, adjacent teeth, and IAN. The proposed method, instead of Pederson, estimated extraction difficulty in four classes: vertical eruption, soft tissue impaction, partial bone impaction, and complete bone impaction. It also assessed IAN injury risk in three levels: low, moderate, and high. For extraction difficulty estimation, the R50+ViT-L/32 model indicated the highest performance with 83.5% accuracy, 66.35% F1 score, and 92.79% AUROC, while the ResNet-34 model showed lower performance with 80.07% accuracy and 63.28% F1 score, and the ResNet-152 model showed lower performance with 82.18% accuracy and 63.23% F1 score. In the IAN injury risk classification, the proposed method gave 81.1% accuracy, 75.55% F1 score, and 90.02% AUROC. Li et al. [35] (2023) proposed a model combining deep learning and super-resolution (SR) technologies to estimate extraction difficulty. A total of 608 panoramic images obtained from two medical centers were used; the mandibular third molar, adjacent teeth, and inferior alveolar nerve regions as ROIs were cropped to 200 × 200 pixels, and then their dimensions were normalized to 800 × 800 pixels. High-resolution images were created from low-resolution images using a GAN-based method for super-resolution, and this process was performed by training the GAN with low–high-resolution pairs of images with Gaussian noise added. Feature extraction was performed with 2048 features obtained from the ResNet152 model, and statistical methods and LASSO regression were used for feature selection to determine the final features. The features were given as input to conventional machine learning models including AdaBoost, Logistic Regression, K-Nearest Neighbor, MLP, and NaiveBayes. Pederson scores were divided into two categories (≤5 and >5) and were used as output classes. However, these categories were not named "easy" or "difficult" in this study; only the scores were used for classification. In the classification performance of extraction difficulty, the Model-SR Logistic Regression machine learning algorithm showed the most optimal algorithm performance with an accuracy of 79.8%, sensitivity of 85.5%, specificity of 60.9%, and AUC of 0.779. The overall AUC of Model-SR was 0.963, which was found to be superior to expert dentists. Trachoo et al. [37] (2024) classified the extraction difficulty of impacted mandibular third molars from 1367 PRs collected retrospectively between 2021 and 2023 as novice, intermediate, and expert, taking into account the Pederson index, according to the level of dentists who can perform the surgical intervention. Images were resized to 300×600 pixels, and data augmentation techniques (zooming, resampling, horizontal flipping) were used. In PRs, images were split in the middle to analyze the right and left teeth separately. The system consisted of a three-stage model: ResNet101V2 performed binary classification to determine the presence of impacted lower third molars and achieved 86.71% accuracy; RetinaNet performed object detection to determine the location of LM3 and showed outstanding performance with 99.28% mAP; and Vision Transformer (ViT) performed multiclass classification to estimate surgical difficulty levels (novice, intermediate, expert) and achieved an average accuracy of 78.99%. Chindanuruks et al. (2024) [36] trained the YOLOv5x model for the Pernambuco Index with 1730 PRs taken in 2021–2023. The images were in .BMP format, labeled with LabelImg, and converted to YOLO format. As a preprocess, the images were resized to 416×416 pixels, and a horizontal flip was applied for data augmentation. The algorithm assessed six radiographic criteria, namely depth (level: 87% accuracy, 85.1% AUC-PRC, mAP@0.5: 87%), ramus relationship (77% accuracy, 76.8% AUC-PRC, mAP@0.5: 77%), angulation (Winter: 84% accuracy, 89.4% AUC-PRC, mAP@0.5: 84%), root number (89% accuracy, 88% AUC-PRC, mAP@0.5: 89%), root curvature (dilacerated: 61% accuracy, 72.2% AUC-PRC, mAP@0.5: 61%) and contact with the second molar (contact: 82% accuracy, 85% AUC-PRC, mAP@0.5: 82%). Surgical difficulty was classified as low, moderate, and high by adding age and body mass index (BMI). The YOLOv5x model used was the version with the highest performance in the series, the overall AUC-ROC score was found to be 85%, 77%, and 74% for low, medium, and high classes, respectively, and the model's agreement with experts was found to be ICC = 0.802.

When the studies in the literature are examined, it can be seen that most of them perform classification after cropping the images. Additionally, preprocessing steps other than resizing are also performed. Single-shot models, such as YOLO11, perform both localization and classification by analyzing the image in one pass, consequently reducing the computational cost. Achieving high results without complex preprocessing and cropping is one of the prominent advantages of the study. PRs are complex images by nature, with anatomical structures that vary according to the person. Different anatomical structures may have various variations such as fillings, missing teeth, screws, plates, wires, artifacts, and superimposition situations. Despite these disadvantages, the third molar position was found to be accurate in almost all images. The results obtained with the pipeline proposed in this study were successful in the automatic calculation of mandibular third molar extraction difficulty, in comparison with other studies. The high precision, recall, F1 score, and mAP values obtained in this study showed that YOLO11 outperformed similar studies with high accuracy and low error rate in Winter, class, and level tasks. In this study, YOLO11, whose performance was tested for the first time in dental diagnosis processes, has an optimized structure compared to previous versions. It offers better overall performance with more parameter control and modern hyperparameter settings [40]. These features of YOLO11 make it a superior model with regard to both speed and accuracy, and it can be favored in AI-supported diagnosis tasks.

Limitations

The fact that this study was conducted only with panoramic radiographs means that clinical findings and other imaging modalities were not integrated. Various factors influencing extraction difficulty, including anatomical challenges, root morphology, bone density, patient age, gender, mouth-opening capacity, body mass index (BMI, kg/m2), proximity to vital structures, and the surgeon's expertise, were not comprehensively assessed. In the future, evaluating these additional parameters using three-dimensional imaging techniques (e.g., CBCT), and using larger datasets obtained from different centers may increase the accuracy and generalizability of the model. The limitations of the developed software and GUI include the possibility of performance degradation in devices with low hardware capacity due to the high computational power required by the YOLO11 model, and the fact that it cannot be generalized for other tooth types or difficulty assessment methods because it focuses only on mandibular third molars and the Pederson difficulty index.

5. Conclusions

This study highlights the effectiveness of YOLO11 models in predicting mandibular third molar extraction difficulty using panoramic radiographs and the Pederson difficulty index. The YOLO11 nano and medium sub-models demonstrated a strong balance between accuracy and efficiency. Their integration into a user-friendly GUI allows for rapid assessment, improving surgical planning and patient management. Future research should incorporate clinical factors and advanced imaging to enhance model accuracy and applicability further.

Author Contributions: Conceptualization, M.Ü.Ö. and M.T.; methodology, M.Ü.Ö., S.A., and M.T.; software, M.Ü.Ö. and S.A.; validation, M.Ü.Ö. and M.T.; formal analysis, M.Ü.Ö. and S.A.; investigation, M.Ü.Ö. and S.A.; resources, M.Ü.Ö. and S.A.; data curation, M.T.; writing—original draft, M.Ü.Ö., S.A., and M.T.; writing—review and editing, M.Ü.Ö., S.A., and M.T.; visualization, M.Ü.Ö.; supervision, M.Ü.Ö. All authors have read and agreed to the published version of the manuscript.

Funding: This work is supported by the Scientific and Technological Research Council of Türkiye grants 2210-C.

Institutional Review Board Statement: This study was conducted at the Faculty of Dentistry, Necmettin Erbakan University, Department of Dentomaxillofacial Radiology, with the approval of the Ethics Committee (numbered:2024/424) and was performed according to the stipulations laid out by the Declaration of Helsinki.

Informed Consent Statement: This study was retrospective, and informed consent was not required since the data were anonymized.

Data Availability Statement: The datasets can be shared with researchers who wish to conduct studies upon reasonable request.

Acknowledgments: This study has been conducted as the outcome of the thesis undertaken by Serap Akdoğan in the Department of Biomedical Engineering at Pamukkale University Graduate School of Natural and Applied Sciences, under the primary supervisor Assist. Muhammet Üsame Öziç and the second supervisor Assoc. Melek Tassoker. The authors are grateful for the support of the Scientific and Technological Research Council of Türkiye.

Conflicts of Interest: The authors declare no conflicts of interest.

Abbreviations

The following abbreviations are used in this manuscript:

AI	Artificial Intelligence
AP	Average Precision
AUC-PRC	Area Under the Precision-Recall Curve
AUROC	Area Under the Receiver Operating Characteristic Curve
BMI	body mass index
CBCT	cone beam computed tomography
CLAHE	Contrast-Limited Adaptive Histogram Equalization
CM	confusion matrix
CNN	convolutional neural network
FN	False Negative
FP	False Positive
F1-S	F1 score
GUI	graphical user interface
ICC	Intraclass Correlation Coefficient
IAN	inferior alveolar nerve
Img	images
Ins	instances
IoU	Intersection over Union
MLP	multilayer perceptron
mAP	mean Average Precision
N/A	Not Applicable
PNG	Portable Network Graphics
PRs	panoramic radiographs
P	precision
R	recall
ROI	region of interest
SR	super-resolution
TP	True Positive
ViT	Vision Transformer
YOLO	You Only Look Once

References

1. Albayati, M.T.; Bede, S.Y. Reliability of two difficulty indexes in predicting the surgical extraction difficulty of impacted mandibular third molars. *J. Oral Med. Oral Surg.* **2023**, *29*, 5. [CrossRef]
2. Kim, J.Y.; Yong, H.S.; Park, K.H.; Huh, J.K. Modified difficult index adding extremely difficult for fully impacted mandibular third molar extraction. *J. Korean Assoc. Oral Maxillofac. Surg.* **2019**, *45*, 309–315. [CrossRef]
3. Bali, A.; Bali, D.; Sharma, A.; Verma, G. Is Pederson Index a True Predictive Difficulty Index for Impacted Mandibular Third Molar Surgery? A Meta-analysis. *J. Maxillofac. Oral Surg.* **2013**, *12*, 359–364. [CrossRef]
4. Njokanma, A.R.; Aborisade, A.; Kuye, O.F.; Amedari, M.I.; Njokanma, A.H. Does Pederson Difficulty Index Accurately Predict the Difficulty of Mandibular Third Molar Extraction? *Niger. J. Basic Clin. Sci.* **2024**, 1–7. [CrossRef]
5. Pederson, G.W. Surgical removal of tooth. In *Oral Surgery*; Pederson, G.W., Ed.; Saunders, WB: Philadelphia, PA, USA, 1988.
6. Pell, G.J. Impacted mandibular third molars, classification and modified technique for removal. *Dent. Dig.* **1933**, *39*, 330–338.
7. Winter, G.B. *Principles of Exodontia as Applied to the Impacted Mandibular Third Molar*; American Medical Book Company: Wilsonville, OR, USA, 1926.
8. Atieh, M.A. Diagnostic accuracy of panoramic radiography in determining relationship between inferior alveolar nerve and mandibular third molar. *J. Oral Maxillofac. Surg.* **2010**, *68*, 74–82. [CrossRef]
9. Zirek, T.; Öziç, M.Ü.; Tassoker, M. AI-Driven localization of all impacted teeth and prediction of winter angulation for third molars on panoramic radiographs: Clinical user interface design. *Comput. Biol. Med.* **2024**, *178*, 108755. [CrossRef]
10. Erturk, M.; Öziç, M.Ü.; Tassoker, M. Deep Convolutional Neural Network for Automated Staging of Periodontal Bone Loss Severity on Bite-wing Radiographs: An Eigen-CAM Explainability Mapping Approach. *J. Imaging Inform. Med.* **2024**, 1–20. [CrossRef]

11. Karakuş, R.; Öziç, M.Ü.; Tassoker, M. AI-Assisted Detection of Interproximal, Occlusal, and Secondary Caries on Bite-Wing Radiographs: A Single-Shot Deep Learning Approach. *J. Imaging Inform. Med.* **2024**, *37*, 3146–3159. [CrossRef]
12. Park, C.; Took, C.C.; Seong, J.-K. Machine learning in biomedical engineering. *Biomed. Eng. Lett.* **2018**, *8*, 1–3. [CrossRef]
13. Pouyanfar, S.; Sadiq, S.; Yan, Y.; Tian, H.; Tao, Y.; Reyes, M.P.; Shyu, M.L.; Chen, S.C.; Iyengar, S.S. A survey on deep learning: Algorithms, techniques, and applications. *ACM Comput. Surv.* **2018**, *51*, 1–36. [CrossRef]
14. Vranckx, M.; Van Gerven, A.; Willems, H.; Vandemeulebroucke, A.; Ferreira Leite, A.; Politis, C.; Jacobs, R. Artificial intelligence (AI)-driven molar angulation measurements to predict third molar eruption on panoramic radiographs. *Int. J. Environ. Res. Public Health* **2020**, *17*, 3716. [CrossRef] [PubMed]
15. Celik, M.E. Deep learning based detection tool for impacted mandibular third molar teeth. *Diagnostics* **2022**, *12*, 942. [CrossRef] [PubMed]
16. Chen, S.-L.; Chou, H.-S.; Chuo, Y.; Lin, Y.-J.; Tsai, T.-H.; Peng, C.-H.; Tseng, A.-Y.; Li, K.-C.; Chen, C.-A.; Chen, T.-Y. Classification of the Relative Position between the Third Molar and the Inferior Alveolar Nerve Using a Convolutional Neural Network Based on Transfer Learning. *Electronics* **2024**, *13*, 702. [CrossRef]
17. Vinayahalingam, S.; Xi, T.; Bergé, S.; Maal, T.; De Jong, G. Automated detection of third molars and mandibular nerve by deep learning. *Sci. Rep.* **2019**, *9*, 9007. [CrossRef]
18. Banar, N.; Bertels, J.; Laurent, F.; Boedi, R.M.; De Tobel, J.; Thevissen, P.; Vandermeulen, D. Towards fully automated third molar development staging in panoramic radiographs. *Int. J. Leg. Med.* **2020**, *134*, 1831–1841. [CrossRef]
19. De Tobel, J.; Radesh, P.; Vandermeulen, D.; Thevissen, P.W. An automated technique to stage lower third molar development on panoramic radiographs for age estimation: A pilot study. *J. Forensic Odonto-Stomatol.* **2017**, *35*, 42.
20. Kwon, D.; Ahn, J.; Kim, C.-S.; Kang, D.O.; Paeng, J.-Y. A deep learning model based on concatenation approach to predict the time to extract a mandibular third molar tooth. *BMC Oral Health* **2022**, *22*, 571. [CrossRef]
21. Milani, O.H.; Atici, S.F.; Allareddy, V.; Ramachandran, V.; Ansari, R.; Cetin, A.E.; Elnagar, M.H. A fully automated classification of third molar development stages using deep learning. *Sci. Rep.* **2024**, *14*, 13082. [CrossRef]
22. Kempers, S.; van Lierop, P.; Hsu, T.-M.H.; Moin, D.A.; Bergé, S.; Ghaeminia, H.; Xi, T.; Vinayahalingam, S. Positional assessment of lower third molar and mandibular canal using explainable artificial intelligence. *J. Dent.* **2023**, *133*, 104519. [CrossRef]
23. Ariji, Y.; Mori, M.; Fukuda, M.; Katsumata, A.; Ariji, E. Automatic visualization of the mandibular canal in relation to an impacted mandibular third molar on panoramic radiographs using deep learning segmentation and transfer learning techniques. *Oral Surg. Oral Med. Oral Pathol. Oral Radiol.* **2022**, *134*, 749–757. [CrossRef] [PubMed]
24. Kim, J.-Y.; Kahm, S.H.; Yoo, S.; Bae, S.-M.; Kang, J.-E.; Lee, S.H. The efficacy of supervised learning and semi-supervised learning in diagnosis of impacted third molar on panoramic radiographs through artificial intelligence model. *Dentomaxillofacial Radiol.* **2023**, *52*, 20230030. [CrossRef] [PubMed]
25. Joo, Y.; Moon, S.-Y.; Choi, C. Classification of the relationship between mandibular third molar and inferior alveolar nerve based on generated mask images. *IEEE Access* **2023**, *11*, 81777–81786. [CrossRef]
26. Zhu, T.; Chen, D.; Wu, F.; Zhu, F.; Zhu, H. Artificial intelligence model to detect real contact relationship between mandibular third molars and inferior alveolar nerve based on panoramic radiographs. *Diagnostics* **2021**, *11*, 1664. [CrossRef]
27. Lo Casto, A.; Spartivento, G.; Benfante, V.; Di Raimondo, R.; Ali, M.; Di Raimondo, D.; Tuttolomondo, A.; Stefano, A.; Yezzi, A.; Comelli, A. Artificial intelligence for classifying the relationship between impacted third molar and mandibular canal on panoramic radiographs. *Life* **2023**, *13*, 1441. [CrossRef]
28. Takebe, K.; Imai, T.; Kubota, S.; Nishimoto, A.; Amekawa, S.; Uzawa, N. Deep learning model for the automated evaluation of contact between the lower third molar and inferior alveolar nerve on panoramic radiography. *J. Dent. Sci.* **2023**, *18*, 991–996. [CrossRef]
29. Maruta, N.; Morita, K.-I.; Harazono, Y.; Anzai, E.; Akaike, Y.; Yamazaki, K.; Tonouchi, E.; Yoda, T. Automatic machine learning-based classification of mandibular third molar impaction status. *J. Oral Maxillofac. Surg. Med. Pathol.* **2023**, *35*, 327–334. [CrossRef]
30. Sukegawa, S.; Matsuyama, T.; Tanaka, F.; Hara, T.; Yoshii, K.; Yamashita, K.; Nakano, K.; Takabatake, K.; Kawai, H.; Nagatsuka, H.; et al. Evaluation of multi-task learning in deep learning-based positioning classification of mandibular third molars. *Sci. Rep.* **2022**, *12*, 684. [CrossRef]
31. Aravena, H.; Arredondo, M.; Fuentes, C.; Taramasco, C.; Alcocer, D.; Gatica, G. Predictive Treatment of Third Molars Using Panoramic Radiographs and Machine Learning. In Proceedings of the 2023 19th International Conference on Wireless and Mobile Computing, Networking and Communications (WiMob), Montreal, QC, Canada, 21–23 June 2023; IEEE: New York, NY, USA, 2023; pp. 123–128.
32. Lei, Y.; Chen, X.; Wang, Y.; Tang, R.; Zhang, B. A Lightweight Knowledge-Distillation-Based Model for the Detection and Classification of Impacted Mandibular Third Molars. *Appl. Sci.* **2023**, *13*, 9970. [CrossRef]
33. Yoo, J.-H.; Yeom, H.-G.; Shin, W.; Yun, J.P.; Lee, J.H.; Jeong, S.H.; Lim, H.J.; Lee, J.; Kim, B.C. Deep learning based prediction of extraction difficulty for mandibular third molars. *Sci. Rep.* **2021**, *11*, 1954. [CrossRef]

34. Lee, J.; Park, J.; Moon, S.Y.; Lee, K. Automated Prediction of Extraction Difficulty and Inferior Alveolar Nerve Injury for Mandibular Third Molar Using a Deep Neural Network. *Appl. Sci.* **2022**, *12*, 475. [CrossRef]
35. Li, W.; Li, Y.; Liu, X. Transfer learning-based super-resolution in panoramic models for predicting mandibular third molar extraction difficulty: A multi-center study. *Med. Data Min.* **2023**, *6*, 20–27. [CrossRef]
36. Chindanuruks, T.; Jindanil, T.; Cumpim, C.; Sinpitaksakul, P.; Arunjaroensuk, S.; Mattheos, N.; Pimkhaokham, A. Development and validation of a deep learning algorithm for the classification of the level of surgical difficulty in impacted mandibular third molar surgery. *Int. J. Oral Maxillofac. Surg.* **2024**. [CrossRef] [PubMed]
37. Trachoo, V.; Taetragool, U.; Pianchoopat, P.; Sukitporn-udom, C.; Morakrant, N.; Warin, K. Deep Learning for Predicting the Difficulty Level of Removing the Impacted Mandibular Third Molar. *Int. Dent. J.* **2024**, *75*, 144–150. [CrossRef] [PubMed]
38. Adamska, P.; Adamski, Ł.J.; Musiał, D.; Tylek, K.; Studniarek, M.; Wychowańński, P.; Kaczoruk-Wieremczuk, M.; Pyrzowska, D.; Jereczek-Fossa, B.A.; Starzyńska, A. Panoramic radiograph–a useful tool to assess the difficulty in extraction of third molars. *Eur. J. Transl. Clin. Med.* **2020**, *3*, 44–52. [CrossRef]
39. Ansari, M.A.M.F.; Mutha, A. Digital Assessment of Difficulty in Impacted Mandibular Third Molar Extraction. *J. Maxillofac. Oral Surg.* **2020**, *19*, 401–406. [CrossRef]
40. Khanam, R.; Hussain, M. YOLOv11: An Overview of the Key Architectural Enhancements. *arXiv* **2024**, arXiv:2410.17725.
41. Gbotolorun, O.M.; Arotiba, G.T.; Ladeinde, A.L. Assessment of factors associated with surgical difficulty in impacted mandibular third molar extraction. *J. Oral Maxillofac. Surg.* **2007**, *65*, 1977–1983. [CrossRef]
42. Prerana, G.; Tantry, D.; Sougata, K.; Sivalanka, S.C.S. Incidence of complications after the surgical removal of impacted mandibular third molars: A single center retrospective study. *J. Acad. Dent. Educ.* **2021**, *7*, 10–17. [CrossRef]
43. Yuasa, H.; Kawai, T.; Sugiura, M. Classification of surgical difficulty in extracting impacted third molars. *Br. J. Oral Maxillofac. Surg.* **2002**, *40*, 26–31. [CrossRef]
44. Kharma, M.Y.; Sakka, S.; Aws, G.; Tarakji, B.; Nassani, M.Z. Reliability of Pederson scale in surgical extraction of impacted lower third molars: Proposal of new scale. *J. Oral Dis.* **2014**, *2014*, 157523. [CrossRef]
45. Parant, M. *Petite Chirurgie de la Bouche*; L'Expansion Scientifique Française: Paris, France, 1963.

Disclaimer/Publisher's Note: The statements, opinions and data contained in all publications are solely those of the individual author(s) and contributor(s) and not of MDPI and/or the editor(s). MDPI and/or the editor(s) disclaim responsibility for any injury to people or property resulting from any ideas, methods, instructions or products referred to in the content.

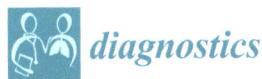

Article

Automated Age Estimation from OPG Images and Patient Records Using Deep Feature Extraction and Modified Genetic–Random Forest

Gulfem Ozlu Ucan [1,*], Omar Abboosh Hussein Gwassi [2], Burak Kerem Apaydin [3] and Bahadir Ucan [4]

[1] Department of Oral and Maxillofacial Radiology, Faculty of Dentistry, Istanbul Gelisim University, Istanbul 34310, Turkey
[2] Electrical and Computer Engineering, School of Engineering and Natural Sciences, Altinbas University, Istanbul 34217, Turkey; 213720043@ogr.altinbas.edu.tr
[3] Department of Oral and Maxillofacial Radiology, Faculty of Dentistry, Pamukkale University, Denizli 20160, Turkey; drkeremapaydin@gmail.com
[4] Department of Communication and Design, Yildiz Technical University, Istanbul 34220, Turkey; bucan@yildiz.edu.tr
* Correspondence: dtgulfemozlu@gmail.com

Abstract: Background/Objectives: Dental age estimation is a vital component of forensic science, helping to determine the identity and actual age of an individual. However, its effectiveness is challenged by methodological variability and biological differences between individuals. Therefore, to overcome the drawbacks such as the dependence on manual measurements, requiring a lot of time and effort, and the difficulty of routine clinical application due to large sample sizes, we aimed to automatically estimate tooth age from panoramic radiographs (OPGs) using artificial intelligence (AI) algorithms. **Methods:** Two-Dimensional Deep Convolutional Neural Network (2D-DCNN) and One-Dimensional Deep Convolutional Neural Network (1D-DCNN) techniques were used to extract features from panoramic radiographs and patient records. To perform age estimation using feature information, Genetic algorithm (GA) and Random Forest algorithm (RF) were modified, combined, and defined as Modified Genetic–Random Forest Algorithm (MG-RF). The performance of the system used in our study was analyzed based on the MSE, MAE, RMSE, and R^2 values calculated during the implementation of the code. **Results:** As a result of the applied algorithms, the MSE value was 0.00027, MAE value was 0.0079, RMSE was 0.0888, and R^2 score was 0.999. **Conclusions:** The findings of our study indicate that the AI-based system employed herein is an effective tool for age detection. Consequently, we propose that this technology could be utilized in forensic sciences in the future.

Keywords: age estimation; dental age estimation; forensic odontology; deep learning; machine learning; forensics; panoramic radiograph

1. Introduction

Identification of individuals represents a crucial area within the discipline of forensic sciences [1,2]. The age of the individual in question carries significant weight in the process of identification [3,4]. In instances of mass disasters, organized crime, and abuse cases, it is imperative to ascertain the age of suspects and victims to facilitate their identification [5]. In the extant literature, the estimation of age in human history and forensic sciences has consistently been highlighted as a research topic, with the objective of developing reliable age estimation techniques for both living and deceased individuals [4].

The term chronological age is used to describe the time that has elapsed since an individual's date of birth. This is calculated by determining the dates of both the individual's birth and death. In the absence of available data regarding the dates of birth and death, the age of an individual can be estimated by examining the biological age of the individual in question. The assessment of biological age is based on the physical development stages of the individual or the changes that occur with aging. This assessment includes the development of various systems such as height, weight, hair, skin, eyes, teeth, bones, and secondary sex characteristics [6–8].

Dental tissues are the most durable part of the skeleton [9]. They are resistant to extreme conditions and are preserved longer than bone [10]. For this reason, teeth are often used in forensic science to estimate age [11]. Even in cases of major disasters, when the victim's body is so mutilated that it cannot be visually identified, the remains of skull bones, jaw bones, and teeth have proven to be the most valuable source of identification [4,12]. Radiographic estimation of age and sex from radiographs of the jaw bones is considered more feasible because it is a simple and less destructive method that can be applied to both deceased and living cases [4,13].

A variety of methods, including morphological, metric, radio morphological, radio metric, histological, and biochemical approaches, can be utilized for age estimation in dental tissues [2,14,15]. However, further research is necessary to ascertain the applicability and reliability of these methods across diverse populations [11]. The classic age estimation methods rely on manual measurements and observer subjectivity, which are time-consuming and prone to observer bias, potentially increasing the workload of forensic experts and introducing subjectivity into the estimation process [16,17].

AI is defined as the capacity of a machine to imitate the cognitive processes and behaviors observed in humans, enabling the completion of tasks that would otherwise require human input. In recent years, the rapid development of AI has facilitated numerous technological advancements that have enhanced the quality of life for many individuals. Furthermore, AI has advanced rapidly in numerous medical domains, garnering significant interest in recent years, particularly within the radiology community. To date, the implementation of AI in dental radiography has demonstrated considerable potential for a multitude of applications. At this point, it can facilitate critical support for clinicians, novice physicians, and students in the decision making process [18].

In recent years, studies based on AI have been conducted with the objective of automating tasks in dentistry. These include caries diagnosis and classification [19–28], automatic diagnosis of dental diseases and conditions of the teeth [29], diagnostic evaluation and segmentation in periapical radiographs [30], periodontal bone loss [31,32], implant planning [33], detection and classification of periapical pathologies [34], cephalometric analysis and automatic detection of anatomical landmarks [35,36], detection of impacted mandibular third molars, and [37] to detecting and classifying impacted maxillary supernumerary teeth [38–42]. Additionally, research has aimed to detect vertical root fractures [43,44], classify osteoporosis [45–47], improve image quality [48–50], identify and classify odontogenic tumors and cysts [51,52], diagnose maxillary sinus pathologies [53–55], identify and classify lymph node metastases [56,57], diagnose patients with Sjogren syndrome [58], and detect oral cancer lesions [59].

AI also offers significant potential in the field of forensic sciences for data analysis and ensuring the proper administration of justice [60]. These models have the potential to be promising tools when identifying victims of mass disasters and as an additional aid in medico-legal situations. In the literature, AI-based models have been reported to show similar accuracy and precision as trained forensic scientists. It has been stated that these models can be promising tools when identifying victims of mass disasters and as an additional aid in medico-legal situations [61].

The advent of deep learning represents a significant milestone in the evolution of AI algorithms. Deep learning is a group of algorithms based on the structure of artificial neural networks and defined as a sub-branch of machine learning. Deep learning algorithms offer significant advantages in processing complex datasets and making sense of problems. These algorithms simplify complex problems by classifying datasets in a hierarchical manner through the use of multilayer artificial neural networks. A typical deep learning system consists of an input layer representing the dataset of the problem, multiple hidden layers, and an output layer. Hidden layers contain links that help to understand the relationships in the dataset. This structure provides more effective results in solving complex problems than classical AI algorithms [62].

Existing classic age estimation methods have been critiqued in the literature for several shortcomings. Observer subjectivity has been identified as a potential source of error in age estimation. Furthermore, manual measurement-based methods are time-consuming and laborious. Additionally, the feasibility of implementing these methods in routine clinical practice has been questioned due to the limited sample sizes typically used. Considering the considerations, the present research endeavors to employ DM-based methodologies for the processing of panoramic radiograph (OPG) images and patient records, with the objective of estimating the age of individuals with the highest estimation rate.

This study utilized the Deep 2D CNN for feature extraction from OPG images and Deep 1D CNN for feature extraction from patient records, hence establishing a dual-feature extraction process resulting in a more robust and comprehensive representation of patient data. Following that, employing a concatenate strategy to merge features from these two approaches enhanced the predictive performance of age estimation models. Furthermore, the study proposes an MG-RF regressor that combines the optimization ability of the GA with RF algorithm. It can minimize overfitting, enhance the detection rate, and utilize genetic indications via chromosomes, affording numerous optimal solutions. The study implemented this innovative methodology specifically for pediatric age estimation, a vital task in both medical and forensic fields. Regarding these advantages, the present work considers this AI-based methodology for age estimation.

The primary objectives of this study were as follows:

- To extract pertinent features from OPG images and patient records, employing innovative approach that combines Deep 2D CNN with a Deep 1D CNN. The extracted features were then concatenated to improve the accuracy of age estimation;
- To achieve the highest coefficient of determination (R^2) for age estimation by leveraging an MG-RF regressor;
- To evaluate the efficiency of the proposed methodology with respect to standard deviation (SD), mean absolute error (MAE), mean square error (MSE), root mean square error (RMSE), and R^2.

2. Related Work

In recent years, AI-based methodologies have been developed with the objective of overcoming these limitations and automating the age estimation process. These approaches yield consistent and reproducible results and facilitate reduced processing times. These approaches are deemed capable of detecting attributes that are not recognizable to human observers and are not feasible for manual computation. Moreover, the substantial benefits in identifying intricate relationships between features facilitate more accurate predictions with diminished error rates [17,63,64]. AI-based approaches in the literature are generally categorized as machine learning, deep learning, or a combination of these two methodologies [17]. The objectives of these studies include numerical age regression [16,17,65–71], staging of teeth [72–74], classification of age groups [75,76], and legal age classification [77].

Galibourg et al. [66] conducted a study with a machine learning approach for numerical age regression. The researchers employed ten machine learning methods, including Random Forest (RF), Support Vector Machine (SVM), Decision Tree (DT), Bayesian Ridge Regression (BRR), K-Nearest Neighbors (KNN), AdaBoost (ADAB), Polynomial Regression (POLYREG), Multi-Layer Perceptron (MLP), Stacking (STACK), and Voting (VOTE). The researchers reported that age estimation using machine learning methods yielded superior results compared to manual methods based on radiographic dental staging from childhood to early adulthood.

In addition, one study employed Scaled-YOLOv4 to detect dental germs with 8023 panoramic radiographs as training data, achieving MAP, EfficientNetV2, and M classifiers for the developmental stages of detected dental germs using 18,485 single-root and 16,313 multi-root images. This approach yielded superior outcomes for multi-root classifications. The MAE between automatic and manual dental age calculations using different methods was 0.274 for single selection, 0.261 for weighted average, and 0.396 for the expected value, with the weighted average demonstrating the most optimal performance [78].

Similarly, Tao et al. [67] employed machine learning for numerical age regression. The researchers employed an MLP for this purpose. It was demonstrated that the proposed system exhibited superior performance compared to the reference manual methods across all performance metrics.

A DL model, designated as DentAge, was developed for the automated estimation of age using panoramic dental X-ray images. This model was trained on a dataset comprising 21,007 images from a private dental center in Slovenia, encompassing subjects ranging in age from 4 to 97 years. The model attained an MAE of 3.12 years across the test dataset, thereby substantiating its efficacy in age estimation under varied dental conditions [79].

Shen et al. [68] employed machine learning for numerical age regression, utilizing RF, SVM, and linear regression (LR). The findings of the study indicated that age estimation accuracy was superior in machine learning methods compared to traditional methods.

De Tobel [72] employed a deep learning approach for staging teeth, with transfer learning (Alex-Net) demonstrating the most effective performance for staging.

Boedi et al. [73] employed the Dense Net machine learning algorithm. The objective of the present study was to ascertain and validate the impact of lower third molar segmentations on automatic tooth development staging. The study's findings led to the conclusion that full tooth segmentation and DenseNet CNN optimization facilitate the accurate allocation of dental stages.

Banar et al. [74] employed a CNN that was similar in structure to the You Only Look Once (YOLO) algorithm, in conjunction with the U-Net CNN and the DenseNet201 CNN. The objective of this study is to automate the staging process in its entirety, utilizing CNN at each stage of the procedure. The results demonstrate that the proposed fully automated approach yields promising outcomes in comparison to manual staging.

In their study, Kim et al. [75] employed a deep learning approach, ResNet 152, for the classification of age groups. The accuracy of the tooth-wise prediction was found to be between 89.05 and 90.27 percent. The performance accuracy was primarily assessed through the use of the majority voting system and area under the curve (AUC) scores. The AUC scores ranged from 0.94 to 0.98 for all age groups, indicating a superior capability.

Dong et al. [76] developed a methodology for identifying tooth maturity stages in fully permanent dentition. This methodology features a YOLOv3-based tooth localization model for detecting and numbering teeth, a symmetric ordinal staging network (SOS-Net) that enhances feature representation while minimizing parameters, and an auxiliary regression branch with adjacent stage-aware (ASA) loss to reduce misclassification. The efficacy of this methodology was evaluated using a private OPG dataset comprising subjects between the ages of 3 and 14 years. The experimental results obtained demonstrated enhanced F1-scores, thereby surpassing contemporary state-of-the-art methodologies in terms of maturity staging and age estimation.

Guo et al. [77] employed the SE-ResNet101 model to ascertain the legal age groups. It was reported that end-to-end CNN models demonstrated superior performance, with accuracy rates of 92.5%, 91.3%, and 91.8% for age thresholds of 14, 16, and 18 years, respectively. To-end CNN models demonstrated superior performance, with accuracy rates of 95.9%, 95.4%, and 95.4% for age thresholds of 14, 16, and 18 years, respectively.

Čular et al. [69] employed a combination of Deep Learning Active Shape Model (ASM), Active Appearance Model (AAM), and Radial Basis Network algorithms for the purpose of numerical age regression. In this study, the researchers proposed a semi-automated system based on deep learning techniques to predict tooth age by analyzing the mandibular right third molar tooth on OPGs.

De Back et al. [70] applied deep learning and Bayesian convolutional neural networks methods for numerical age regression. The system achieved a concordance correlation coefficient of ccc = 0.91 in the validation set.

A three-step framework for estimating dental age in children aged 3 to 15 was also developed. This framework includes the following elements: the employment of a YOLOv3 network for tooth localization and numbering, the achievement of a mean average precision, and the establishment of a novel SOS-Net for accurate tooth development staging based on a modified Demirjian method. The result of these efforts was an average accuracy of 82.97% for full dentition. In addition, a dental age assessment was conducted through a single-group meta-analysis, yielding an MAE of 0.72 years when excluding third molars [80].

Wallraff et al. [71] employed the ResNet18 algorithm. In this study, a supervised regression-based deep learning method for automatic age estimation of adolescents aged 11 to 20 years was proposed as a means of reducing the estimation error. In an initial investigation, the proposed methodology demonstrated a mean absolute error (MAE) of 1.08 years and an error rate (ER) of 17.52% on the test dataset, exhibiting superior performance compared to the predictions of dental experts.

In their study, Vila-Blanco et al. [65] employed Rotated R-CNN algorithms to propose a novel, fully automatic methodology for age and gender estimation. The method initially employs a modified CNN to detect teeth and extract oriented bounding boxes for each tooth. These boxes are then fed into a second CNN module, designed to produce probability distributions of age and gender per tooth. Finally, an uncertainty-sensitive approach is used to aggregate these estimated distributions, resulting in an improvement in the absolute error rate.

3. Materials and Methods

This study was approved by the Pamukkale University Non-Interventional Clinical Research Ethics Committee (E-60116787-020-202083/26 April 2022). The study was conducted in accordance with the principles set forth in the Declaration of Helsinki.

In this study, feature extraction is individually performed using the proposed Deep 2D CNN and Deep 1D CNN. In addition, MG-RF is proposed for estimating the age. The proposed methodologies estimate age through the sequence of processes shown in Figure 1. Initially, the dataset was loaded. Subsequently, pre-processing was undertaken to make the data easier to interpret and use. This process also assisted in eliminating the duplicates or inconsistencies in the data that could otherwise negatively impact the prediction rate of the model. Preprocessing the data also assisted in ensuring that there were no missing or incorrect data due to bugs or human error. Following this, feature extraction was performed for eliminating the redundant data. Deep 2D CNN was used to extract the features from OPG images. Simultaneously, Deep ID CNN was utilized to extract features from patient records. These features were individually extracted and then concatenated to attain suitably efficient features for better age estimation using MG-RF. Finally, performance metrics were utilized to validate the effectiveness of the proposed system in comparison to existing methods.

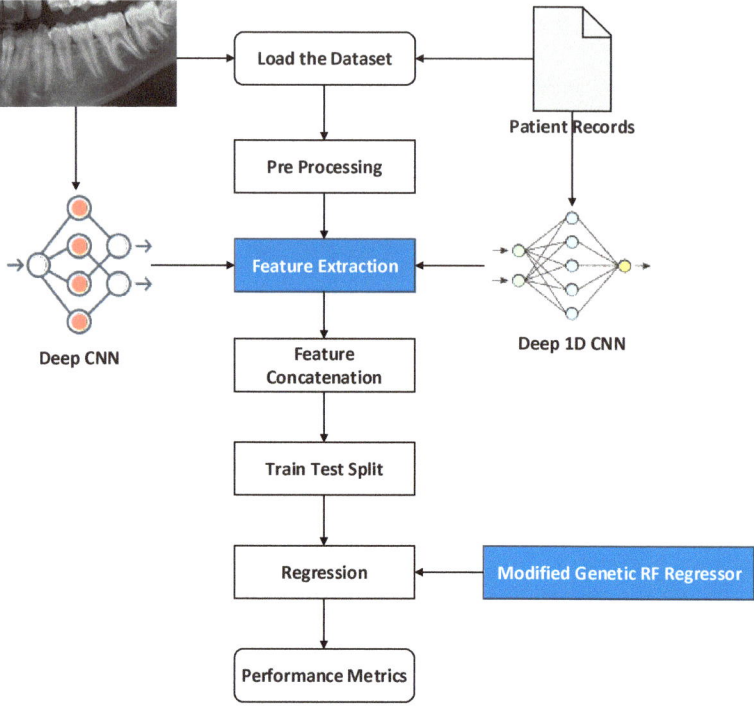

Figure 1. Overall view of the proposed system. Feature extraction is a key step in machine learning and data analysis, that is colored to emphasize its role on transferring data in between Deep CNN and Deep 1D CNN. Modified random forest regression is a type of supervised learning algorithm that employs an ensemble approach to tackle regression tasks.

3.1. Dataset Description

The present study included all systemically healthy patients between the ages of 6 and 15 years who had undergone an OPG in the correct position, yielding an OPG free of artifacts and distortions that was clearly evaluable, and who did not have any dental deficiencies and dental restorations. The archive of the Department of Oral, Dental and Maxillofacial Radiology, Faculty of Dentistry, Pamukkale University, was the source of the data. The dataset was created between 1 March 2020 and 1 March 2022. The patients' chronological age was calculated by subtracting the date of birth from the date of the OPGs.

OPGs were obtained with a digital orthopantomograph (OP200D; Instrumentarium Company, Imaging Unit, Tuusula, Finland) with exposure values between 66 kVp, 2.5 mA, and 13.4 s and 60 kVp, 6.3 mA, and 14.1 s. The OPGs were subsequently evaluated using AI algorithms.

The dataset consists of OPGs and corresponding patient records intended for research purposes and utilized in real-time applications. It includes patients within a specific age range, as indicated by the average ages of males and females, highlighting a focus on a particular developmental stage. Both genders are represented, and images are selected based on clinical relevance, such as the presence of dental conditions or anomalies, ensuring that only high-quality OPGs with sufficient diagnostic value are included. The distribution of images in the dataset, which consists of orthopantomogram (OPG) images and patient records, is characterized by the features of 275 male and 346 female patients, suggesting a minimum of 621 images if one image per patient is assumed. Out of 275 male patients, the average age is 10.94, while out of 346 female, average age is 11.1.

3.2. Preprocessing

The preprocessing pipeline for patient data comprises several essential steps to ensure high-quality input for DL models. Initially, data cleaning is performed to eliminate any missing information, followed by the application of a normalization approach, such as min–max scaling for OPG images and Z-score method for patient records (numeric data). The min–max technique is applied to adjust the pixel intensity values of images, transforming the data into a specified range, generally as [0, 1]. The Z-score method is employed to convert numerical data into a standard normal distribution, thereby facilitating more efficient analysis. Consequently, this step enhances the quality of the input image, leading to an improved prediction accuracy.

3.3. Feature Extraction: Deep Two-Dimensional Convolution Neural Network and Deep One-Dimensional Convolution Neural Network

Recently, DL has gained paramount significance in the medical domain, as it possesses the capability for handling huge data. Thus, this study employed two Deep CNN models to perform feature extraction. The Deep 2D CNN model was applied to extract features from OPG images, while Deep 1D CNN was utilized for extracting features from the patient records. After extracting individual features, these were concatenated and fed into the trained model for age estimation.

3.3.1. Deep 2D CNN: Deep Two-Dimensional Convolutional Neural Network

Deep 2D CNN is a standard CNN and has obtained use in extensive application areas of deep CNN. It has numerous advantages. The CNNs possess the capability to integrate the feature extraction and classification process into one learning body. It can also learn to perform feature optimization during the training stage from raw input. Deep CNN are sparsely associated with connected weights and could process many inputs with high computational efficacy. These are also immune to trivial conversions in input data inclusive of translation, skewing, scaling, and distortion. Deep CNNs could also adapt to varied input sizes. Generally, Deep 2D CNN is employed on images, and its overall architecture is shown in Figure 2, which comprises numerous layers, such as batch normalization, maxpooling, dropout, flatten, and dense layers. It is called 2D CNN, with kernel slides with two data dimensions.

Feature extraction from OPG images is performed by Deep 2D CNN based on the below procedure.

1. Input Layer

Features from pre-processed data are declared as an input of Deep 2D CNN and are given by Equation (1).

$$X = [x_1, x_2, x_3, \ldots, x_{numF}] \tag{1}$$

In Equation (1), represents the feature count per window after computation. To enhance the speed of model's convergence, min–max normalization is used (as shown in

Equation (2)), by which values in the individual data dimension are linearly converted. Then, they are normalized to a range of [0, 1].

$$x = \frac{x - \min}{\max - \min} \quad (2)$$

In Equation (2), represents minimum of individual column, while represents the maximum of the individual column.

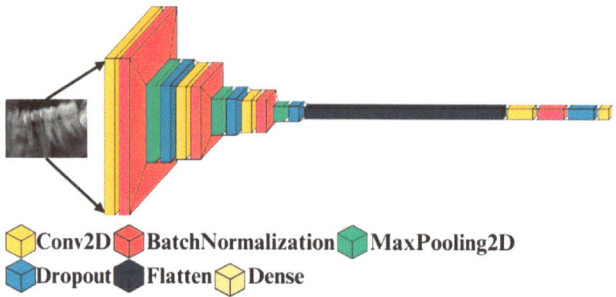

Figure 2. Overall architecture of Deep 2D CNN.

2. Convolution layer

The output from the feature map residing on the unit of the convolution layer is given by Equation (3).

$$x_i^{l,j} = \sigma\left(b_j + \sum_{a=1}^{m} w_a^j x_{i+a-1}^{l-1,j}\right) \quad (3)$$

where represents the bias for feature map, size of kernel is indicated by, indicates the weight of feature map, represents filter-index, and represents activation function.

3. Maxpooling layer

The pooling layer gives descending aggregation measurements for the adjacent outcome that could minimize the dimension as well as the output sensitivity, accomplishing scale invariant feature maintenance. Maxpooling is the pooling function utilized in this study that divides the convolutional layer's output features into various partitions and determines the maximum in the individual partition. The output of this layer is given by Equation (4).

$$x_i^{l,j} = \max_{pos=1}^{r}\left(x_{(i-1)*T_{ps}}^{l-1,j}\right) \quad (4)$$

In Equation (4), indicates pooling stride, and represents the pooling size.

4. Training the model

Deep CNN comprises numerous layers, such as Conv2D, batch normalization, maxpooling 2D, dropout, flatten, and dense layers. Then, input is mapped into the feature space of the hidden layer. Finally, the dense layer integrates varied features of local structure learned from the lower layer for performing final prediction. This study used a single pair of a convolution layer and a maxpooling 2D layer. Subsequently, the 2D data are flattened into 1D data; in this way, the overall neural network is completed with a dense layer and is given by Equation (5).

$$f(x) = \text{argmax}_{cls}\left(\frac{e^{x^{l-1}w_j}}{\sum_{n=1}^{N} e^{x^{l-1}w_{ps}}}\right) \quad (5)$$

In Equation (5), indicates class label, represents features of a sample, indicates layer index, and indicates the class count. Further, forward propagations are processed in accordance with Equations (3) and (5). The information proliferates forward from the input layer by the hidden layer to the output layer and thereby accomplishes the output of the overall network. Moreover, an iteration of forward propagation affords the network error value. Cross-entropy cost function computes the error value as given in Equation (6).

$$L(y) = -\frac{1}{n}\sum_x [y \ln a + (1-y)\ln(1-a)] \quad (6)$$

In Equation (6), indicates sample, represents total training samples, and indicates actual value, while represents predicted value. The overall algorithm of Deep 2D CNN is given in Algorithm 1.

Algorithm 1: Deep 2D CNN

1 Input: OPG Images
2 Output: Features
3 **STEP 1**: Sliding Window Process
4 **STEP 2**: sef ← Extract Shadow Features
5 **STEP 3**: Normalize sef using equation (2)
6 regularization feature data, size = 64 Units–128 Units
7 repeat:
8 **STEP 4**: Forward Propagation
9 cdf ← Convolution2D(sef);
10 mp ← Max_pooling(cdf);
11 fc ← Fully_connected(mp);
12 class label ← relu(fc);
13 **STEP 5**: Backward Propagation
14 conduct backward propagation with Adam;
15 Until wi convergences;// wi: weight
16 **STEP 6**: Use the trained network to predict the features

---

Initially, OPG images are taken as input. Then, the sliding window process is performed. Following this, the shadow features are extracted. Then, these features are normalized and regularized using Equation (2). Subsequently, forward and backward propagation is performed until the weight converges. Finally, the trained model is used for predicting features.

3.3.2. Deep 1D CNN: Deep One-Dimensional Convolutional Neural Network

Deep 2D CNN is an altered version of Deep 1D CNN, which has gained interest in recent times. It requires minimum computational requirements and is suited for low-cost and real-time applications. Though mainstream models mostly rely on 2D convolution, the main idea of 1D CNN is almost the same. The main variation is that 2D convolution operates with information of the matrix, wherein 1D convolution operates with 1D vector information and can be expressed by the following:

$$x_l = conv1d(w_{l-1}, x_{l-1}) + b_l \quad (7)$$

In Equation (7), represents the results, and indicates bias.

Non-linear functions are added to fit the actual function in a better way. So, the overall outcome is indicated as follows:

$$y_l = f(x_l) \quad (8)$$

In Equation (8), represents ReLU activation functions or sigmoid functions.

In CNNs, there exists a significant concept called receptive fields, which represents the region where input data could be viewed by features of the CNN. When (3 × 1) kernel size is utilized, the initial hidden layer can view the three characteristic original data values, and the subsequent hidden layer can view five characteristic original data values. Thus, utilizing two (3 × 1) convolution kernels instead of single convolution kernel having size (5 × 1) could minimize the parameters while confirming that a similar receptive area is attained. In accordance with this idea, the block below was framed using numerous small kernels for extracting features.

3.3.3. Feature Concatenation

After features were extracted from OPG images and patient records, they were concatenated, and these features were fed into train and test split for age estimation. The total number of OPG images was 622, and total number of records was also 622. Out of 622 OPG images, 60 images were extracted, while out of 622 patient records, 15 features were extracted. Upon concatenating, a total of 75 features were obtained.

3.4. Regression-MG-RF (Modified Genetic–Random Forest)

Generally, GA (Genetic Algorithm) is a general-purpose and optimization search method relying on genetic theory and the natural selection of Darwin in biological systems. In this algorithm, the population individually is called a chromosome, which relates to a resolution for a specific issue. The individual chromosome indicates a combination of DT (Decision Tree), so the length of an individual chromosome indicates total DT, and when DT possesses a value of 1, DT is retained, while value 0 represents that DT is denounced. On the other hand, RF adds additional randomness to model while developing trees. Rather than searching a significant feature during node split, it searches the suitable feature within a random feature subset. This leads to extensive diversity and a better model. Due to such advantages, this study considered GA and RF together as MG-RF to estimate age by the specific, distinct process shown in Figure 3.

Initially, features are normalized, wherein the numeric column values in the dataset are changed to common form without distorting variations in value ranges. This assists in solving the learning challenges of a model. After this, feature ranking is performed using RF for considering important features. Following this, Compact Genetic Algorithm (cGA) is initialized. Subsequently, multiple RF models are created with chromosomes. Then, the fitness value is evaluated using the selection, crossover, and mutation processes of GA. These operations transform the chromosome's initial population, improving the quality. The selection represents the process that chooses parents that mate and then reunite for developing offspring for the succeeding generation. This is vital for the convergence of GA, based on which it can obtain the best solutions. The selection process uses fitness for controlling chromosome evolution. Maximum fitness affords more chances to select optimal solutions, whereas crossover involves the integration of the genetic material as well as the elite position chosen for the crossover operation. Further, mutation is employed in a chromosome at the individual position. Finally, the fitness value is assessed, and the current feature is recorded. Then, the feature subset is evaluated. For a specific issue, the fitness function improves the chromosome quality as a solution. Hence, it assists in attaining better age estimation. The overall algorithm of GA is shown in Algorithm 2.

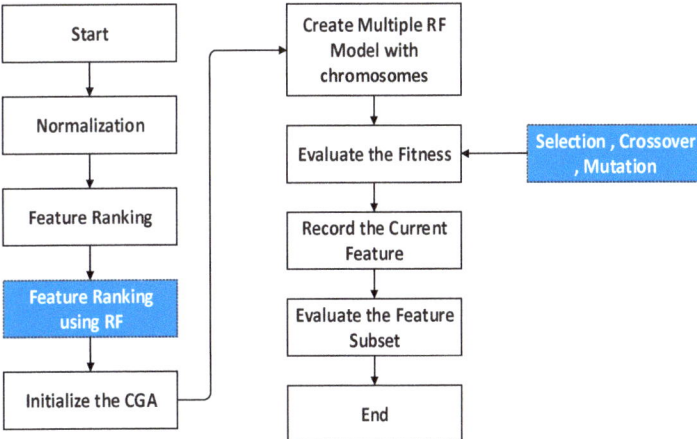

Figure 3. Overall workflow of Modified Genetic–Random Forest.

Algorithm 2: Genetic algorithm

1 Input: (it, n, GA Parameters)
2 **STEP 1:** begin
3 **STEP 2:** Initialize c = 0 and i = 0,
4 **STEP 3:** Generation: generate random n solutions;
5 **STEP 4:** Compute Fitness(s) and Generation c;
6 **STEP 5:** While fitness not reached compute for i iterations do
7 Generation c + 1 evolve(Generation c);
8 **STEP 6:** fitness computeFitness (s) and Generation c;
9 i = i + 1;
10 end
11 return (solution fitness)
12 end

At first, the parameters are initialized. Then, random solutions are generated. Subsequently, fitness and generation are computed. When a suitable fitness value is not found, iterations are performed until the best fitness solution is attained. After finding this value, the best parameters are attained through the use of the obtained best fitness value. The algorithm corresponding to this process is shown in Algorithm 3.

Algorithm 3: Modified fitness computation

1 Input: Dataset(D), Chromosome
2 Output: MAE of the Random Forests
3 **STEP 1:** begin
4 **STEP 2:** Ds—Dataset;
5 **STEP 3:** Compute kvalues, num_trees, mtry by decoding (Chromosome);
6 Dc—decompose the set as (Ds, kvalues);
7 **STEP 4:** Fitnessmodel—RF fit(Dc,num_trees,mtry);
8 **STEP 5:** Rank the feature using RF Regressor
9 **STEP 6:** MAE—evaluate(model)
10 **STEP 7:** return (MAE);
11 end

Initially, the dataset and chromosome are taken as input. Then, they are computed by decoding. Following this, the sets are decomposed. Subsequently, the fitness model is determined. After this, the features are ranked using an RF regressor. Finally, the MAE of a model is assessed. Lastly, the best parameters are attained from GA, as shown in Table 1.

Table 1. Best parameters from GA.

Best Parameters from Genetic Algorithm	
max_depth'	[10]
max_features'	[sqrt]
min_samples_leaf'	[4]
min_samples_split'	[10]
n_estimators'	[600]

After extraction of the best parameters, the optimized solution is obtained based on Algorithm 4.

Algorithm 4: Optimized Random Forest

1 Input: minK, maxK, minNTree, maxNTree, treeIncrement, RF best, RF fit
2 Output: Optimized RF
3 **STEP 1:** begin
4 **STEP 2:** Compute computeFitness(s) and Generation c;
5 **STEP 3:** Evaluate fitness and return fitness,
6 **STEP 4:** MAE (Fit RF best)
7 **STEP 5:** Fit RF best = Optimized RF
8 **STEP 6:** Optimized RF(D) = solution
9 end

At first, the input is considered. Then, the fitness value is computed. Following this, the fitness value is evaluated and returned. Subsequently, the fitness value is assessed to determine the solution. After this, the hyperparameters for RF are attained, as shown in Table 2.

Table 2. Hyperparameters for RF.

Hyperparameters For RF	
'max_depth'	[10, 20, 30, 40, 50, 60, 70, 80, 90, 100, None]
'max_features'	['auto', 'sqrt']
'min_samples_leaf'	[1, 2, 4]
'min_samples_split'	[2, 5, 10]
'n_estimators'	[200, 400, 600, 800, 1000, 1200, 1400, 1600, 1800, 2000]

The main stages involved in the outcome of the optimized RF are summarized below.

Step 1: Modified genetic RF

MG-RF is trained, and the fitness value is evaluated with GA. In this phase, the classes obtained are optimized in accordance with GA, and this attains the input for RF that calculates the fitness of individual trees in a forest. Iteration continues until the optimized trees are determined.

Step 2: Fitness calculation

In this stage, the overall fitness of trees is assessed based on the values attained through decoding the chromosomes. The decomposed class obtained from phase 2 is assessed for its fitness value with ranked features corresponding to MAE score.

Step 3: Optimized RF

The optimized RF is attained from integration of GA (with the assistance of selection, crossover, and mutation processes) and multiple class decompositions.

Step 4: Termination

The operation is terminated after obtaining the optimal RF.

Step 5: Outcome

This stage involves predicted data for estimating age.

Hyperparameter tuning exerts a substantial influence on the performance of deep learning DL models. The integration of the GA with the RF algorithm not only enhances the predictive accuracy but also improves interpretability. The GA method was used to adjust the hyperparameters of the Random Forest to improve its regression accuracy.

Additionally, GA was designed to optimize dental age estimation, and the population size was set at 20 individuals, allowing for a diverse representation of potential solutions. The algorithm was run for 50 generations, providing ample opportunity for the population to evolve and improve over time. The fitness function utilized was the MSE, calculated on validation data, ensuring that the solutions were evaluated based on their predictive accuracy. To select individuals for reproduction, tournament selection was employed, which enhanced the chances of selecting high-quality solutions. The crossover rate was set at 0.8, thereby facilitating a robust exchange of genetic material between parent solutions, while a mutation rate of 0.1 introduced variability and aided in the prevention of premature convergence. This structured approach was designed to effectively navigate the solution space and achieve optimal results.

The following Table 3 describes the number of layers and size of the kernel utilized in the Deep 2D CNN and Deep 1D CNN architecture. Accordingly, the Deep 2D CNN analyses the OPG images with four convolutional layers, with progressively increasing filter counts, followed by maxpooling and fully connected layers. The Deep 1D CNN processes patient records with three convolutional layers, each generating a 128-unit feature vector as output. The output features from each network are then combined in a fusion layer. Following that, the outcome is fed into an MG-RF regressor to enhance the predictive accuracy.

Table 3. Components in Deep CNN architecture.

Model	Component	Details
Deep 2D CNN	Input Layer	Input size: (224, 224, 3) (Resized OPG Images)
	Convolutional Layers	Conv1: 32 filters, kernel size (3 × 3), ReLU Conv2: 64 filters, kernel size (3 × 3), ReLU Conv3: 128 filters, kernel size (3 × 3), ReLU Conv4: 256 filters, kernel size (3 × 3), ReLU
	Pooling Layers	Maxpooling after each convolutional block, pool size (2 × 2)
	Fully Connected Layer	Dense layer: 512 units, ReLU activation
	Output Layer	Dense layer: 128 units (feature vector), Linear activation
Deep 1D CNN	Input Layer	Input size: Variable (Patient Records)
	Convolutional Layers	Conv1: 16 filters, kernel size (5), ReLU Conv2: 32 filters, kernel size (3), ReLU Conv3: 64 filters, kernel size (3), ReLU
	Pooling Layers	Global Maxpooling layer after final convolutional layer
	Fully Connected Layer	Dense layer: 256 units, ReLU activation
	Output Layer	Dense layer: 128 units (feature vector), Linear activation
Feature Fusion	Concatenation Layer	Combines 128-unit outputs from both Deep 2D CNN and Deep 1D CNN
Modified Genetic-RF	Feature Input	256 features (128 from Deep 2D CNN + 128 from Deep 1D CNN)
	Regressor	Random Forest with Genetic Algorithm optimization: - Number of Trees: 100 Maximum Depth: Optimized by Genetic Algorithm- Split Criterion: Mean Squared Error

4. Results

This study utilized the OPG images and patient records within the dataset. A real-time dataset was considered for this research work. Some sample OPG images from the dataset are shown in Figure 4. Out of 275 males, the average age was 10.94, while out of 346 females, the average age was 11.1.

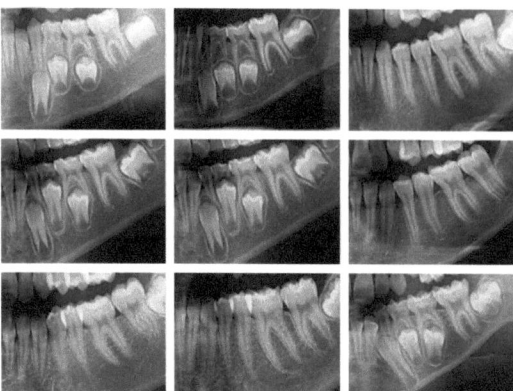

Figure 4. Sample OPGs from the dataset.

4.1. Performance Metrics

The metrics considered for analysis of the proposed methods are discussed in this section.

4.1.1. SD (Standard Deviation)

Standard deviation represents the computation of dispersion or variation on a particular set of values. Minimum standard deviation denotes that values incline to be close to the mean of set, whereas maximum standard deviation denotes that values are extended on a wide range, as given by Equation (9).

$$\sigma = \frac{\sqrt{\sum(x_i - \mu)^2}}{N} \qquad (9)$$

In Equation (9), σ indicates standard deviation, N represents the population size, μ indicates mean of the population, and x_i denotes the individual value from the population.

4.1.2. MAE (Mean Absolute Error)

This is an assessment metric of a model utilized with regression models. The MAE of a model in terms of the test set could be indicated as the mean of the absolute values corresponding to the individual errors of prediction upon cases of the test set, afforded by Equation (10).

$$\text{MAE(Mean Absolute Error)} = \frac{\sum_{i=1}^{n} |\text{predicted value} - \text{actual value}|}{n} \qquad (10)$$

In Equation (10), n represents the overall data points.

4.1.3. MSE (Mean Square Error)

This explores the closeness of a set of regression lines and points, as given in Equation (11).

$$\text{MSE} = \frac{1}{n}\sum_{i=1}^{n}(\text{observed values} - \text{predicted values}) \qquad (11)$$

4.1.4. R^2 (Coefficient of Determination)

The coefficient of determination refers to computation of the goodness of model fit. In regression, R^2 indicates the statistical computation of the degree to which regression predictions determine the actual data points. When $R^2 = 1$, it means that the regression estimations perfectly fit the corresponding data, as given by Equation (12).

$$R^2 = 1 - \frac{\text{Sum(squares of the residuals)}}{\text{Total sum of the squares}} \qquad (12)$$

4.1.5. RMSE (Root Mean Square Error)

The RMSE is the ideal accuracy calculation that only compares model configurations or prediction errors of diverse models for specific variables. It is given by Equation (13).

$$\text{RMSE} = \frac{\sqrt{\sum_{i=1}^{N}(\text{actual time series observation} - \text{predicted time series observation})^2}}{N} \qquad (13)$$

In Equation (13), N represents overall non-missing data-points, and i indicates the variable.

4.2. Performance Analysis

In this study, the performance of the proposed system was evaluated based on the mean MSE, MAE, RMSE, and R^2 values calculated during the implementation of the code. The efficacy of a system is gauged by its maximum prediction rate and minimum error rate. In this regard, the maximum R^2 score serves as a measure of the proposed system's effectiveness. In this study, the MSE value of the proposed system was 0.00027, the MAE value was 0.0079, the RMSE value was 0.0888, and the R^2 score was 0.999. This is shown in Figure 5. A comparative analysis of the predicted and actual values is presented in graphical form in Figures 6 and 7.

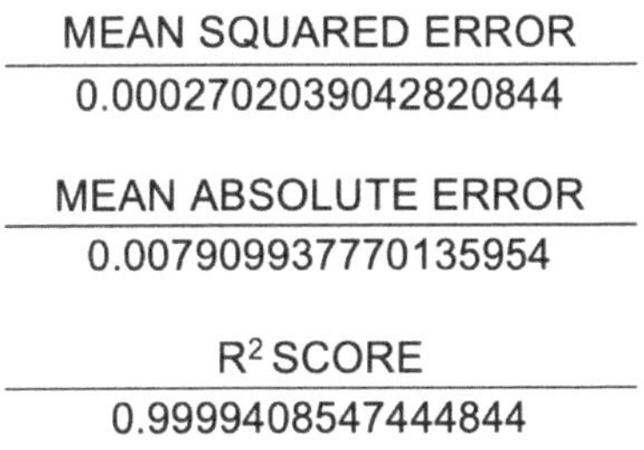

MEAN SQUARED ERROR
0.0002702039042820844

MEAN ABSOLUTE ERROR
0.007909937770135954

R^2 SCORE
0.9999408547444844

Figure 5. Analysis of the proposed system with respect to metrics. In statistics, the mean squared error of an estimator (of a procedure for estimating an unobserved quantity) measures the average of the squares of the errors—that is, the average squared difference between the estimated values and the true value. Mean absolute error is a measure of errors between paired observations expressing the same phenomenon. R-squared (R^2) score is defined as a number that tells you how well the independent variable(s) in a statistical model explains the variation in the dependent variable.

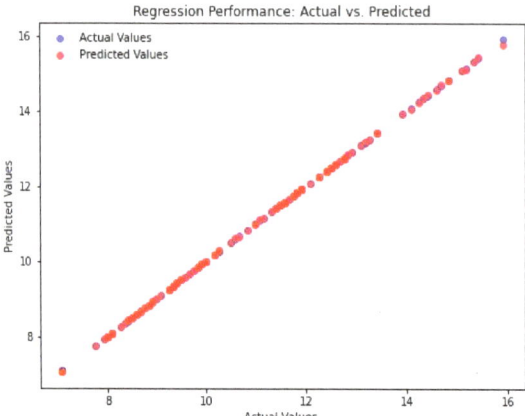

Figure 6. Actual vs. predicted values for proposed model.

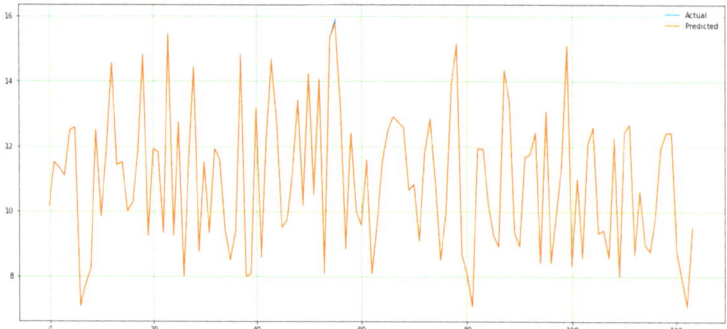

Figure 7. Plot showing variation degree between the actual and predicted values.

Figure 6 presents a scatter plot, which is a graphical representation of the relationship between actual and predicted values in regression analysis, thereby indicating the performance of the model. A model that functions optimally aligns points along the diagonal, where the predicted value is equivalent to the actual value. This is referred to as "Regression Performance of Actual vs. Predicted". The figure includes an x-axis, which represents actual values, and a y-axis, which represents predicted values. Blue points denote actual values, while red points represent predicted values. The substantial overlap of red points with the blue points, indicating strong model accuracy, is evident in the figure. This overlap is further demonstrated by the majority of red points aligning with the diagonal line y = x without bias, suggesting a high degree of model accuracy.

5. Discussion

In the field of forensic science, the determination of an individual's age is of paramount importance. Consequently, the methodology employed must be both reliable and accurate. This indicates that the degree of accuracy should be high, and the mean discrepancy between dental age and chronological age should be as minimal as feasible [66].

An existing study [78] employed a two-stage approach with the efficientNetV2 model for automatic dental age estimation. It obtained outcomes with MAE 0.274, MSE 0.261, and expected value 0.396. Similarly, another study [81] implemented the estimation of age using an ML approach only on OPG images. The model performance was analyzed with InceptionV4 and achieved MAE metrics of 3.1 and an R^2 value of 95.5%. Another existing study [79] implemented the DentAge model based on a DL approach for predicting chorological age. It used a transfer learning strategy for training the model with gradient descent features. It attained an MAE of 3.12 years and MAE of 1.94 for the age group between 10 and 20.

However, the current study employed DL models such as Deep 2D CNN for spatial features from OPG images and Deep 1D CNN for extracting sequential data from patient records. Moreover, an MG-RF regressor was employed to enhance the predictive accuracy and obtained a low MAE of 0.0079, RMSE of 0.0888, and R^2 of 0.999. Hence, the proposed model indicates efficiency in automatically predicting dental age estimation and is suitable for the forensic field.

The age estimation methods that have been documented in the existing literature are based on the evaluation of specific indicators that assess the stage of dental development that the individual has reached. The earliest known studies on this subject are dated to the 19th century [17]. One of the earliest methods based on dental indicators is the Schour and Massler method, which was developed in 1941. This method involves the morphological evaluation of tooth development through the use of diagrams that illustrate the expected developmental stages of deciduous and permanent teeth [82]. Subsequently, Nolla et al. [83] developed a ten-stage chart for age estimation, which was considered an important milestone in the field of age estimation, prompting the rapid development of new methods [11,17,83–85]. Currently, in the literature, the most commonly used methods for age estimation in children are reported to be the Willems and Demirjian methods [66].

Demirjian et al. [84] developed a method that can be used as a universal tool for assessing dental maturity and estimating dental age in children. Demirjian's method is the first in the literature to provide visualization of the stages of tooth development, descriptive criteria, radiographic examples of each stage, and selection rules for decision making at borderline stages. In the Willems method, the stages of tooth development described in the Demirjian method are used to estimate tooth age by means of maturity tables that provide the age in years directly [11,84,85].

The classical methods that have been introduced in the literature have been developed through the analysis of large datasets comprising a large number of participants. However, these methods have several shortcomings, including the fact that results are often population-specific and rely on time-consuming manual procedures that are susceptible to observer subjectivity [16,86].

A further limitation of classical manual radiologic tooth age estimation techniques is that they lack the requisite number of stages to enable the closest possible monitoring of the growth process. Another disadvantage is the difficulty in selecting a method that allows researchers to distinguish teeth that are not sufficiently differentiated in terms of developmental stage [16].

The objective of the research was to estimate the age of patients from a real-time dataset comprising patient records and OPG images using AI-based methodologies. This study employed Deep CNN with 1D and 2D architectures for feature extraction and an MG-RF method for estimating age. The proposed system was evaluated by examining the discrepancies between the actual and predicted values. The results demonstrated a strong correlation between the two variables. Furthermore, the performance of this system was evaluated in comparison to that of the conventional system in terms of MAE, RMSE, MSE, SD, and R^2 score. The analytical outcomes revealed that the proposed system outperformed the conventional system, exhibiting an SD rate of 0.0004, an MAE rate of 0.0079, an MSE rate of 0.00027, an RMSE value of 0.0888, and an R^2 value of 0.9999.

The performance of the reference methods and machine learning algorithms utilized in the study conducted by Galibourg et al. [66] was evaluated with analogous metrics to those employed in our study, namely R^2, MAE, RMSE, and SD. The researchers reported that age estimation with machine learning methods demonstrated superior performance compared to manual methods based on radiographic tooth staging from childhood to early adulthood. The results of the study are presented in Table 4, along with a comparison to the findings of our study.

Table 4. Comparison of the findings of Galibourg et al.'s [66] study with the findings of our study.

Methods	SD	MAE	MSE	RMSE	R^2
Demirjian	−0.705	1.108	1.981	1.406	0.816
Willems	−0.220	0.928	1.418	1.190	0.868
BRR	−0.002	0.812	1.030	1.014	0.904
SVM	0.016	0.729	0.901	0.949	0.916
DT	−0.012	0.758	0.973	0.985	0.910
RF	−0.007	0.731	0.885	0.940	0.918
KNN	0.009	0.738	0.921	0.959	0.915
MLP	−0.041	0.742	0.907	0.952	0.916
POLYREG	−0.008	0.735	0.913	0.955	0.915
ADAB	−0.025	0.796	1.001	1.000	0.907
STACK	−0.013	0.733	0.904	0.950	0.916
VOTE	0.068	0.770	0.995	0.984	0.908
The proposed method	0.0004	0.0079	0.00027	0.0888	0.9999

The study of Galibourg et al. [66] was carried out with a methodology based entirely on machine learning. The Demirjian and Willems methods were used as the explanatory system in the training of the machine learning system. These methods focus on the left seven mandibular permanent teeth for age estimation.

Our study was carried out with the aim of performing age estimation on OPG sections containing the left seven mandibular permanent teeth in a fully automatic manner without any explanatory system. From the radiographs and patient records that constitute the dataset of our study, feature extraction was performed using 1D-DCNN and 2D-DCNN architecture from deep learning methods. In the regression step, RF and GA methods were modified and combined, and age estimation was performed.

When our study is compared with the study of Galibourg et al. [66], in terms of performance, it is observed that our study has a superior performance than the manual predictions and all machine learning approaches evaluated in the related study. In addition, it was found that the MAE value decreased significantly with the system used in our study. It is thought that the reason for the decrease in the MAE value may be due to the use of deep learning algorithms in the feature extraction step of our study due to the perception by deep learning algorithms of various age-related indicators that cannot be detected by the human eye, and thus, more information is transferred to the MG-RF algorithm. In the MG-RF step, the RF algorithm reduces the similarity between individual trees as a methodology. For this reason, the robustness of the final model was increased by the selection of the point of departure from a random subset of the input features at each step in the tree-building process. In addition, in our study, it is thought that the integration of four different approaches into the system together with the use of machine learning techniques following deep learning processes resulted in a significant decrease in the error rate and a significant increase in the performance of the system.

In our study, age estimation was performed completely automatically without using any explanatory reference system. The fact that our method eliminates the disadvantages of exposure to human interpretation and the subjectivity of human observers by automating the age estimation task can be argued as a distinct advantage of our study. In addition, the fact that no explanatory system is used and that it is an automatic method makes our study easy to use, fast, and reproducible.

Tao et al. [67] proposed a machine learning-based approach to improve the accuracy of tooth age estimation in 2020 using a dataset of 1636 OPGs of 787 male and 849 female individuals aged 11 to 19 years. In the study, tooth age estimation was considered as a regression problem.

In the methodology of the study, manual measurements were first performed using the Demirjian method and the Willems method. The attributes were determined by entering the real ages of the patients into the system. Then, the MLP algorithm, which is a feed-forward artificial neural network from machine learning approaches, was trained with these features, and experiments were conducted. The performance of the proposed system was evaluated using MAE, MSE, and RMSE metrics. It was reported that the proposed system outperformed the reference manual methods in terms of all performance metrics [67]. The findings of the study and the findings of our study are presented in Table 5.

Table 5. Comparison of the findings of Tao et al.'s study [67] with the findings of our study.

Male	RMSE	MSE	MAE	Female	RMSE	MSE	MAE
Demirjian	1.596	2.548	1.307	Demirjian	1.677	2.812	1.364
Willems	1.602	2.556	1.291	Willems	1.788	3.196	1.407
MLP	1.332	1.775	0.990	MLP	1.617	2.616	1.261
The proposed method	0.8888	0.00027	0.0079	The proposed method	0.8888	0.00027	0.0079

The findings of our study, as indicated by the RMSE, MSE, and MAE metrics, demonstrate significantly enhanced performance in comparison to the results obtained for both female and male groups in the study conducted by Tao et al. [67]. This discrepancy may be attributed to the fact that the group under examination in our study comprises younger individuals (6–15 years old) as well as the variations in the age distribution of these individuals. Given that age indicators of growth and development decline with age, it is a well-established fact that studies in the field of age estimation obtain more accurate results with younger study populations [17].

In our study, it is thought that the combination of deep learning and machine learning methods significantly enhanced the performance. The use of deep learning techniques allows for the establishment of connections that are not discernible to the human eye, thereby enabling the inclusion of age indicators that cannot be calculated manually in the system under study. It can be proposed that this may be the source of the observed improvement in the system's performance. Furthermore, we employed an automated system that is not contingent on any explanatory framework. Therefore, our method has the advantages of being fast, repeatable, and less susceptible to human interpretation.

In their 2021 study, Shen et al. [68] employed a series of machine learning systems to estimate age. The dataset utilized in the study comprised 748 OPGs of 356 female and 392 male individuals between the ages of 5 and 13. The study employed a methodology based on random forest (RF), support vector machines (SVM), and linear logistic regression (LR). The machine learning models were trained with the manually realized Cameriere method as an explanatory system and gender information. The target value was set to the subject's chronological age. The accuracy of the proposed systems for estimating age was evaluated based on the following metrics: R^2, ME, RMSE, MSE, and MAE. The results were then compared with those obtained using the European and Chinese formulas of the Cameriere method, which were employed in the training of the system. The findings of the study and the findings of our study are shown in Table 6 [68].

Table 6. Comparison of the findings of Shen et al.'s [68] study with the findings of our study.

Methods	MAE	MSE	RMSE	R^2
LR	0.553	0.488	0.698	0.909
SVM	0.489	0.392	0.625	0.925
RF	0.495	0.389	0.623	0.928
Cameriere Method (European Formula)	0.846	0.755	0.869	-
Cameriere Method (Chinese Formula)	0.812	0.89	0.943	-
The proposed method	0.0079	0.0002	0.0888	0.9999

The performance of the systems proposed in the study is comparable to that observed in our own study in terms of the R^2 value. It is, however, noteworthy that the error rates of the systems proposed by Shen et al. are significantly higher than those observed in our study with respect to the other performance metrics evaluated. It is thought that this discrepancy may be attributed to the utilization of deep convolutional neural networks in the feature extraction phase of the present study, the incorporation of certain age indicators that cannot be discerned by the human eye, and the combination of numerous techniques.

In 2017, Čular et al. [69] conducted a study utilizing OPGs of 203 individuals between the ages of 10 and 25. In this study, the researchers proposed a semi-automated system based on deep learning techniques to estimate tooth age by examining the mandibular right third molar on OPGs. The researchers employed two statistical computer vision models, namely the Active Shape Model (ASM) and the Active Appearance Model (AAM), which have been extensively utilized in face recognition, gender estimation, and medical image interpretation and feature extraction in previous studies, to extract the features describing the right mandibular wisdom teeth selected for this investigation. In the training set, the images were manually segmented. In the study, the extracted features were presented as input to an artificial neural network, specifically the Radial Basis Network, and age estimation was performed as the output. The findings of the age estimation performance of the study were evaluated using the mean absolute error (MAE) in years. The findings of that study indicated that the system demonstrated superior performance when AAM feature extraction was employed. Although AGM was reported to perform better in this study, it was reported that the age estimation performance of the system was adversely affected when AAM and ASM were applied together [69].

The researchers noted that the MAE value of less than 3 years represents a promising preliminary result. Should the prediction error be reduced in future studies, the system proposed in their study may prove a viable option for use within the scope of forensic sciences. Furthermore, the researchers indicated that the system proposed in their study offers two key advantages: minimal user input and the ability to function without the input of an experienced dentist [69]. The findings of the study and the findings of our study are shown in Table 7.

Table 7. Comparison of the findings of Čular et al.'s [69] study with the findings of our study.

	MAE	SD
AAM	2.481	2.148
AGM	2.283	2.168
The proposed method	0.0079	0.0004

A direct comparison between our study and that of Čular et al. [69] is not feasible due to differences in methodology and age group. As there is a greater number of age indicators of growth and development in younger individuals within the existing literature, the MAE value is typically reported to be lower in studies involving this age group. The present study focuses on individuals between the ages of 6 and 15. Accordingly, the lower MAE value observed in our study relative to that reported by Čular et al. is an anticipated outcome.

In contrast to the present study, the fact that our study does not entail a manual step such as segmentation over radiographs while estimating age can be demonstrated as an advantage of the system utilized in our study. Furthermore, as our study employed OPG sections encompassing the left seven mandibular permanent teeth, the third molars, which are the most common congenitally missing teeth, were not required, thus conferring another advantage to our study.

In 2021, Wallraff et al. [71] conducted a study on automatic age estimation to reduce the estimation error, which is a disadvantage of traditional manual age estimation methods. In this study, the researchers proposed a deep learning system based on supervised regression to perform age estimation. The study was conducted on 14,000 OPGs of individuals between the ages of 11 and 20. The system proposed in the study uses raw OPGs as input. Images do not need to be pre-processed and cropped. The researchers reported that the focus of this study was individuals 11–20 years of age, as teeth develop in a predictable pattern during the first two decades of life. Radiographs in the dataset that were affected by various external factors, such as low-contrast images, diseases, and jaw malpositions, were not excluded. In this study, age estimation was considered as a regression problem, and the ResNet18 algorithm was used as the network architecture in the proposed system. The MAE of the proposed system was reported to be 1.08, with an SD of +1.41 and an error rate of 17.52%. The researchers stated that the dataset in their study provided comprehensive data for the age range of 11–20 years and that individuals aged 0–20 years should be included in the proposed system in the future [71].

As indicated in the literature, age-related indicators tend to decline as growth and development progress, resulting in lower error rates in studies that examine younger age groups. In the study conducted by Wallraff et al. [71], individuals below the age of 11 were excluded from the analysis. A comparison of our study with that of Wallraff et al. revealed a significantly lower MAE value for our study. It is postulated that this finding is attributable to the fact that our study focused on younger individuals.

In their 2020 study, Vila-Blanco et al. proposed a method based on deep learning algorithms for fully automatic age estimation from OPGs. This method was designed to overcome the limitations of traditional methods, which are affected by observer subjectivity and time-consuming manual operations. The study was conducted on OPGs of 2289 individuals from a Spanish population with an age range of 4.5 to 89 years. Only OPGs of the requisite quality were included in the study. In contrast to other studies in the literature, this study did not exclude OPGs with any of the following: orthodontic brackets or appliances, dentures, implants, restorative materials, fillings, endodontic treatment, foreign bodies such as caries, missing teeth, residual tooth roots, or earrings and external elements such as distorted or blurred images. The images in question were identified as defective within the system. In this study, convolutional neural networks from deep learning algorithms were employed as the methodology. Two distinct network architectures, namely DANet and DASNet, were devised for the purposes of this study. These architectures were designed and trained specifically for the purpose of age estimation in the context of this study [16].

The results of the study indicate a strong correlation between the DANet and DASNet systems and age. The coefficient of determination was $R^2 = 0.87$ for DANet and $R^2 = 0.90$ for DASNet. In the assessment of the data across all age groups, MAE was found to be 2.84 years. As the age of the individuals decreased, the MAE value was found to be

0.78 years for DANet and 0.75 years for DASNet in the group of individuals younger than 15 years.

In contrast to the methodology employed by Vila-Blanco et al. [16], our study utilized an OPG section encompassing seven left mandibular permanent teeth as the input data for the system. In the study conducted by Vila-Blanco et al. [16], the raw OPGs were utilized as the input data, and no exclusion criteria were employed. However, radiographs with inadequate acquisition quality were designated as defective and submitted to the system. The present study was conducted using high-quality radiographs of individuals without any dental or bony pathology. It is believed that this contributed to the success of the system used in our study.

With regard to the age group under examination, our study encompasses a much younger population than that considered by Vila-Blanco et al. Given that developmental age indicators are more prevalent in younger age groups, it may be posited that the superior performance of the Vila-Blanco et al. study can be attributed to the findings of our study. Moreover, the integration of deep learning and machine learning methodologies is believed to be a contributing factor to the enhanced performance of the system in our study.

A series of ablation experiments was conducted to assess the contribution of the components utilized in our study to the overall model performance and to enhance interpretability. Upon evaluating the method proposed in the current study, it was observed that the highest performance was achieved with a low mean absolute error (MAE) of 0.0079 and a high R^2 of 0.999. These findings underscore the efficacy of the proposed method and underscore the critical role of feature fusion. Table 8 provides a comprehensive overview of the performance of various experimental configurations, facilitating a nuanced evaluation of the proposed work using performance metrics.

Table 8. Ablation experiment result.

Experiment Configuration	MAE	MSE	RMSE	R^2
Proposed Method (Full)	0.0079	0.0002	0.0888	0.9999
Without Deep 2D CNN	0.0125	0.0008	0.1414	0.9985
Without Deep 1D CNN	0.0113	0.0006	0.1225	0.9989
Without Feature Concatenation	0.0150	0.0012	0.1732	0.9978
Using Only Deep 2D CNN	0.0132	0.0009	0.1500	0.9982
Using Only Deep 1D CNN	0.0148	0.0011	0.1667	0.9979

6. Conclusions

The application of AI methodologies has the potential to significantly reduce the time required for the resolution of complex problems. Moreover, these systems provide consistent and reproducible high-performance results.

The proposed systems with deep learning algorithms show exceptional performance due to their capacity to distinguish features that are imperceptible to the human eye and to discern the relationships between these features. However, the underlying logic behind the outstanding performance of these systems has not yet been fully elucidated, which constitutes a disadvantage for the interpretability of these systems. As in other studies in this area, interpretability is a limitation in our study. In order to address this limitation, a series of ablation experiments was conducted with the objective of enhancing interpretability. To increase interpretability and enhance the efficiency and reliability of real-world applications, in future work, we will use methodologies such as Class Activation Maps (CAM) to gain real-time insights into model predictions, interactive dashboards integrating SHAP and LIME visualizations, and Deep LIFT and Integrated Gradients to provide more understandable explanations of deep model predictions.

The present study focuses on individuals aged 6–15 years. In the field of forensic sciences, accurate age estimation is paramount, particularly in cases involving legal issues related to age and identification of elderly individuals. This represents a limitation of the present study. In subsequent studies, efforts will be directed towards the development of automatic age estimation methods for study populations that include individuals belonging to older age groups.

In conclusion, contemporary AI-based techniques in the field of forensic sciences have reached a point where they are capable of providing substantial assistance to human analysts. It is of significant importance to conduct future studies that will test the potential of these techniques to supplant human analysts and to elucidate the reasons behind their performance.

Author Contributions: Conceptualization, G.O.U. and B.K.A.; methodology, O.A.H.G.; software, O.A.H.G. and B.U.; validation, G.O.U. and O.A.H.G.; formal analysis G.O.U. and O.A.H.G.; investigation, G.O.U. and B.K.A.; resources, G.O.U.; data curation, G.O.U.; writing—original draft preparation G.O.U.; writing—review and editing, O.A.H.G., B.K.A., and B.U.; visualization, B.U.; supervision, B.K.A. All authors have read and agreed to the published version of the manuscript.

Funding: This research received no external funding.

Institutional Review Board Statement: This study was approved by the Pamukkale University Non-Interventional Clinical Research Ethics Committee (E-60116787-020-202083). The study was conducted in accordance with the principles set forth in the Declaration of Helsinki.

Informed Consent Statement: Not applicable.

Data Availability Statement: Data are available from the corresponding author upon reasonable request.

Acknowledgments: This study is derived from the author's (G.O.U.) residency thesis, "The Determination of Individuals' Dental Ages Through Panoramic Radiographs Using Artificial Intelligence Algorithms", under the supervision of (B.K.A.) and completed at Pamukkale University's Faculty of Dentistry.

Conflicts of Interest: The authors declare no conflicts of interest.

References

1. Senn, D.R.; Stimson, P.G. *Forensic Dentistry*; CRC Press: Boca Raton, FL, USA, 2010.
2. Apaydin, B.; Yasar, F. Accuracy of the demirjian, willems and cameriere methods of estimating dental age on turkish children. *Niger. J. Clin. Pract.* **2018**, *21*, 257. [CrossRef] [PubMed]
3. Limdiwala, P.; Shah, J. Age estimation by using dental radiographs. *J. Forensic Dent. Sci.* **2013**, *5*, 118. [CrossRef] [PubMed]
4. Khanagar, S.B.; Albalawi, F.; Alshehri, A.; Awawdeh, M.; Iyer, K.; Alsomaie, B.; Aldhebaib, A.; Singh, O.G.; Alfadley, A. Performance of Artificial Intelligence Models Designed for Automated Estimation of Age Using Dento-Maxillofacial Radiographs—A Systematic Review. *Diagnostics* **2024**, *14*, 1079. [CrossRef] [PubMed]
5. Han, M.; Du, S.; Ge, Y.; Zhang, D.; Chi, Y.; Long, H.; Yang, J.; Yang, Y.; Xin, J.; Chen, T.; et al. With or without human interference for precise age estimation based on machine learning? *Int. J. Legal. Med.* **2022**, *136*, 821–831. [CrossRef] [PubMed]
6. Garn, S.M.; Lewis, A.B.; Kerewsky, R.S. Genetic, Nutritional, and Maturational Correlates of Dental Development. *J. Dent. Res.* **1965**, *44*, 228–242. [CrossRef] [PubMed]
7. Noble, H.W. The Estimation of Age from the Dentition. *J. Forensic Sci. Soc.* **1974**, *14*, 215–221. [CrossRef]
8. Huda, T.F.J.; Bowman, J.E. Age determination from dental microstructure in juveniles. *Am. J. Phys. Anthropol.* **1995**, *97*, 135–150. [CrossRef]
9. Graham, E.A. Economic, Racial, and Cultural Influences on the Growth and Maturation of Children. *Pediatr. Rev.* **2005**, *26*, 290–294. [CrossRef] [PubMed]
10. Schmeling, A.; Grundmann, C.; Fuhrmann, A.; Kaatsch, H.J.; Knell, B.; Ramsthaler, F.; Reisinger, W.; Riepert, T.; Ritz-Timme, S.; Rösing, F.W.; et al. Criteria for age estimation in living individuals. *Int. J. Legal. Med.* **2008**, *122*, 457–460. [CrossRef]
11. Willems, G. A review of the most commonly used dental age estimation techniques. *J. Forensic Odontostomatol.* **2001**, *19*, 9–17. [PubMed]

12. Celik, S.; Zeren, C.; Çelikel, A.; Yengil, E.; Altan, A. Applicability of the Demirjian method for dental assessment of southern Turkish children. *J. Forensic Leg. Med.* **2014**, *25*, 1–5. [CrossRef] [PubMed]
13. Uzuner, F.D.; Kaygısız, E.; Darendeliler, N. Defining Dental Age for Chronological Age Determination. In *Post Mortem Examination and Autopsy—Current Issues From Death to Laboratory Analysis*; InTech: Nappanee, IN, USA, 2018. [CrossRef]
14. Sakuma, A.; Saitoh, H.; Suzuki, Y.; Makino, Y.; Inokuchi, G.; Hayakawa, M.; Yajima, D.; Iwase, H. Age Estimation Based on Pulp Cavity to Tooth Volume Ratio Using Postmortem Computed Tomography Images. *J. Forensic Sci.* **2013**, *58*, 1531–1535. [CrossRef] [PubMed]
15. Ge, Z.-P.; Ma, R.-H.; Li, G.; Zhang, J.-Z.; Ma, X.-C. Age estimation based on pulp chamber volume of first molars from cone-beam computed tomography images. *Forensic Sci. Int.* **2015**, *253*, 133.e1–133.e7. [CrossRef]
16. Vila-Blanco, N.; Carreira, M.J.; Varas-Quintana, P.; Balsa-Castro, C.; Tomas, I. Deep Neural Networks for Chronological Age Estimation from OPG Images. *IEEE Trans. Med. Imaging* **2020**, *39*, 2374–2384. [CrossRef] [PubMed]
17. Milošević, D.; Vodanović, M.; Galić, I.; Subašić, M. Automated estimation of chronological age from panoramic dental X-ray images using deep learning. *Expert. Syst. Appl.* **2022**, *189*, 116038. [CrossRef]
18. Putra, R.H.; Doi, C.; Yoda, N.; Astuti, E.R.; Sasaki, K. Current applications and development of artificial intelligence for digital dental radiography. *Dentomaxillofacial Radiol.* **2022**, *51*, 20210197. [CrossRef] [PubMed]
19. Devito, K.L.; de Souza Barbosa, F.; Filho, W.N.F. An artificial multilayer perceptron neural network for diagnosis of proximal dental caries. *Oral. Surg. Oral. Med. Oral. Pathol. Oral. Radiol. Endodontol.* **2008**, *106*, 879–884. [CrossRef] [PubMed]
20. Choi, J.; Eun, H.; Kim, C. Boosting Proximal Dental Caries Detection via Combination of Variational Methods and Convolutional Neural Network. *J. Signal Process Syst.* **2018**, *90*, 87–97. [CrossRef]
21. Lee, J.H.; Kim, D.H.; Jeong, S.N.; Choi, S.H. Detection and diagnosis of dental caries using a deep learning-based convolutional neural network algorithm. *J. Dent.* **2018**, *77*, 106–111. [CrossRef]
22. Geetha, V.; Aprameya, K.S.; Hinduja, D.M. Dental caries diagnosis in digital radiographs using back-propagation neural network. *Health Inf. Sci. Syst.* **2020**, *8*, 8. [CrossRef]
23. Yu, Y.; Li, Y.-J.; Wang, J.-M.; Lin, D.-H.; Ye, W.-P. Tooth Decay Diagnosis using Back Propagation Neural Network. In Proceedings of the 2006 International Conference on Machine Learning and Cybernetics, Dalian, China, 13–16 August 2006; IEEE: Piscataway, NJ, USA, 2006; pp. 3956–3959. [CrossRef]
24. Li, W.; Kuang, W.; Li, Y.; Li, Y.J.; Ye, W.P. Clinical X-Ray Image Based Tooth Decay Diagnosis using SVM. In Proceedings of the 2007 International Conference on Machine Learning and Cybernetics, Hong Kong, China, 19–22 August 2007; IEEE: Piscataway, NJ, USA, 2007; pp. 1616–1619. [CrossRef]
25. Ali, R.B.; Ejbali, R.; Zaied, M. Detection and Classification of Dental Caries in X-ray Images Using Deep Neural Networks. In Proceedings of the Eleventh International Conference on Software Engineering Advances (ICSEA), Rome, Italy, 21–25 August 2016.
26. Singh, P.; Sehgal, P. Automated caries detection based on Radon transformation and DCT. In Proceedings of the 2017 8th International Conference on Computing, Communication and Networking Technologies (ICCCNT), Delhi, India, 3–5 July 2017; IEEE: Piscataway, NJ, USA, 2017; pp. 1–6. [CrossRef]
27. Szabó, V.; Szabó, B.T.; Orhan, K.; Veres, D.S.; Manulis, D.; Ezhov, M.; Sanders, A. Validation of artificial intelligence application for dental caries diagnosis on intraoral bitewing and periapical radiographs. *J. Dent.* **2024**, *147*, 105105. [CrossRef]
28. El-Gayar, M.M. Hybrid Transfer Learning for Diagnosing Teeth Using Panoramic X-rays. *Int. J. Adv. Comput. Sci. Appl.* **2024**, *15*, 228–232. [CrossRef]
29. Orhan, K.; Belgin, C.A.; Manulis, D.; Golitsyna, M.; Bayrak, S.; Aksoy, S.; Sanders, A.; Önder, M.; Ezhov, M.; Shamshiev, M.; et al. Determining the reliability of diagnosis and treatment using artificial intelligence software with panoramic radiographs. *Imaging Sci. Dent.* **2023**, *53*, 199. [CrossRef] [PubMed]
30. Ari, T.; Sağlam, H.; Öksüzoğlu, H.; Kazan, O.; Bayrakdar, I.Ş.; Duman, S.B.; Çelik, Ö.; Jagtap, R.; Futyma-Gąbka, K.; Różyło-Kalinowska, I.; et al. Automatic Feature Segmentation in Dental Periapical Radiographs. *Diagnostics* **2022**, *12*, 3081. [CrossRef] [PubMed]
31. Lin, P.L.; Huang, P.Y.; Huang, P.W. Automatic methods for alveolar bone loss degree measurement in periodontitis periapical radiographs. *Comput. Methods Programs Biomed.* **2017**, *148*, 1–11. [CrossRef]
32. Lin, P.L.; Huang, P.W.; Huang, P.Y.; Hsu, H.C. Alveolar bone-loss area localization in periodontitis radiographs based on threshold segmentation with a hybrid feature fused of intensity and the H-value of fractional Brownian motion model. *Comput. Methods Programs Biomed.* **2015**, *121*, 117–126. [CrossRef] [PubMed]
33. Kurt Bayrakdar, S.; Orhan, K.; Bayrakdar, I.S.; Bilgir, E.; Ezhov, M.; Gusarev, M.; Shumilov, E. A deep learning approach for dental implant planning in cone-beam computed tomography images. *BMC Med. Imaging* **2021**, *21*, 86. [CrossRef]
34. Orhan, K.; Bayrakdar, I.S.; Ezhov, M.; Kravtsov, A.; Özyürek, T. Evaluation of artificial intelligence for detecting periapical pathosis on cone-beam computed tomography scans. *Int. Endod. J.* **2020**, *53*, 680–689. [CrossRef]

35. Gupta, A.; Kharbanda, O.P.; Sardana, V.; Balachandran, R.; Sardana, H.K. Accuracy of 3D cephalometric measurements based on an automatic knowledge-based landmark detection algorithm. *Int. J. Comput. Assist. Radiol. Surg.* **2016**, *11*, 1297–1309. [CrossRef] [PubMed]
36. Gupta, A.; Kharbanda, O.P.; Sardana, V.; Balachandran, R.; Sardana, H.K. A knowledge-based algorithm for automatic detection of cephalometric landmarks on CBCT images. *Int. J. Comput. Assist. Radiol. Surg.* **2015**, *10*, 1737–1752. [CrossRef]
37. Orhan, K.; Bilgir, E.; Bayrakdar, I.S.; Ezhov, M.; Gusarev, M.; Shumilov, E. Evaluation of artificial intelligence for detecting impacted third molars on cone-beam computed tomography scans. *J. Stomatol. Oral Maxillofac. Surg.* **2021**, *122*, 333–337. [CrossRef] [PubMed]
38. Vinayahalingam, S.; Xi, T.; Bergé, S.; Maal, T.; de Jong, G. Automated detection of third molars and mandibular nerve by deep learning. *Sci Rep.* **2019**, *9*, 9007. [CrossRef] [PubMed]
39. Fukuda, M.; Ariji, Y.; Kise, Y.; Nozawa, M.; Kuwada, C.; Funakoshi, T.; Muramatsu, C.; Fujita, H.; Katsumata, A.; Ariji, E. Comparison of 3 deep learning neural networks for classifying the relationship between the mandibular third molar and the mandibular canal on panoramic radiographs. *Oral Surg Oral Med. Oral Pathol. Oral Radiol.* **2020**, *130*, 336–343. [CrossRef] [PubMed]
40. Jaskari, J.; Sahlsten, J.; Järnstedt, J.; Mehtonen, H.; Karhu, K.; Sundqvist, O.; Hietanen, A.; Varjonen, V.; Mattila, V.; Kaski, K. Deep Learning Method for Mandibular Canal Segmentation in Dental Cone Beam Computed Tomography Volumes. *Sci. Rep.* **2020**, *10*, 5842. [CrossRef] [PubMed]
41. Kwak, G.H.; Kwak, E.-J.; Song, J.M.; Park, H.R.; Jung, Y.-H.; Cho, B.-H.; Hui, P.; Hwang, J.J. Automatic mandibular canal detection using a deep convolutional neural network. *Sci. Rep.* **2020**, *10*, 5711. [CrossRef] [PubMed]
42. Kuwada, C.; Ariji, Y.; Fukuda, M.; Kise, Y.; Fujita, H.; Katsumata, A.; Ariji, E. Deep learning systems for detecting and classifying the presence of impacted supernumerary teeth in the maxillary incisor region on panoramic radiographs. *Oral Surg. Oral Med. Oral Pathol. Oral Radiol.* **2020**, *130*, 464–469. [CrossRef] [PubMed]
43. Johari, M.; Esmaeili, F.; Andalib, A.; Garjani, S.; Saberkari, H. Detection of vertical root fractures in intact and endodontically treated premolar teeth by designing a probabilistic neural network: An ex vivo study. *Dentomaxillofac. Radiol.* **2017**, *46*, 20160107. [CrossRef]
44. Fukuda, M.; Inamoto, K.; Shibata, N.; Ariji, Y.; Yanashita, Y.; Kutsuna, S.; Nakata, K.; Katsumata, A.; Fujita, H.; Ariji, E. Evaluation of an artificial intelligence system for detecting vertical root fracture on panoramic radiography. *Oral Radiol.* **2020**, *36*, 337–343. [CrossRef] [PubMed]
45. Chu, P.; Bo, C.; Liang, X.; Yang, J.; Megalooikonomou, V.; Yang, F.; Huang, B.; Li, X.; Ling, H. Using Octuplet Siamese Network for Osteoporosis Analysis on Dental Panoramic Radiographs. In Proceedings of the 2018 40th Annual International Conference of the IEEE Engineering in Medicine and Biology Society (EMBC), Honolulu, HI, USA, 18–21 July 2018; IEEE: Piscataway, NJ, USA; pp. 2579–2582. [CrossRef]
46. Lee, K.S.; Jung, S.K.; Ryu, J.J.; Shin, S.W.; Choi, J. Evaluation of Transfer Learning with Deep Convolutional Neural Networks for Screening Osteoporosis in Dental Panoramic Radiographs. *J. Clin. Med.* **2020**, *9*, 392. [CrossRef] [PubMed]
47. Lee, J.S.; Adhikari, S.; Liu, L.; Jeong, H.G.; Kim, H.; Yoon, S.J. Osteoporosis detection in panoramic radiographs using a deep convolutional neural network-based computer-assisted diagnosis system: A preliminary study. *Dentomaxillofac. Radiol.* **2019**, *48*, 20170344. [CrossRef] [PubMed]
48. Liang, K.; Zhang, L.; Yang, H.; Yang, Y.; Chen, Z.; Xing, Y. Metal artifact reduction for practical dental computed tomography by improving interpolation-based reconstruction with deep learning. *Med. Phys.* **2019**, *46*, pp.823–834. [CrossRef] [PubMed]
49. Minnema, J.; Minnema, J.; van Eijnatten, M.; van Eijnatten, M.; Hendriksen, A.A.; Hendriksen, A.A.; Liberton, N.; Liberton, N.; Pelt, D.M.; Pelt, D.M.; et al. Segmentation of dental cone-beam CT scans affected by metal artifacts using a mixed-scale dense convolutional neural network. *Med. Phys.* **2019**, *46*, 5027–5035. [CrossRef] [PubMed]
50. Hegazy, M.A.A.; Cho, M.H.; Cho, M.H.; Lee, S.Y. U-net based metal segmentation on projection domain for metal artifact reduction in dental CT. *Biomed. Eng. Lett.* **2019**, *9*, 375–385. [CrossRef]
51. Flores, A.; Rysavy, S.; Enciso, R.; Okada, K. Non-invasive differential diagnosis of dental periapical lesions in cone-beam CT. In Proceedings of the 2009 IEEE International Symposium on Biomedical Imaging: From Nano to Macro, Boston, MA, USA, 28 June–1 July 2009; IEEE: Piscataway, NJ, USA; pp. 566–569. [CrossRef]
52. Okada, K.; Rysavy, S.; Flores, A.; Linguraru, M.G. Noninvasive differential diagnosis of dental periapical lesions in cone-beam CT scans. *Med. Phys.* **2015**, *42*, 1653–1665. [CrossRef] [PubMed]
53. Murata, M.; Ariji, Y.; Ohashi, Y.; Kawai, T.; Fukuda, M.; Funakoshi, T.; Kise, Y.; Nozawa, M.; Katsumata, A.; Fujita, H.; et al. Deep-learning classification using convolutional neural network for evaluation of maxillary sinusitis on panoramic radiography. *Oral Radiol.* **2019**, *35*, 301–307. [CrossRef]
54. Kuwana, R.; Ariji, Y.; Fukuda, M.; Kise, Y.; Nozawa, M.; Kuwada, C.; Muramatsu, C.; Katsumata, A.; Fujita, H.; Ariji, E. Performance of deep learning object detection technology in the detection and diagnosis of maxillary sinus lesions on panoramic radiographs. *Dentomaxillofac. Radiol.* **2021**, *50*, 20200171. [CrossRef]

55. Kim, Y.; Lee, K.J.; Sunwoo, L.; Choi, D.; Nam, C.-M.; Cho, J.; Kim, J.; Bae, Y.J.; Yoo, R.-E.; Choi, B.S.; et al. Deep Learning in Diagnosis of Maxillary Sinusitis Using Conventional Radiography. *Investig. Radiol.* **2019**, *54*, 7–15. [CrossRef] [PubMed]
56. Kann, B.H.; Aneja, S.; Loganadane, G.V.; Kelly, J.R.; Smith, S.M.; Decker, R.H.; Yu, J.B.; Park, H.S.; Yarbrough, W.G.; Malhotra, A.; et al. Pretreatment Identification of Head and Neck Cancer Nodal Metastasis and Extranodal Extension Using Deep Learning Neural Networks. *Sci. Rep.* **2018**, *8*, 14036. [CrossRef]
57. Ariji, Y.; Fukuda, M.; Kise, Y.; Nozawa, M.; Yanashita, Y.; Fujita, H.; Katsumata, A.; Ariji, E. Contrast-enhanced computed tomography image assessment of cervical lymph node metastasis in patients with oral cancer by using a deep learning system of artificial intelligence. *Oral Surg. Oral Med. Oral Pathol. Oral Radiol.* **2019**, *127*, 458–463. [CrossRef]
58. Kise, Y.; Ikeda, H.; Fujii, T.; Fukuda, M.; Ariji, Y.; Fujita, H.; Katsumata, A.; Ariji, E. Preliminary study on the application of deep learning system to diagnosis of Sjögren's syndrome on CT images. *Dentomaxillofac. Radiol.* **2019**, *48*, 20190019. [CrossRef]
59. Keser, G.; Pekiner, F.N.; Bayrakdar, İ.Ş.; Çelik, Ö.; Orhan, K. A deep learning approach to detection of oral cancer lesions from intra oral patient images: A preliminary retrospective study. *J. Stomatol. Oral Maxillofac. Surg.* **2024**, *125*, 101975. [CrossRef] [PubMed]
60. Chinnikatti, S.K. Artificial Intelligence in Forensic Science. *Forensic. Sci. Addict. Res.* **2018**, 2. [CrossRef]
61. Khanagar, S.B.; Vishwanathaiah, S.; Naik, S.; Al-Kheraif, A.A.; Divakar, D.D.; Sarode, S.C.; Bhandi, S.; Patil, S. Application and performance of artificial intelligence technology in forensic odontology—A systematic review. *Leg. Med.* **2021**, *48*, 101826. [CrossRef]
62. Goodfellow, I.; Bengio, Y.; Courville, A. *Deep Learning*; MIT Press: Cambridge, MA, USA, 2016.
63. Kahm, S.H.; Kim, J.Y.; Yoo, S.; Bae, S.M.; Kang, J.E.; Lee, S.H. Application of entire dental panorama image data in artificial intelligence model for age estimation. *BMC Oral Health* **2023**, *23*, 1007. [CrossRef]
64. Kazimierczak, W.; Wajer, R.; Wajer, A.; Kiian, V.; Kloska, A.; Kazimierczak, N.; Janiszewska-Olszowska, J.; Serafin, Z. Periapical Lesions in Panoramic Radiography and CBCT Imaging—Assessment of AI's Diagnostic Accuracy. *J. Clin. Med.* **2024**, *13*, 2709. [CrossRef] [PubMed]
65. Vila-Blanco, N.; Varas-Quintana, P.; Aneiros-Ardao, Á.; Tomás, I.; Carreira, M.J. XAS: Automatic yet eXplainable Age and Sex determination by combining imprecise per-tooth predictions. *Comput. Biol. Med.* **2022**, *149*, 106072. [CrossRef]
66. Galibourg, A.; Cussat-Blanc, S.; Dumoncel, J.; Telmon, N.; Monsarrat, P.; Maret, D. Comparison of different machine learning approaches to predict dental age using Demirjian's staging approach. *Int. J. Legal. Med.* **2021**, *135*, 665–675. [CrossRef]
67. Tao, J.; Wang, J.; Wang, A.; Xie, Z.; Wang, Z.; Wu, S.; Hassanien, A.E.; Xiao, K. Dental Age Estimation: A Machine Learning Perspective. In *Advances in Intelligent Systems and Computing*; Springer: Berlin/Heidelberg, Germany, 2020; Volume 921, pp. 722–733. [CrossRef]
68. Shen, S.; Liu, Z.; Wang, J.; Fan, L.; Ji, F.; Tao, J. Machine learning assisted Cameriere method for dental age estimation. *BMC Oral Health* **2021**, *21*, 641. [CrossRef] [PubMed]
69. Cular, L.; Tomaic, M.; Subasic, M.; Saric, T.; Sajkovic, V.; Vodanovic, M. Dental age estimation from panoramic X-ray images using statistical models. In *International Symposium on Image and Signal Processing and Analysis, ISPA*; IEEE Computer Society: Washington, DC, USA, 2017; pp. 25–30. [CrossRef]
70. De Back, W.; Seurig, S.; Wagner, S.; Marré, B.; Roeder, I.; Scherf, N. Forensic Age Estimation with Bayesian Convolutional Neural Networks Based on Panoramic Dental X-Ray Imaging. *Proc. Mach. Learn. Res.* **2019**, 1–4.
71. Wallraff, S.; Vesal, S.; Syben, C.; Lutz, R.; Maier, A. Age Estimation on Panoramic Dental X-ray Images using Deep Learning. In *Informatik Aktuell*; Springer Science and Business Media Deutschland GmbH: Berlin, Germany, 2021; pp. 186–191. [CrossRef]
72. De Tobel, J.; Radesh, P.; Vandermeulen, D.; Thevissen, P.W. An automated technique to stage lower third molar development on panoramic radiographs for age estimation: A pilot study. *J. Forensic Odontostomatol.* **2017**, *35*, 42–54.
73. Merdietio Boedi, R.; Banar, N.; De Tobel, J.; Bertels, J.; Vandermeulen, D.; Thevissen, P.W. Effect of Lower Third Molar Segmentations on Automated Tooth Development Staging using a Convolutional Neural Network. *J. Forensic Sci.* **2020**, *65*, 481–486. [CrossRef]
74. Banar, N.; Bertels, J.; Laurent, F.; Boedi, R.M.; De Tobel, J.; Thevissen, P.; Vandermeulen, D. Towards fully automated third molar development staging in panoramic radiographs. *Int. J. Legal. Med.* **2020**, *134*, 1831–1841. [CrossRef] [PubMed]
75. Kim, S.; Lee, Y.H.; Noh, Y.K.; Park, F.C.; Auh, Q.S. Age-group determination of living individuals using first molar images based on artificial intelligence. *Sci. Rep.* **2021**, *11*, 1073. [CrossRef]
76. Dong, W.; You, M.; He, T.; Dai, J.; Tang, Y.; Shi, Y.; Guo, J. An automatic methodology for full dentition maturity staging from OPG images using deep learning. *Appl. Intell.* **2023**, *53*, 29514–29536. [CrossRef]
77. Guo, Y.-C.; Han, M.; Chi, Y.; Long, H.; Zhang, D.; Yang, J.; Yang, Y.; Chen, T.; Du, S. Accurate age classification using manual method and deep convolutional neural network based on orthopantomogram images. *Int. J. Legal. Med.* **2021**, *135*, 1589–1597. [CrossRef]

78. Kokomoto, K.; Kariya, R.; Muranaka, A.; Okawa, R.; Nakano, K.; Nozaki, K. Automatic dental age calculation from panoramic radiographs using deep learning: A two-stage approach with object detection and image classification. *BMC Oral Health* **2024**, *24*, 143. [CrossRef] [PubMed]
79. Bizjak, Ž.; Robič, T. DentAge: Deep learning for automated age prediction using panoramic dental X-ray images. *J. Forensic Sci.* **2024**, *69*, 2069–2074. [CrossRef]
80. Shi, Y.; Ye, Z.; Guo, J.; Tang, Y.; Dong, W.; Dai, J.; Miao, Y.; You, M. Deep learning methods for fully automated dental age estimation on orthopantomograms. *Clin. Oral Investig.* **2024**, *28*, 198. [CrossRef]
81. Oliveira, W.; Albuquerque Santos, M.; Burgardt, C.A.P.; Anjos Pontual, M.L.; Zanchettin, C. Estimation of human age using machine learning on panoramic radiographs for Brazilian patients. *Sci. Rep.* **2024**, *14*, 19689. [CrossRef] [PubMed]
82. Schour, I.; Massler, M. The development of the Human Dentition. *J. Am. Dent. Assoc.* **1941**, *28*, 1153–1160.
83. Nolla, C.M. The development of the permanent teeth. *J. Dent. Child.* **1960**, *27*, 254–266.
84. Demirjian, A.; Goldstein, H.; Tanner, J.M. A new system of dental age assessment. *Hum. Biol.* **1973**, *45*, 211–227. [PubMed]
85. Demirjian, A.; Goldstein, H. New Systems for Dental Maturity Based on Seven and Four Teeth. *Ann. Hum. Biol.* **1976**, *3*, 411–421. [CrossRef]
86. Kapoor, P.; Jain, V. Comprehensive Chart for Dental Age Estimation (DAEcc8) based on Demirjian 8-teeth method: Simplified for operator ease. *J. Forensic Leg. Med.* **2018**, *59*, 45–49. [CrossRef] [PubMed]

Disclaimer/Publisher's Note: The statements, opinions and data contained in all publications are solely those of the individual author(s) and contributor(s) and not of MDPI and/or the editor(s). MDPI and/or the editor(s) disclaim responsibility for any injury to people or property resulting from any ideas, methods, instructions or products referred to in the content.

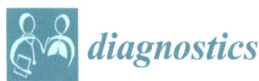 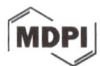

Article

Artificial Intelligence for Tooth Detection in Cleft Lip and Palate Patients

Can Arslan [1,*], Nesli Ozum Yucel [1], Kaan Kahya [1], Ezgi Sunal Akturk [2] and Derya Germec Cakan [1]

[1] Department of Orthodontics, Faculty of Dentistry, Yeditepe University, Istanbul 34728, Turkey
[2] Department of Orthodontics, Hamidiye Faculty of Dental Medicine, University of Health Sciences, Istanbul 34668, Turkey
* Correspondence: dt.canarslan@gmail.com

Abstract: Introduction: Cleft lip and palate patients often present with unique anatomical challenges, making dental anomaly detection and numbering particularly complex. The accurate identification of teeth in these patients is crucial for effective treatment planning and long-term management. Artificial intelligence (AI) has emerged as a promising tool for enhancing diagnostic precision, yet its application in this specific patient population remains underexplored. **Objectives:** This study aimed to evaluate the performance of an AI-based software in detecting and numbering teeth in cleft lip and palate patients. The research focused on assessing the system's sensitivity, precision, and specificity, while identifying potential limitations in specific anatomical regions and demographic groups. **Methods:** A total of 100 panoramic radiographs (52 males, 48 females) from patients aged 6 to 15 years were analyzed using AI software. Sensitivity, precision, and specificity were calculated, with ground truth annotations provided by four experienced orthodontists. The AI system's performance was compared across age and gender groups, with particular attention to areas prone to misidentification. **Results:** The AI system demonstrated high overall sensitivity (0.98 ± 0.03) and precision (0.96 ± 0.04). No statistically significant differences were found between age groups ($p > 0.05$), but challenges were observed in the maxillary left region, which exhibited higher false positive and false negative rates. These findings were consistent with the prevalence of unilateral left clefts in the study population. **Conclusions:** The AI system was effective in detecting and numbering teeth in cleft lip and palate patients, but further refinement is required for improved accuracy in the cleft region, particularly on the left side. Addressing these limitations could enhance the clinical utility of AI in managing complex craniofacial cases.

Keywords: artificial intelligence; cleft lip and palate; tooth detection; tooth numbering

1. Introduction

The early detection and accurate classification of dental anomalies in individuals with cleft lip and palate is crucial for effective treatment planning and improved patient outcomes. Early identification of dental abnormalities allows for timely intervention and customized treatment strategies, which can significantly enhance the overall quality of care and long-term outcomes for these patients. Individuals with cleft lip and palate often exhibit a range of dental anomalies, including missing teeth, ectopic eruption, and malformed tooth structure [1]. The presence of such anomalies complicates the identification of teeth, particularly in the cleft region, and can impede the delivery of comprehensive dental care [2]. Artificial intelligence (AI) encompasses a wide range of computational methods and technologies designed to mimic human intelligence. Among these, convolutional neural networks (CNNs) are a specific type of deep learning model that excel in image analysis tasks [3–5]. Advancements in AI have shown promise in automating and enhancing the identification and classification of dental features, offering a potential solution to streamline the diagnostic process [6–8].

In fixed prosthodontics, AI-based techniques have demonstrated the ability to accurately detect and classify dental margins, a critical step in the design and fabrication of dental restorations. Similarly, in removable prosthodontics, convolutional neural networks have been used to classify dental arches, providing valuable insights for treatment planning [9]. Moreover, AI has been applied in various other areas of dentistry, from diagnostic dentistry and patient management to orthodontics and radiology, offering improved efficiencies, precision, and patient-centric care. However, the successful integration of AI in routine dental practice faces several challenges, including limited data availability, lack of methodological rigor, and practical concerns around the value and usefulness of these solutions [10].

Nonetheless, the potential of AI-based software to enhance the identification and classification of dental anomalies in cleft lip and palate patients is promising [11]. By automating and optimizing the diagnostic process, AI-based tools could ultimately lead to more personalized, predictive, and preventive dental care, ultimately improving the quality of life for individuals with this complex craniofacial condition [12–18].

Panoramic radiographs are critical for the initial diagnosis of dental abnormalities in cleft lip and palate patients. However, interpreting these radiographs can be challenging, even for experienced clinicians, due to the anatomical complexity and presence of dental anomalies [15]. Several studies have explored the use of AI-based programs for tooth detection and numbering on panoramic radiographs, reporting that deep convolutional neural network systems demonstrate high sensitivity and precision in these tasks [16–18]. To the best of our knowledge, no studies to date have investigated the application of AI-based software for tooth detection and numbering specifically in individuals with cleft lip and palate. This study aims to evaluate the performance of an artificial-intelligence-based application in identifying and classifying teeth in patients with this craniofacial condition. The null hypothesis of this study is that the performance of the AI-based software in detecting and numbering teeth in cleft lip and palate patients does not differ significantly from expert ground truth annotations, irrespective of age or gender.

2. Materials and Methods

This retrospective study examined a set of panoramic radiographs from individuals in mixed dentition with cleft lip and palate, obtained from the archives of the Yeditepe University Faculty of Dentistry, Department of Orthodontics, taken from March 2019 to June 2024. A power analysis was conducted using the G*Power 3.1.9.7. (G*Power, Düsseldorf, Germany) software protocol [19]. Based on sensitivity and specificity values from a reference study [18], with a 95% confidence level ($1 - \alpha$), 95% test power ($1 - \beta$), sensitivity of 0.9559, and specificity of 0.9652, the minimum sample size required for this study was calculated to be 90 participants. Therefore, a total of 100 (52 males, 48 females) individuals in mixed dentition (mean age 8.18 ± 2.24 years) with unilateral or bilateral cleft lip and palate were included in this study. To assess the impact of age-related differences in dental development, these patients were divided into three groups: 6–7 years, 8–9 years, and 10 years and older. These groups were selected due to the significant dental changes that occur during the mixed dentition period.

Panoramic radiographs that exhibited artifacts related to metal superposition, positioning errors, movement, or image distortion were excluded from the analysis. Radiographs of patients with additional severe craniofacial anomalies or those who had undergone surgical interventions affecting dental structures were also excluded. However, radiographs that displayed typical cleft-associated dental anomalies such as missing, rotated, or supernumerary teeth in the cleft region were included to ensure the study's focus on cleft-related dental challenges. Ethical approval was obtained from the Non-Interventional Clinical Research Ethics Committee of Yeditepe University (Approval Number: 202311Y0694). The study was conducted in accordance with the principles of the Declaration of Helsinki.

All panoramic radiographs were obtained using the Morita Veraviewepocs (Morita Corp., Kyoto, Japan) and subsequently uploaded to the Diagnocat software (DC, Diagnocat

LLC, San Francisco, CA, USA, https://diagnocat.com/ accessed on 24 November 2024). A radiologic report for each radiograph was generated, which served as the basis for the automatic evaluation (Figure 1). Teeth detection and numbering were performed according to the FDI notation and analyzed by five different orthodontists. In this study, ground truth annotations, manual identification, and the labeling of the correct positions and numbering of teeth, were provided by one orthodontist with 20 years of experience, two with 10 years of experience, and two with 4 years of experience. These annotations served as the reference standard for evaluating the performance of the AI-based software.

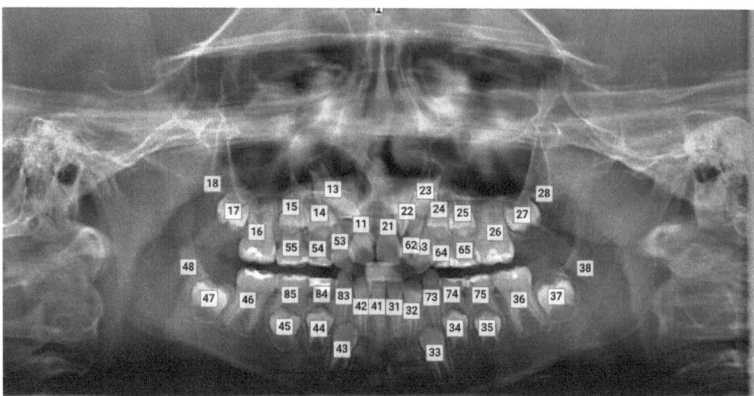

Figure 1. Teeth detection and numbering by the software.

The commercially available AI system used in this study, Diagnocat, is based on deep learning methods, specifically CNNs, which are a type of deep learning architecture designed to process and analyse visual data by identifying patterns and features within images. In the context of dental imaging, these networks are trained to detect and number teeth by recognizing anatomical structures in panoramic radiographs. Diagnocat includes various specialized modules, such as region of interest (ROI) localization and tooth localization and numeration, which enhance its diagnostic capabilities. These modules are supported by state-of-the-art CNN architectures trained on extensive datasets of cone beam computed tomography (CBCT) scans and panoramic radiographs.

To assess the success of the AI model in tooth detection and numbering, the following procedures and metrics, based on two prior studies in the literature [17,18], were employed:

Initially, the true positive (TP), false positive (FP), true negative (TN), and false negative (FN) rates were calculated:

- True Positive (TP): The model correctly detects and identifies teeth.
- False Positive (FP): The model detects teeth correctly but assigns the wrong number.
- False Negative (FN): The model fails to detect or incorrectly identifies teeth.
- True Negative (TN): The model correctly identifies areas where no teeth are present.

Using these values, the following metrics were calculated:

- Sensitivity: $TP/(TP + FN)$
- Precision: $TP/(TP + FP)$
- F1 Score: $2TP/(2TP + FP + FN)$
- False Discovery Rate: $FP/(FP + TP)$
- False Negative Rate: $FN/(FN + TP)$
- Error: Instances where the model incorrectly identifies a tooth in an irrelevant anatomical region where no tooth is present.

Statistical Analysis

The data were analyzed using IBM SPSS version 23.0 software (IBM Corp., Armonk, NY, USA). The normality of the data distribution was evaluated using the Shapiro–Wilk and Kolmogorov–Smirnov tests. For comparisons between two independent groups, an independent samples *t*-test was employed for normally distributed variables, while the Mann–Whitney U test was used for non-normally distributed variables. For comparisons among three or more groups, one-way ANOVA was applied for normally distributed variables, with post hoc comparisons performed using Duncan and Tamhane tests. For non-normally distributed variables, the Kruskal–Wallis test was utilized, with post hoc comparisons conducted using the Dunn test. The results of the analyses are presented as mean ± standard deviation for normally distributed variables, and median for non-normally distributed variables. A significance level of $p < 0.05$ was considered statistically significant.

3. Results

A total of 100 patients with cleft lip and palate (52 males, 48 females) were included in this study. Among the male patients, 30 (57.7%) had unilateral clefts, with 21 (40.4%) on the left side and 9 (17.3%) on the right side, while 22 (42.3%) had bilateral clefts. Among the female patients, 29 (60.4%) had unilateral clefts, with 19 (39.6%) on the left side and 10 (20.8%) on the right side, and 19 (39.6%) had bilateral clefts. Table 1 summarizes the descriptive statistics for the variables studied across all patients included in the study.

Table 1. The descriptive statistics for the variables studied across all patients included in the study.

	Mean ± SD	Median (Min–Max)
True Positive	31.78 ± 4.96	33 (20–43)
False Positive	1.17 ± 1.31	1 (0–5)
False Negative	0,81 ± 1.02	1 (0–6)
True Negative	0.51 ± 0.69	0 (0–3)
Errors	1.03 ± 1.08	1 (0–4)
Sensitivity	0.98 ± 0.03	0.97 (0.83–1)
Precision	0.96 ± 0.04	0.97 (0.83–1)
F1 Score	0.97 ± 0.03	0.97 (0.86–1)
False Discovery Rate	0.04 ± 0.04	0.03 (0–0.17)
False Negative Rate	0.02 ± 0.03	0.03 (0–0.17)

SD, Standard Deviation.

3.1. Intraclass Correlation Coefficient (ICC)

The consistency between evaluators was assessed using the intraclass correlation coefficient (ICC). The ICC values indicated strong reliability, with intra-rater reliability ranging between 0.96 and 1, and inter-rater reliability ranging from 0.95 to 0.98. To assess intra-rater reliability, each evaluator randomly selected and re-evaluated 25 panoramic radiographs 15 days after the initial assessment. This high level of agreement confirms the accuracy and reliability of the ground truth annotations, which served as the gold standard for evaluating the AI system's performance in tooth detection and numbering.

3.2. Sensitivity and Precision Across Age Groups

With the ground truth annotations established as the reference standard, the AI system's sensitivity and precision were evaluated across the three age groups (Table 2). Sensitivity values were consistently high across all groups, with no statistically significant differences observed between the age groups ($p = 0.840$). Similarly, precision values showed no statistically significant differences among the groups ($p = 0.172$).

Table 2. Comparison of the AI system's sensitivity, precision, and specificity across the three age groups.

	Age Group			Test Statistics	p *
	6–7 Years	8–9 Years	10 and More Years		
True Positive	33.86 ± 4.38	31.67 ± 3.51	26.63 ± 5.97	23.810	<0.001 *
	35 (22–41) [c]	32 (24–38) [b]	25 (20–43) [a]		
False Positive	1 ± 1.27	1.19 ± 1.27	1.56 ± 1.5	1.859	0.395
	1 (0–5)	1 (0–4)	1.5 (0–4)		
False Negative	0.83 ± 0.85	0.83 ± 1.23	0.69 ± 0.87	0.660	0.719
	1 (0–3)	0.5 (0–6)	0 (0–2)		
	36 (25–43) [c]	33 (28–39) [b]	27 (20–45) [a]		
True Negative	0.48 ± 0.63	0.57 ± 0.77	0.44 ± 0.63	0.293	0.864
	0 (0–2)	0 (0–3)	0 (0–2)		
Errors	0.83 ± 0.96	1.26 ± 1.27	0.94 ± 0.68	2.354	0.308
	1 (0–3)	1 (0–4)	1 (0–2)		
Sensitivity	0.98 ± 0.02	0.97 ± 0.04	0.98 ± 0.03	0.349	0.840
	0.97 (0.92–1)	0.99 (0.83–1)	1 (0.92–1)		
	0 (0–0.07)	0 (0–0.12)	0 (0–0.08)		
Precision	0.97 ± 0.04	0.96 ± 0.04	0.94 ± 0.05	3.521	0.172
	0.97 (0.83–1)	0.97 (0.86–1)	0.94 (0.85–1)		
F1 Score	0.97 ± 0.03	0.97 ± 0.03	0.96 ± 0.03	2.727	0.256
	0.97 (0.89–1)	0.98 (0.86–1)	0.96 (0.91–1)		
False Discovery Rate	0.03 ± 0.04	0.04 ± 0.04	0.06 ± 0.05	3.521	0.172
	0.03 (0–0.17)	0.03 (0–0.14)	0.06 (0–0.15)		
False Negative Rate	0.02 ± 0.02	0.03 ± 0.04	0.02 ± 0.03	0.349	0.840
	0.03 (0–0.08)	0.01 (0–0.17)	0 (0–0.08)		

* p = Kruskal–Wallis test; mean ± standard deviation; median (minimum–maximum) [a–c]: groups with the same letter have no statistically significant difference.

3.3. True Positive, False Positive, and False Negative Rates

Comparisons of true positive, false positive, and false negative rates between groups are shown in Table 2. The true positive rates, correctly representing detected teeth, showed significant variation between the age groups ($p < 0.001$). The older group exhibited significantly lower true positive rates compared to the younger groups, likely due to the complexity of dental structures in older patients. The false positive rate, which reflects the incorrect detection of teeth, showed no statistically significant differences across the age groups ($p = 0.395$). However, tooth number 21 had the highest false positive rate at 16%, while tooth number 62 had the highest false negative rate at 11%. This finding is particularly important, as it aligns with the fact that the majority of our patient population had unilateral left clefts, where the AI system may face more challenges in detecting teeth. Similarly, the false negative rate was consistent across age groups ($p = 0.719$).

3.4. F1 Score and Error Rate

The F1 score, a metric combining sensitivity and precision, was calculated for all age groups (Table 2). The F1 score remained consistently high across all groups, with no statistically significant differences observed between the age groups ($p = 0.256$). Similarly, the error rate, which reflects instances where the model falsely identifies teeth in non-dental regions, did not show significant differences between the age groups ($p = 0.308$).

3.5. Gender Comparisons

Gender comparisons for sensitivity, precision, and F1 score are presented in Table 3, with no statistically significant differences observed between male and female participants ($p = 0.119$, $p = 0.441$, and $p = 0.827$, respectively). However, although not statistically significant, there was a notable difference in the false negative rates between genders ($p = 0.079$), with males showing slightly higher values compared to females.

Table 3. Gender comparisons for sensitivity, precision, and F1 score.

	Gender				Test Statistics	p *
	Male		Female			
	Mean ± SD	Median (Min–Max)	Mean ± SD	Median (Min–Max)		
True Positive	31.58 ± 5.21	33 (20–43)	32 ± 4.71	33 (22–41)	1195.5	0.716
False Positive	1.08 ± 1.23	1 (0–4)	1.27 ± 1.4	1 (0–5)	1155.5	0.503
False Negative	1.02 ± 1.21	1 (0–6)	0.58 ± 0.71	0 (0–2)	1013	0.079
True Negative	0.44 ± 0.61	0 (0–2)	0.58 ± 0.77	0 (0–3)	1152	0.448
Errors	1.02 ± 1.06	1 (0–4)	1.04 ± 1.11	1 (0–4)	1246	0.988
Sensitivity	0.97 ± 0.04	0.97 (0.83–1)	0.98 ± 0.02	1 (0.92–1)	1035	0.119
Precision	0.96 ± 0.04	0.97 (0.85–1)	0.96 ± 0.05	0.97 (0.83–1)	1140	0.441
F1 Score	0.97 ± 0.03	0.97 (0.86–1)	0.97 ± 0.03	0.98 (0.89–1)	1216.5	0.827
False Discovery Rate	0.04 ± 0.04	0.03 (0–0.15)	0.04 ± 0.05	0.03 (0–0.17)	1140	0.441
False Negative Rate	0.03 ± 0.04	0.03 (0–0.17)	0.02 ± 0.02	0 (0–0.08)	1035	0.119

* p = Mann–Whitney U test; mean ± standard deviation; median (minimum–maximum); $p > 0.05$.

3.6. Age and Gender-Specific Performance

The performance of the AI system was further analyzed by dividing the participants by gender and age groups (Tables 4 and 5). The results indicate that some significant differences were observed across different age and gender groups:

- The 6–7 years age group: Female participants showed a significantly lower false negative rate ($p = 0.0004$) and higher sensitivity ($p = 0.0006$) compared to males.
- The 8–9 years age group: Male participants exhibited higher precision ($p = 0.0036$) and a lower false discovery rate ($p = 0.0036$) than females.
- The 10+ years age group: No significant differences were observed between males and females in this age group.

Table 4. Comparison of variables by gender within each age group.

Age Group		Male		Female		Test Statistics	p
		Mean ± SD	Median (Min–Max)	Mean ± SD	Median (Min–Max)		
6–7 years	True Positive	33.29 ± 4.21	34 (26–39)	34.24 ± 4.54	35 (22–41)	181.5	0.425 *
	False Positive	1 ± 0.94	1 (0–3)	1 ± 1.47	0 (0–5)	184.5	0.444 *
	False Negative	1.29 ± 0.85	1 (0–3)	0.52 ± 0.71	0 (0–2)	107	**0.004** *
	True Negative	0.53 ± 0.62	0 (0–2)	0.44 ± 0.65	0 (0–2)	192.5	0.555 *
	Errors	0.59 ± 0.71	0 (0–2)	1 ± 1.08	1 (0–3)	172.5	0.270 *
	Sensitivity	0.96 ± 0.02	0.97 (0.92–1)	0.98 ± 0.02	1 (0.94–1)	110	**0.006** *
	Precision	0.97 ± 0.03	0.97 (0.9–1)	0.97 ± 0.05	1 (0.83–1)	189	0.527 *
	F1 Score	0.97 ± 0.02	0.97 (0.91–1)	0.98 ± 0.03	0.99 (0.89–1)	140	0.059 *
	False Discovery Rate	0.03 ± 0.03	0.03 (0–0.1)	0.03 ± 0.05	0 (0–0.17)	189	0.527 *
	False Negative Rate	0.04 ± 0.02	0.03 (0–0.08)	0.02 ± 0.02	0 (0–0.06)	110	**0.006** *
8–9 years	True Positive	32.57 ± 3.69	33 (24–38)	30.58 ± 3.02	30 (25–37)	140	**0.046** *
	False Positive	0.87 ± 1.18	0 (0–4)	1.58 ± 1.3	1 (0–4)	138.5	**0.034** *
	False Negative	1 ± 1.54	0 (0–6)	0.63 ± 0.68	1 (0–2)	212	0.858 *
	True Negative	0.43 ± 0.66	0 (0–2)	0.74 ± 0.87	1 (0–3)	176.5	0.230 *
	Errors	1.35 ± 1.3	1 (0–4)	1.16 ± 1.26	1 (0–4)	199.5	0.618 *
	Sensitivity	0.97 ± 0.05	1 (0.83–1)	0.98 ± 0.02	0.97 (0.94–1)	218.5	1.000 *
	Precision	0.97 ± 0.04	1 (0.86–1)	0.95 ± 0.04	0.97 (0.86–1)	137.5	**0.036** *
	F1 Score	0.97 ± 0.04	0.99 (0.86–1)	0.96 ± 0.02	0.97 (0.91–0.99)	139.5	**0.045** *
	False Discovery Rate	0.03 ± 0.04	0 (0–0.14)	0.05 ± 0.04	0.03 (0–0.14)	137.5	**0.036** *
	False Negative Rate	0.03 ± 0.05	0 (0–0.17)	0.02 ± 0.02	0.03 (0–0.06)	218.5	1.000 *
10 and more years	True Positive	27.25 ± 6.77	25 (20–43)	24.75 ± 1.89	25.5 (22–26)	22.5	0.854 *
	False Positive	1.58 ± 1.62	1.5 (0–4)	1.5 ± 1.29	1.5 (0–3)	24	1.000 *
	False Negative	0.67 ± 0.89	0 (0–2)	0.75 ± 0.96	0.5 (0–2)	22.5	0.839 *
	True Negative	0.33 ± 0.49	0 (0–1)	0.75 ± 0.96	0.5 (0–2)	18	0.394 *
	Errors	1 ± 0.74	1 (0–2)	0.75 ± 0.5	1 (0–1)	19.5	0.543 *
	Sensitivity	0.98 ± 0.03	1 (0.93–1)	0.97 ± 0.04	0.98 (0.92–1)	22	0.789 *
	Precision	0.94 ± 0.06	0.95 (0.85–1)	0.95 ± 0.04	0.94 (0.9–1)	24	1.000 *
	F1 Score	0.96 ± 0.03	0.96 (0.91–1)	0.96 ± 0.02	0.96 (0.93–0.98)	0.166	0.870 **
	False Discovery Rate	0.06 ± 0.06	0.05 (0–0.15)	0.05 ± 0.04	0.06 (0–0.1)	24	1.000 *
	False Negative Rate	0.02 ± 0.03	0 (0–0.07)	0.03 ± 0.04	0.02 (0–0.08)	22	0.789 *

* Mann–Whitney U test; ** independent samples *t*-test; mean ± standard deviation; median (minimum–maximum).

Table 5. Comparison of variables across age groups within each gender.

Gender		Age Group			Test Statistics	p
		6–7 Years	8–9 Years	10 and More Years		
Male	True Positive	33.29 ± 4.21	32.57 ± 3.69	27.25 ± 6.77	9.868	**0.007** *
		34 (26–39) [a]	33 (24–38) [a]	25 (20–43) [b]		
	False Positive	1 ± 0.94	0.87 ± 1.18	1.58 ± 1.62	1.795	0.408 *
		1 (0–3)	0 (0–4)	1.5 (0–4)		
	False Negative	1.29 ± 0.85	1 ± 1.54	0.67 ± 0.89	4.516	0.105 *
		1 (0–3)	0 (0–6)	0 (0–2)		
		36 (30–42)	35 (28–39)	28 (20–45)		
	True Negative	0.53 ± 0.62	0.43 ± 0.66	0.33 ± 0.49	0.744	0.689 *
		0 (0–2)	0 (0–2)	0 (0–1)		
	Errors	0.59 ± 0.71	1.35 ± 1.3	1 ± 0.74	4.067	0.131 *
		0 (0–2)	1 (0–4)	1 (0–2)		
	Sensitivity	0.96 ± 0.02	0.97 ± 0.05	0.98 ± 0.03	3.805	0.149 *
		0.97 (0.92–1)	1 (0.83–1)	1 (0.93–1)		
		0 (0–0.07)	0 (0–0.07)	0 (0–0.04)		
	Precision	0.97 ± 0.03	0.97 ± 0.04	0.94 ± 0.06	1.853	0.396 *
		0.97 (0.9–1)	1 (0.86–1)	0.95 (0.85–1)		
	F1 Score	0.97 ± 0.02	0.97 ± 0.04	0.96 ± 0.03	2.287	0.319 *
		0.97 (0.91–1)	0.99 (0.86–1)	0.96 (0.91–1)		
	False Discovery Rate	0.03 ± 0.03	0.03 ± 0.04	0.06 ± 0.06	1.853	0.396 *
		0.03 (0–0.1)	0 (0–0.14)	0.05 (0–0.15)		
	False Negative Rate	0.04 ± 0.02	0.03 ± 0.05	0.02 ± 0.03	3.805	0.149 *
		0.03 (0–0.08)	0 (0–0.17)	0 (0–0.07)		
Female	True Positive	34.24 ± 4.54	30.58 ± 3.02	24.75 ± 1.89	17.548	**<0.001** *
		35 (22–41) [b]	30 (25–37) [a]	25.5 (22–26) [a]		
	False Positive	1 ± 1.47	1.58 ± 1.3	1.5 ± 1.29	3.798	0.150 *
		0 (0–5)	1 (0–4)	1.5 (0–3)		
	False Negative	0.52 ± 0.71	0.63 ± 0.68	0.75 ± 0.96	0.566	0.753 *
		0 (0–2)	1 (0–2)	0.5 (0–2)		
		36 (25–43)	33 (29–39)	27 (24–30)		
	True Negative	0.44 ± 0.65	0.74 ± 0.87	0.75 ± 0.96	1.543	0.462 *
		0 (0–2)	1 (0–3)	0.5 (0–2)		
	Errors	1 ± 1.08	1.16 ± 1.26	0.75 ± 0.5	0.160	0.923 *
		1 (0–3)	1 (0–4)	1 (0–1)		

Table 5. Cont.

Gender		Age Group			Test Statistics	p
		6–7 Years	8–9 Years	10 and More Years		
Female	Sensitivity	0.98 ± 0.02	0.98 ± 0.02	0.97 ± 0.04	0.943	0.624 *
		1 (0.94–1)	0.97 (0.94–1)	0.98 (0.92–1)		
		0 (0–0.06)	0.03 (0–0.12)	0.02 (0–0.08)		
	Precision	0.97 ± 0.05	0.95 ± 0.04	0.95 ± 0.04	4.822	0.090 *
		1 (0.83–1)	0.97 (0.86–1)	0.94 (0.9–1)		
	F1 Score	0.98 ± 0.03	0.96 ± 0.02	0.96 ± 0.02	7.435	**0.024 ***
		0.99 (0.89–1)	0.97 (0.91–0.99)	0.96 (0.93–0.98)		
	False Discovery Rate	0.03 ± 0.05	0.05 ± 0.04	0.05 ± 0.04	4.822	0.090 *
		0 (0–0.17)	0.03 (0–0.14)	0.06 (0–0.1)		
	False Negative Rate	0.02 ± 0.02	0.02 ± 0.02	0.03 ± 0.04	0.943	0.624 *
		0 (0–0.06)	0.03 (0–0.06)	0.02 (0–0.08)		

* Kruskal–Wallis test; mean ± standard deviation; median (minimum–maximum) [a,b]: groups with the same letter have no statistically significant difference.

4. Discussion

This study evaluated the performance of an artificial intelligence-based system in detecting and numbering teeth in patients with cleft lip and palate. Overall, the AI system demonstrated high sensitivity (0.98 ± 0.03) and precision (0.96 ± 0.04), confirming its reliability in tooth detection across a wide patient cohort. Based on the findings of this study, the null hypothesis was rejected. While the commercially available AI system, Diagnocat, demonstrated overall high performance comparable to expert ground truth annotations, specific challenges were identified, particularly in the maxillary left region. These findings indicate that the AI-based software requires further refinement to address limitations in the cleft region.

Several studies have evaluated the use of AI systems for tooth detection and numbering, particularly focusing on panoramic radiographs and CBCTs [20–22]. In many of these studies, AI systems have demonstrated high sensitivity and precision, generally ranging from 0.90 to 0.95 [23]. These findings align with a growing body of research highlighting the potential of AI in various dental diagnostic tasks, including tooth identification and lesion detection [23]. The accuracy and consistency of the AI system presented here suggest that it can be a useful tool in assisting clinicians with dental numbering and detection, even in patients with complex conditions such as cleft lip and palate.

Moreover, the AI system's performance across different age groups was also evaluated, which is crucial given the developmental changes in dentition, particularly in patients with cleft lip and palate. Analyzing mixed dentition presents unique challenges for clinicians due to the rapid developmental changes and variations in tooth eruption patterns [24]. One of the significant findings of this study is the lack of statistically significant differences in the AI system's performance across different age groups. This, consistent with the existing literature, suggests that the AI model can effectively detect and number teeth in patients of varying ages, despite the rapid developmental changes that occur during the mixed dentition period [25]. Notably, in younger age groups, where dental development is still ongoing, the AI system performed with similar accuracy as in older age groups, such as those aged 10 and above. These findings highlight the potential applicability of AI systems in managing mixed dentition cases, where manual tooth detection can be more challenging due to the transitory nature of the dental arch.

Additionally, gender-based differences were identified, particularly in the younger age groups. Female participants in the 6–7 age group showed significantly higher sensitivity and lower false negative rates compared to their male counterparts. This suggests that the AI system may be more efficient in detecting teeth in female patients within this age range. In contrast, the 8–9 age group showed higher precision values for male participants, although the clinical significance of this remains unclear. These findings point to the possibility that anatomical or developmental factors, such as tooth eruption patterns or growth differences, may influence the performance of AI systems in different genders and age groups [26,27]. Further investigation is needed to better understand these gender-based disparities and their implications for the clinical application of AI-based dental imaging technologies.

The AI system's consistent performance across different age groups aligns with the findings of Kim et al. [25], who also reported successful AI performance across varying patient ages. These studies suggest that age-related factors do not significantly affect AI performance. Our results further reinforce the idea that the AI model is robust in detecting and numbering teeth across a wide range of ages.

While the AI system demonstrated high overall performance in tooth detection and numbering, there are potential limitations that warrant further consideration. The study findings suggest that the AI model may face challenges in accurately identifying teeth in the maxillary left region, which exhibited higher false positive and false negative rates across all age groups. This may be attributed to the higher prevalence of cleft anomalies on the left side, as reported in the literature [28]. Among the individuals included in this study, unilateral left clefts were more common, consistent with previous research indicating that cleft lip and palate cases are predominantly unilateral and more frequently affect the left side [29]. Specifically, tooth number 21 had the highest false positive rate (16%), while tooth number 62 had the highest false negative rate (11%). These teeth are located in the regions most affected by cleft anomalies, particularly in patients with left-sided clefts, further emphasizing the challenges AI faces in accurately detecting and numbering teeth in these areas.

Additionally, the observed gender-based differences, particularly in the younger age groups, suggest that the AI system may not be equally effective in detecting teeth across all patient populations. These findings indicate the need for the further refinement and customization of AI algorithms to better address the unique dental characteristics and developmental variations seen in cleft lip and palate patients. While the overall performance of the AI system is promising, the limitations highlighted in this study underscore the importance of continued research and validation to ensure the technology can be applied effectively and equitably across diverse patient demographics [30,31].

The AI system's consistent performance across different age and gender groups observed in this study may reflect the robustness of Diagnocat's training process. As a commercially available tool, Diagnocat has been trained by its developers using diverse datasets to optimize its accuracy and generalizability. However, since the specifics of the training data, including demographic distributions, are proprietary, further studies could explore how variations in training datasets might influence AI performance in populations with unique anatomical challenges, such as cleft lip and palate patients.

5. Conclusions

This study demonstrates the strong potential of artificial intelligence (AI) to detect and number teeth in patients with cleft lip and palate, with the AI system showing high sensitivity and precision overall. The system performed well across various age groups, proving its robustness in managing the unique dental challenges that these patients present. Future improvements focused on the cleft area could further elevate its clinical utility, leading to better diagnosis and management in this population.

Author Contributions: C.A.: Conceptualization, methodology, supervision, collecting data, writing—original draft, reviewing and editing the manuscript; N.O.Y.: Collecting data, writing—original draft; K.K.: Conceptualization collecting data, data analysis; E.S.A.: Writing—original draft, reviewing and editing the manuscript, D.G.C.: Methodology, data analysis. All authors have read and agreed to the published version of the manuscript.

Funding: This research received no external funding.

Institutional Review Board Statement: The study was conducted in accordance with the Declaration of Helsinki, and approved by the Ethics Committee of Yeditepe University (Approval Number and Date: 202311Y0694, 11 October 2024).

Informed Consent Statement: Informed consent was obtained from all subjects involved in the study.

Data Availability Statement: The data presented in this study are available on request from the corresponding author.

Conflicts of Interest: The authors declare no conflicts of interest.

References

1. Shetye, P.R. Update on treatment of patients with cleft—Timing of orthodontics and surgery. *Semin. Orthod.* **2016**, *22*, 45–51. [CrossRef]
2. Zreaqat, M.H.; Hassan, R.; Hanoun, A. Cleft Lip and Palate Management from Birth to Adulthood: An Overview. In *Insights into Various Aspects of Oral Health*; IntechOpen: Rijeka, Croatia, 2017.
3. Orhan, K.; Aktuna Belgin, C.; Manulis, D.; Golitsyna, M.; Bayrak, S.; Aksoy, S.; Sanders, A.; Önder, M.; Ezhov, M.; Shamshiev, M.; et al. Determining the reliability of diagnosis and treatment using artificial intelligence software with panoramic radiographs. *Imaging Sci. Dent.* **2023**, *53*, 199–207. [CrossRef] [PubMed]
4. Ezhov, M.; Gusarev, M.; Golitsyna, M.; Yates, J.M.; Kushnerev, E.; Tamimi, D.; Aksoy, S.; Shumilov, E.; Sanders, A.; Orhan, K. Clinically applicable artificial intelligence system for dental diagnosis with CBCT. *Sci. Rep.* **2021**, *11*, 15006. [CrossRef] [PubMed]
5. Estai, M.; Tennant, M.; Gebauer, D.; Brostek, A.; Vignarajan, J.; Mehdizadeh, M.; Saha, S. Deep learning for automated detection and numbering of permanent teeth on panoramic images. *Dentomaxillofac. Radiol.* **2022**, *51*, 20210296. [CrossRef]
6. Hung, K.; Montalvao, C.; Tanaka, R.; Kawai, T.; Bornstein, M.M. The use and performance of artificial intelligence applications in dental and maxillofacial radiology: A systematic review. *Dentomaxillofac. Radiol.* **2020**, *49*, 20190107. [CrossRef]
7. Hiraiwa, T.; Ariji, Y.; Fukuda, M.; Kise, Y.; Nakata, K.; Katsumata, A.; Fujita, H.; Ariji, E. A deep learning artificial intelligence system for assessment of root morphology of the mandibular first molar on panoramic radiography. *Dentomaxillofac. Radiol.* **2019**, *48*, 20180218. [CrossRef]
8. Lee, J.S.; Adhikari, S.; Liu, L.; Jeong, H.G.; Kim, H.; Yoon, S.J. Osteoporosis detection in panoramic radiographs using a deep convolutional neural network-based computer-assisted diagnosis system: A preliminary study. *Dentomaxillofac. Radiol.* **2019**, *48*, 20170344. [CrossRef]
9. Hendi KDAl Alyami, M.H.; Alkahtany, M.; Dwivedi, A.; Alsaqour, H.G. Artificial intelligence in prosthodontics. *Bioinformation* **2024**, *20*, 238–242. [CrossRef]
10. Schwendicke, F.; Samek, W.; Krois, J. Artificial Intelligence in Dentistry: Chances and Challenges. *J. Dent. Res.* **2020**, *99*, 769–774. [CrossRef]
11. Kuwada, C.; Ariji, Y.; Kise, Y.; Fukuda, M.; Nishiyama, M.; Funakoshi, T.; Takeuchi, R.; Sana, A.; Kojima, N.; Ariji, E. Deep-learning systems for diagnosing cleft palate on panoramic radiographs in patients with cleft alveolus. *Oral Radiol.* **2023**, *39*, 349–354. [CrossRef]
12. Ahmed, N.; Abbasi, M.S.; Zuberi, F.; Qamar, W.; Halim, M.S.B.; Maqsood, A.; Alam, M.K. Artificial Intelligence Techniques: Analysis, Application, and Outcome in Dentistry-A Systematic Review. *Biomed. Res. Int.* **2021**, *2021*, 9751564. [CrossRef] [PubMed]
13. Chen, Y.W.; Stanley, K.; Att, W. Artificial intelligence in dentistry: Current applications and future perspectives. *Quintessence Int.* **2020**, *51*, 248–257. [PubMed]
14. Thurzo, A.; Urbanová, W.; Novák, B.; Czako, L.; Siebert, T.; Stano, P.; Mareková, S.; Fountoulaki, G.; Kosnáčová, H.; Varga, I. Where Is the Artificial Intelligence Applied in Dentistry? Systematic Review and Literature Analysis. *Healthcare* **2022**, *10*, 1269. [CrossRef] [PubMed]
15. De Mulder, D.; Cadenas de Llano-Pérula, M.; Willems, G.; Jacobs, R.; Dormaar, J.T.; Verdonck, A. An optimized imaging protocol for orofacial cleft patients. *Clin. Exp. Dent. Res.* **2018**, *4*, 152–157. [CrossRef]
16. Zadrożny, Ł.; Regulski, P.; Brus-Sawczuk, K.; Czajkowska, M.; Parkanyi, L.; Ganz, S.; Mijiritsky, E. Artificial Intelligence Application in Assessment of Panoramic Radiographs. *Diagnostics* **2022**, *12*, 224. [CrossRef]
17. Tuzoff, D.V.; Tuzova, L.N.; Bornstein, M.M.; Krasnov, A.S.; Kharchenko, M.A.; Nikolenko, S.I.; Sveshnikov, M.M.; Bednenko, G.B. Tooth detection and numbering in panoramic radiographs using convolutional neural networks. *Dentomaxillofac. Radiol.* **2019**, *48*, 20180051. [CrossRef]

18. Bilgir, E.; Bayrakdar, İ.Ş.; Çelik, Ö.; Orhan, K.; Akkoca, F.; Sağlam, H.; Odabaş, A.; Aslan, A.F.; Ozcetin, C.; Kıllı, M.; et al. An artificial intelligence approach to automatic tooth detection and numbering in panoramic radiographs. *BMC Med. Imaging* **2021**, *21*, 124. [CrossRef]
19. Faul, F.; Erdfelder, E.; Lang, A.G.; Buchner, A. G*Power 3: A flexible statistical power analysis program for the social, behavioral, and biomedical sciences. *Behav. Res. Methods* **2007**, *39*, 175–191. [CrossRef]
20. Song, I.-S.; Shin, H.-K.; Kang, J.-H.; Kim, J.-E.; Huh, K.-H.; Yi, W.-J.; Lee, S.-S.; Heo, M.-S. Deep learning-based apical lesion segmentation from panoramic radiographs. *Imaging Sci. Dent.* **2022**, *52*, 351–357. [CrossRef]
21. Orhan, K.; Bilgir, E.; Bayrakdar, I.S.; Ezhov, M.; Gusarev, M.; Shumilov, E. Evaluation of artificial intelligence for detecting impacted third molars on cone-beam computed tomography scans. *J. Stomatol. Oral Maxillofac. Surg.* **2021**, *122*, 333–337. [CrossRef]
22. Miki, Y.; Muramatsu, C.; Hayashi, T.; Zhou, X.; Hara, T.; Katsumata, A.; Fujita, H. Classification of teeth in cone-beam CT using deep convolutional neural network. *Comput. Biol. Med.* **2017**, *80*, 24–29. [CrossRef] [PubMed]
23. Maganur, P.C.; Vishwanathaiah, S.; Mashyakhy, M.; Abumelha, A.S.; Robaian, A.; Almohareb, T.; Almutairi, B.; Alzahrani, K.M.; Binalrimal, S.; Marwah, N.; et al. Development of Artificial Intelligence Models for Tooth Numbering and Detection: A Systematic Review. *Int. Dent. J.* **2024**, *74*, 917–929. [CrossRef] [PubMed]
24. Proffit, W.R.; Frazier-Bowers, S.A. Mechanism and control of tooth eruption: Overview and clinical implications. *Orthod. Craniofac. Res.* **2009**, *12*, 59–66. [CrossRef]
25. Kim, Y.-R.; Choi, J.-H.; Ko, J.; Jung, Y.-J.; Kim, B.; Nam, S.-H.; Chang, W.-D. Age Group Classification of Dental Radiography without Precise Age Information Using Convolutional Neural Networks. *Healthcare* **2023**, *11*, 1068. [CrossRef]
26. Bianchi, I.; Oliva, G.; Vitale, G.; Bellugi, B.; Bertana, G.; Focardi, M.; Grassi, S.; Dalessandri, D.; Pinchi, V. A Semi-Automatic Method on a Small Italian Sample for Estimating Sex Based on the Shape of the Crown of the Maxillary Posterior Teeth. *Healthcare* **2023**, *11*, 845. [CrossRef]
27. Zhou, Y.; Jiang, F.; Cheng, F.; Li, J. Detecting representative characteristics of different genders using intraoral photographs: A deep learning model with interpretation of gradient-weighted class activation mapping. *BMC Oral Health* **2023**, *23*, 327. [CrossRef]
28. Carinci, F.; Scapoli, L.; Palmieri, A.; Zollino, I.; Pezzetti, F. Human genetic factors in nonsyndromic cleft lip and palate: An update. *Int. J. Pediatr. Otorhinolaryngol.* **2007**, *71*, 1509–1519. [CrossRef]
29. Putri, F.A.; Pattamatta, M.; Anita, S.E.S.; Maulina, T. The Global Occurrences of Cleft Lip and Palate in Pediatric Patients and Their Association with Demographic Factors: A Narrative Review. *Children* **2024**, *11*, 322. [CrossRef]
30. Almoammar, K.A. Harnessing the Power of Artificial Intelligence in Cleft Lip and Palate: An In-Depth Analysis from Diagnosis to Treatment, a Comprehensive Review. *Children* **2024**, *11*, 140. [CrossRef]
31. Hwang, J.J.; Jung, Y.H.; Cho, B.H.; Heo, M.S. An overview of deep learning in the field of dentistry. *Imaging Sci. Dent.* **2019**, *49*, 1–7. [CrossRef]

Disclaimer/Publisher's Note: The statements, opinions and data contained in all publications are solely those of the individual author(s) and contributor(s) and not of MDPI and/or the editor(s). MDPI and/or the editor(s) disclaim responsibility for any injury to people or property resulting from any ideas, methods, instructions or products referred to in the content.

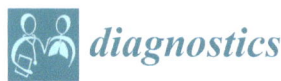
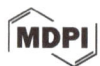

Article

Evaluation of a Vendor-Agnostic Deep Learning Model for Noise Reduction and Image Quality Improvement in Dental CBCT

Wojciech Kazimierczak [1,2,3,*], Róża Wajer [1,2], Oskar Komisarek [4], Marta Dyszkiewicz-Konwińska [5], Adrian Wajer [6], Natalia Kazimierczak [3], Joanna Janiszewska-Olszowska [7] and Zbigniew Serafin [8]

[1] Department of Radiology and Diagnostic Imaging, Collegium Medicum, Nicolaus Copernicus University in Torun, Jagiellońska 13-15, 85-067 Bydgoszcz, Poland
[2] Department of Radiology and Diagnostic Imaging, University Hospital No. 1 in Bydgoszcz, Marii Skłodowskiej—Curie 9, 85-094 Bydgoszcz, Poland
[3] Kazimierczak Private Medical Practice, Dworcowa 13/u6a, 85-009 Bydgoszcz, Poland
[4] Department of Otolaryngology, Audiology and Phoniatrics, Collegium Medicum, Nicolaus Copernicus University in Torun, Jagiellońska 13-15, 85-067 Bydgoszcz, Poland
[5] Department of Diagnostic Imaging, Poznan University of Medical Sciences, 61-701 Poznań, Poland
[6] Dental Primus, Poznańska 18, 88-100 Inowrocław, Poland
[7] Department of Interdisciplinary Dentistry, Pomeranian Medical University in Szczecin, Al. Powstańców Wlkp. 72, 70-111 Szczecin, Poland
[8] Faculty of Medicine, Bydgoszcz University of Science and Technology, Kaliskiego 7, 85-796 Bydgoszcz, Poland
* Correspondence: wojtek.kazimierczak@gmail.com

Abstract: Background/Objectives: To assess the impact of a vendor-agnostic deep learning model (DLM) on image quality parameters and noise reduction in dental cone-beam computed tomography (CBCT) reconstructions. Methods: This retrospective study was conducted on CBCT scans of 93 patients (41 males and 52 females, mean age 41.2 years, SD 15.8 years) from a single center using the inclusion criteria of standard radiation dose protocol images. Objective and subjective image quality was assessed in three predefined landmarks through contrast-to-noise ratio (CNR) measurements and visual assessment using a 5-point scale by three experienced readers. The inter-reader reliability and repeatability were calculated. Results: Eighty patients (30 males and 50 females; mean age 41.5 years, SD 15.94 years) were included in this study. The CNR in DLM reconstructions was significantly greater than in native reconstructions, and the mean CNR in regions of interest 1-3 (ROI1-3) in DLM images was 11.12 ± 9.29, while in the case of native reconstructions, it was 7.64 ± 4.33 ($p < 0.001$). The noise level in native reconstructions was significantly higher than in the DLM reconstructions, and the mean noise level in ROI1-3 in native images was 45.83 ± 25.89, while in the case of DLM reconstructions, it was 35.61 ± 24.28 ($p < 0.05$). Subjective image quality assessment revealed no statistically significant differences between native and DLM reconstructions. Conclusions: The use of deep learning-based image reconstruction algorithms for CBCT imaging of the oral cavity can improve image quality by enhancing the CNR and lowering the noise.

Keywords: cone-beam computed tomography; deep learning model; image quality; noise reduction; dental imaging; oral diagnosis

1. Introduction

Cone-beam computed tomography (CBCT) has emerged as a valuable dental imaging tool because of its ability to provide precise three-dimensional reconstruction of the dentomaxillofacial region. CBCT surpasses the limitations of conventional two-dimensional dental imaging, facilitating accurate insight into the multiplanar details of maxillofacial bony structures and adjacent soft tissues. A spatial resolution of less than 100 μm significantly surpasses the imaging capabilities of conventional computed tomography (CT), allowing for precise diagnosis and measurements [1–3]. Such precision is desired in implant procedure planning, cephalometry, and endodontics. Although relatively recently introduced (2000s) for broader commercial use, CBCT has already proven its value in a wide range of dental applications, including implant planning, periodontology, temporomandibular joint (TMJ) imaging, orthodontics, and oral and maxillofacial surgery [4,5].

However, the application of CBCT as an imaging modality has limitations. Despite the exceptional image quality achieved in phantom studies, patient studies should be conducted in accordance with ALADIP (As Low as Diagnostically Acceptable being Indication-oriented and Patient-specific) principles [6]. This approach, inter alia, aims to prevent excessive tube setting and thus may lead to a greater number of artifacts and excessive noise. In the case of CBCT, there is a significant variation in image quality, specifically regarding contrast resolution and the level of noise, across various CBCT machines and settings used during acquisition, accompanied by a broad spectrum of radiation doses administered to patients [7]. CBCT artifacts are induced by discrepancies between mathematical models and actual imaging processes [8]. Noise, an unwanted disturbance in a signal, can significantly impair the quality of the images produced by CBCT units. Noise manifests as inconsistent attenuation values in projection images, causing errors in the computed attenuation coefficient and reducing low-contrast resolution, affecting the differentiation of low-density tissues [9,10]. Both artifacts and noise may simulate or obscure pathologies, leading to misdiagnoses and potentially worsening patient outcomes. Additionally, noise is inherently associated with the dose delivered during examinations, demonstrating an inversely proportional relationship [11]. Therefore, it is reasonable to seek noise and artifact reduction, as their application may have an impact on reducing the radiation dose delivered during CBCT and improving its diagnostic accuracy.

To date, several studies have demonstrated the efficacy of deep learning-based image reconstruction algorithms in reducing noise and improving image quality in CBCT scans. For instance, iterative reconstruction (IR) techniques have been shown to significantly enhance image quality in conventional CT and CBCT imaging [12–18]. Recent advancements in vendor-specific DLRs, such as TrueFidelity™ by GE Healthcare and AiCE by Canon Medical Systems, have further improved diagnostic accuracy and reduced radiation doses [19–21]. However, the limitation of these approaches is their vendor-specific nature, which restricts their use to specific scanners. Our study explored the potential of a vendor-agnostic DLM to overcome these limitations. The solution appears to be a vendor-agnostic deep learning model (DLM) that works in the image postprocessing domain and does not require projection data. The term vendor-agnostic refers to the fact that the program is not limited to specific CT or CBCT machine manufacturers and can be applied across different platforms [22]. Previous studies have already proven that vendor-agnostic DLMs can both reduce image noise and provide high diagnostic accuracy comparable to vendor-specific DLRs [23–26]. Hypothetically, they could also positively affect the quality parameters of dental CBCT images, thereby increasing their diagnostic value for the evaluation of common pathological and dental lesions.

The aim of this study was to assess objective and subjective image quality parameters of standard dental CBCT and DLM-reconstructed images.

2. Materials and Methods

2.1. Population

The study population consisted of 93 patients (41 males and 52 females aged 15–72 years, SD 15.8; median 41.2). All CBCT scans were acquired at a single private orthodontic center. All patients were referred for CBCT scans by orthodontists and dental surgeons between January and September 2023. The primary indication was suspicion of periapical lesions on the basis of the OPG and single-tooth X-rays. The main study inclusion criterion was images obtained using the standard radiation dose and image quality protocol. Images burdened by motion artifacts were excluded from the study.

2.2. Image Acquisition and Postprocessing

All scans were performed using a Hyperion X9 PRO 13 × 10 (MyRay, Imola, Italy). One standard, marked as the "Regular" setting of the apparatus, was used (90 kV, 36 mAs, CTDI/Vol 4.09 mGy, and 13 cm field of view). All images were reconstructed at a slice thickness of 0.3 mm. After scanning, the images were anonymized and exported for further analysis. The deep learning and denoised reconstructions were obtained with the use of ClariCT.AI software (ClariPI, Seoul, Republic of Korea).

2.3. Objective Image Quality

To assess the objective image quality, a radiologist with 2 years of craniofacial CT assessment placed square regions of interest (ROIs) at:

1. Periapical region of tooth 15 within the maxillary bone,
2. Periapical region of tooth 33 within the mandible,
3. The spongious bone of the mandible in the mental foramen area,
4. Muscles of the tongue.

The ROIs were carefully placed in homogeneous tissues (spongious bone of periapical regions, mandible, and tongue musculature) to avoid artifacts and lesions (e.g., cysts, enostoses, and endodontic materials). The contrast-to-noise ratio (CNR) was evaluated using ImageJ software v. 1.41 (National Institutes of Health, Bethesda, MD, USA). ROIs were automatically propagated between the native and DLM reconstructions to maximize the objectivity of the results. The CNR calculation formula presented by Koivisto [27] was adopted:

$$CNR = (S_{R1\text{-}3,L} - S_T)/N$$

where $S_{R1\text{-}3,L}$ is the mean signal at the anatomical landmark or periapical lesion, S_T is the mean signal in the background (tongue), and N is the average standard deviation (SD) in the anatomical landmark and background ROI (tongue).

The CNRs of the specified anatomical landmarks were compared to evaluate the effectiveness of the AI denoising tool.

2.4. Subjective Image Quality

Subjective image quality was assessed by a radiologist and two dentists (all readers with >5 years of experience in craniofacial CT assessment) who were blinded to patient details and the use of the AI denoising tool. The images were evaluated on a five-point scale (1 = poor, 5 = excellent), considering factors such as noise, sharpness, and visibility of anatomical structures as follows:

Level 5—excellent delineation of structures and excellent image quality;
Level 4—clear delineation of structures and good image quality;
Level 3—anatomical structures still fully assessable in all parts and acceptable image quality;
Level 2—structures identifiable with adequate image quality;
Level 1—anatomical structures not identifiable, images with no diagnostic value.

Image quality assessment was performed in the following predefined anatomical regions: the alveolar recess of the maxillary sinuses, the apical area of tooth 15, and the apical area of tooth 33.

To enhance the repeatability and objectivity of the qualitative analyses, an illustration was created to depict representative images evaluated according to the aforementioned scale (Figure 1). In cases of metal artifacts or missing teeth, the opposite side of the dental arch was assessed (e.g., severe artifacts in the apical area of tooth 15–tooth 25 were evaluated).

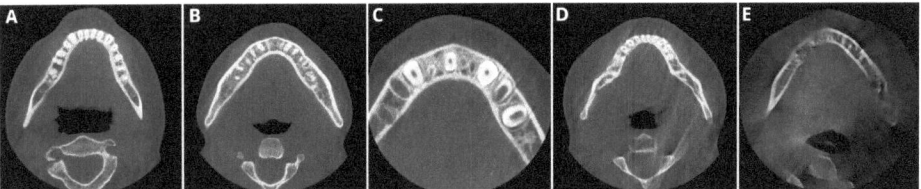

Figure 1. Qualitative image analysis: (**A**)—(5 points) excellent delineation of structures and excellent image quality; (**B**)—(4 points) clear delineation of structures and good image quality; (**C**)—(3 points) anatomical structures still fully assessable in all parts and acceptable image quality; (**D**)—(2 points) structures identifiable in adequate image quality; (**E**)—(1 point) anatomical structures not identifiable, image of no diagnostic value.

Agreement between all the readers' ratings of the subjective image quality of the native and DLM-reconstructed images was assessed.

Subjective image quality analysis was performed on a dedicated console using iRYS Viewer version 6.2 (MyRay, Imola, Italy) software. The window width and center were predefined at 1048 and 4096, respectively.

2.5. Error Study

Fifteen randomly selected subjects were re-examined by the same author one month after the initial analysis. The ICC for subjective image quality analyses was calculated to assess the agreement between examinations.

2.6. Sample Size Calculation

The post hoc power analysis was conducted to determine adequacy of study sample. A two-tailed paired-sample t-test was used since CNR measurements were taken from the same patients under both conditions (native and DLM reconstructions). The effect size (Cohen's d) for paired samples was assessed with pooled SD of mean CNR values in DLM and native reconstructions. Power analysis was conducted with G*Power software (version 3.1) [28]. The following assumptions were made: α error probability: 0.05, Power $(1 - \beta)$: 0.80.

2.7. Statistical Evaluation

Inter-rater agreement was assessed using Fleiss' Kappa. Differences between native and DLM reconstructions were analyzed using paired t-tests. A power analysis was conducted to determine the appropriate sample size for detecting significant differences in noise levels between the two reconstruction methods. Statistical significance was set at $p < 0.05$ [27]. Statistical analyses were conducted using R software version 4.3.2 [29].

3. Results

3.1. Population

The authors screened a total of 93 CBCT scans. Out of these, 13 scans were excluded, as they did not meet the inclusion criteria. Therefore, CBCT scans from 80 patients (30 males and 50 females; mean age 41.45 years, SD 15.94 years) were included in the final analysis (80/93 screened patients). The application of eligibility criteria is presented in Figure 2.

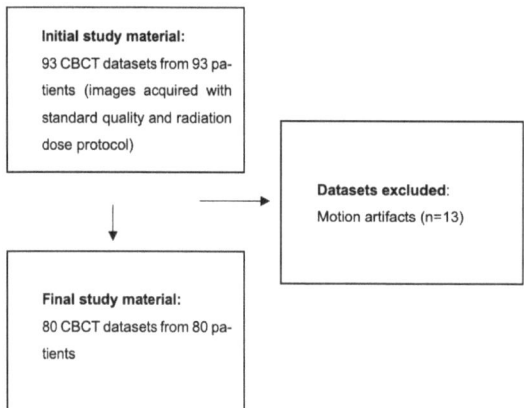

Figure 2. Flow-chart presenting application of eligibility criteria in study material.

3.2. Objective Image Quality

Figure 3 shows the sample ROI position with the corresponding signal and SD values.

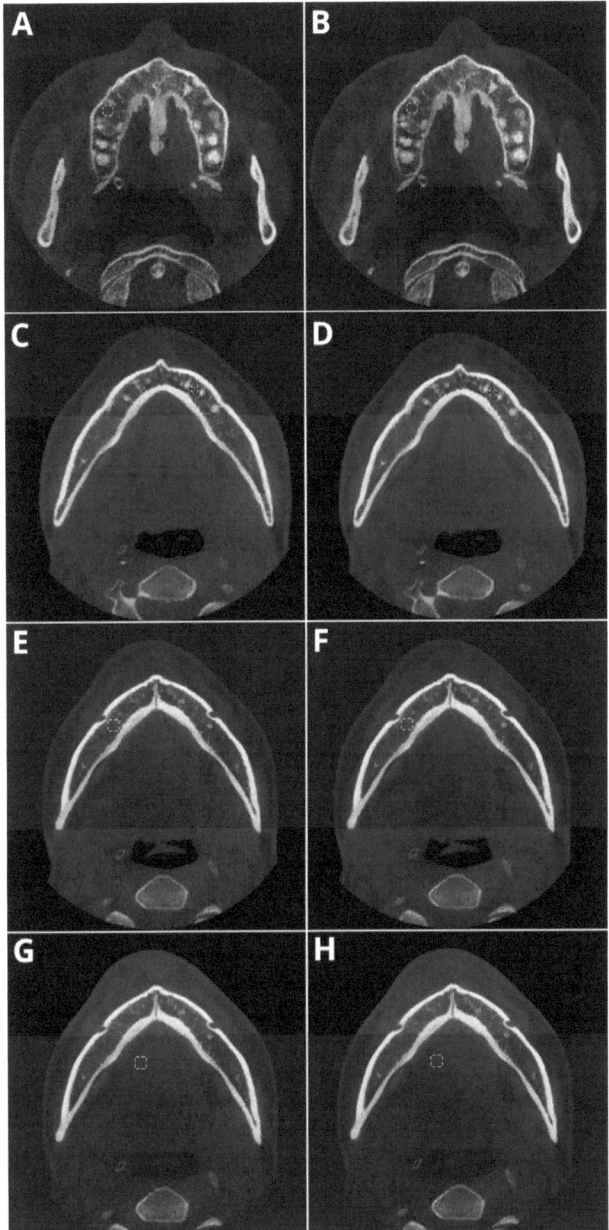

Figure 3. The sample ROI (yellow circle) positions and values in the native (**A,C,E,G**) and DLM (**B,D,F,H**) reconstructions were as follows: (**A,B**), tooth 15, mean signal 227.748, 227.267 and SD 179.793, 170,854, respectively; (**C,D**), tooth 33, mean signal 418.06, 417.462 and SD 136.493, 129,878, respectively; (**E,F**), mental foramen, mean signal 336.191, 330.893 and SD 111.672, 89.153, respectively; and (**G,H**), tongue musculature, mean signal 96.336, 95.785 and SD 38.251, 26.848, respectively.

The average signal measured in the regions of interest (ROIs) in three locations (periapical area of teeth 15 and 33 and spongious bone of the mandible in the area of the mental foramen) showed slightly lower mean values in DLM images than in native reconstructions. However, the difference was not statistically significant ($p > 0.05$). Table 1 summarizes the results of the objective image quality assessment. Graphical representation of the mean signal calculations in Figure 4.

Table 1. Results of the objective image quality assessment.

	Parameter	Native	DLM	p
Signal	Tooth 15	341 ± 197.60	339.91 ± 194.93	$p = 0.961$
	Tooth 33	448.33 ± 232.01	452.84 ± 249.1	$p = 0.906$
	Mental foramen	456.15 ± 235.78	454.46 ± 238.97	$p = 0.964$
	Mean ROI_{1-3}	415.3 ± 178.11	415.74 ± 181.75	$p = 0.988$
Noise		45.83 ± 25.89	35.61 ± 24.28	$p = 0.011$ *
CNR	Tooth 15	5.62 ± 5.19	8.28 ± 8.25	$p = 0.016$ *
	Tooth 33	8.58 ± 5.45	12.42 ± 8.76	$p = 0.001$ *
	Mental foramen	8.63 ± 5.81	12.29 ± 9.02	$p = 0.003$ *
	Mean ROI_{1-3}	7.64 ± 4.33	11.12 ± 9.29	$p < 0.001$ *

The signal and CNR are given as the means ± standard deviations. DLM—deep learning model reconstruction; ROI—region of interest; CNR—contrast-to-noise ratio. *—statistically significant difference.

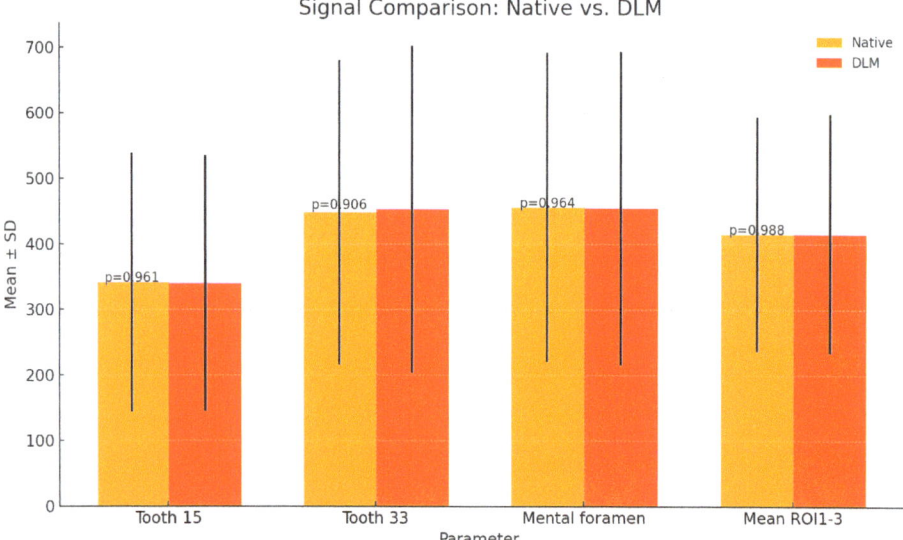

Figure 4. Results of the mean signal calculations (mean values error bars represent SDs). No statistically significant differences were found ($p > 0.05$).

There was a statistically significant difference between noise levels on both types of reconstructions ($p = 0.011$). Figure 5 illustrates mean noise levels.

The CNR in DLM reconstructions was significantly higher than that in native reconstructions across all examined locations ($p < 0.05$), as shown in Figure 6. The mean CNR in ROI_{1-3} in DLM images was 11.12 ± 9.29, while in the case of native reconstructions, it was 7.64 ± 4.33 (Table 1).

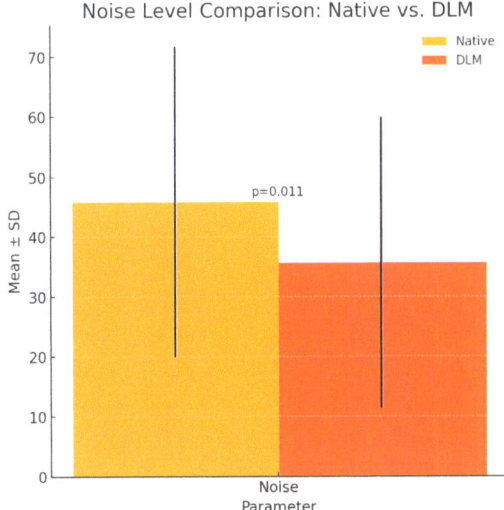

Figure 5. Results of noise calculations in ROIs 1–3 (mean values error bars represent SDs). *p* values shown on graphs. There was a statistically significant difference ($p = 0.011$).

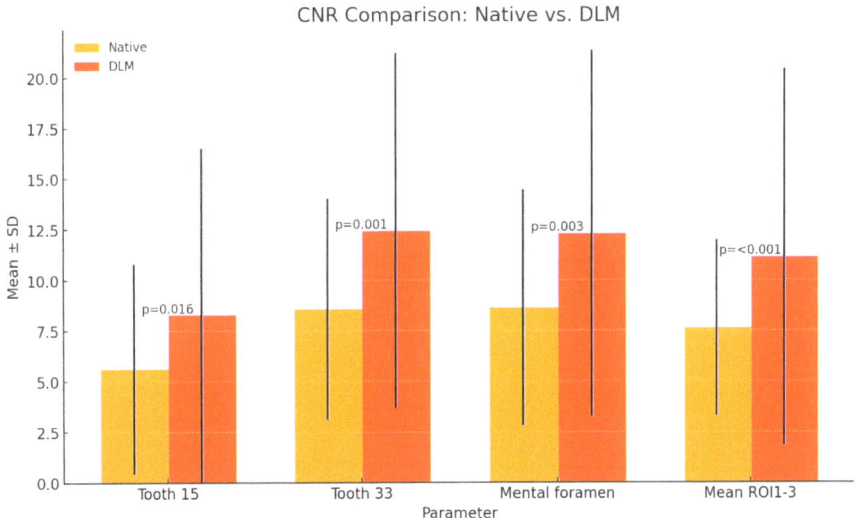

Figure 6. Results of CNR calculations (mean values, error bars represent SDs). *p* values shown on graphs.

3.3. Subjective Image Quality

The results of the subjective image quality assessments are summarized in Table 2. The data in the table represent the mean ratings of all readers. Overall, subjective image quality was lowest for the apical area of tooth 15 in both the native and DLM reconstructions. The highest mean scores were given to the apical area of tooth 33 in both the evaluated reconstructions. The differences between the mean ratings for both types of reconstructions were slight and not statistically significant ($p > 0.05$), ICC = 0.753. Figure 7 presents the results of the subjective image quality assessments.

Table 2. Results of the subjective image quality assessment.

Region	Native			DLM			p
	Reader 1	Reader 2	Reader 3	Reader 1	Reader 2	Reader 3	
Maxillary Sinus	3.25	3.26	3.36	3.34	3.25	3.55	0.350
Apex 15	3.23	3.25	3.48	3.18	3.25	3.40	0.674
Apex 33	3.49	3.46	3.52	3.55	3.45	3.66	0.529

DLM—deep learning model. p—Wilcoxon paired test.

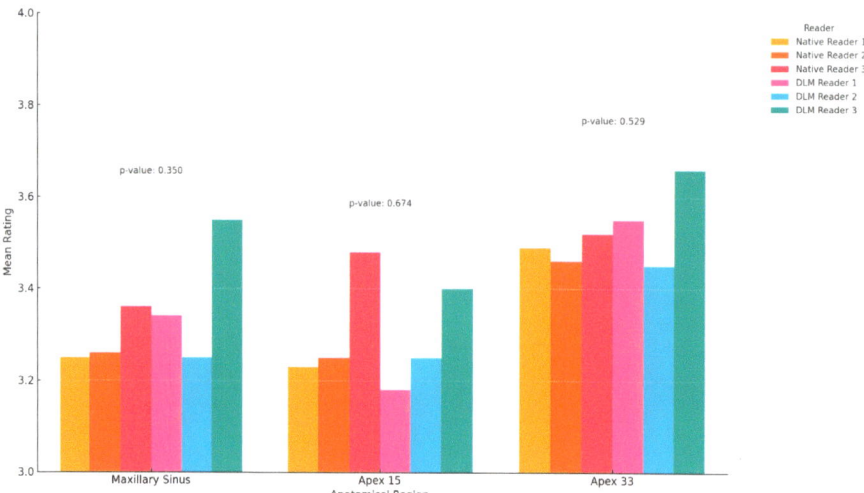

Figure 7. Results of subjective image quality assessments (mean values).

Inter-reader agreement for subjective image quality assessments was evaluated using Fleiss' Kappa. The results indicated moderate to substantial agreement among the three readers, with Kappa values ranging from 0.536 to 0.628 for native reconstructions and 0.540 to 0.628 for DLM reconstructions (Table 3).

Table 3. Inter-reader agreement for subjective image quality assessment.

Region	Reconstruction	ICC	Interpretation
Alveolar recess of maxillary sinus	Native	0.536	Moderate Agreement
	DLM	0.552	Moderate Agreement
Apex 15	Native	0.628	Substantial Agreement
	DLM	0.628	Moderate Agreement
Apex 33	Native	0.541	Moderate Agreement
	DLM	0.540	Moderate Agreement

DLM—deep learning model; ICC—interclass correlation coefficient.

3.4. Error Study

Analysis of the repeatability of subjective image quality analysis carried out by the reader demonstrated excellent concordance (ICC = 0.841).

3.5. Sample Size

A power analysis was conducted to determine the appropriate sample size required to detect significant differences in noise levels between native and DLM reconstructions. Pooled SD of mean CNR values of DLM and native images was 7.25. The calculated Cohen's d was 0.48.

The analysis indicated that a sample size of 34 subjects per group was sufficient to achieve a power of 0.8, with an effect size (Cohen's d) of 0.48 and a significance level of 0.05. This sample size ensures that the study is adequately powered to detect meaningful differences in objective image quality parameters.

4. Discussion

The aim of this study was to assess the image quality parameters of standard dental CBCT images and images reconstructed using DLM algorithms. Our study revealed that DLM reconstructions had slightly greater mean signal values than native reconstructions, although this difference was not statistically significant. However, the CNR was significantly higher in the DLM reconstructions than in the native reconstructions. Noise levels were also statistically significantly lower in the DLM reconstructions than in the native reconstructions. This indicates that the evaluated DLM algorithm improves the contrast between the anatomical structures in CBCT images. The results of the subjective image quality analysis performed by three readers blinded to the type of reconstruction showed no statistically significant differences.

Surprisingly, although the differences were statistically insignificant, the results of the subjective image quality assessments showed mixed results in the evaluation of the selected anatomical structures. The mean scores for all readers of the alveolar recess of the maxillary sinus and the apical area of tooth 33 were both greater for DLM reconstructions than for native reconstructions. However, the ratings for the apical area of tooth 15 were greater in native reconstructions than in DLM reconstructions. In our opinion, this indicates a clear convergence in the quality of both reconstructions and high repeatability of readers in quality assessment. Upon re-evaluation by the readers, after the results of the analyses were obtained, some of the DLM reconstructions showed poorer delineation of structures, which might have influenced the image quality ratings of both periapical areas. However, combined with reduced noise levels, excessive smoothing of the very thin structures worsened the delineation of structures, for example, the periodontal ligament. This phenomenon might have an impact on the visualization of critical CBCT-indicated structures, such as the root canal or alveolar bone, where spatial resolution is key [30–32]. Similar results were shown by Ylisiurua et al. [33], who reported that deep learning algorithms enhanced the visualization of soft tissues but degraded the visualization of bones and teeth. The authors subjectively noted a significant decrease in resolution and concluded that the images resembled images reconstructed with "soft-tissue kernels" used with CT scanners. Since CBCT is used mainly in the diagnosis of bones and teeth, such over-smoothing of the details may compromise diagnostic accuracy. Future studies focused on evaluating the delineation of such structures may answer the question of whether DLM algorithms significantly reduce the value of the examination in assessing submillimeter structures.

Our findings suggest that although the quantitative improvements are noticeable, the qualitative assessment of these changes may require a higher threshold to achieve significance. We must emphasize that the evaluated DLM was not designed for CBCT imaging. The purpose of the program was to reduce additional image noise in CT images. Therefore, the results of our study should be regarded as a scientifically driven attempt to explore the impact of this tool on a domain similar to CT. The results are similar to our previous study evaluating the effects of applying the same vendor-agnostic DLM to CBCT images of TMJs [34]. The study showed significantly better objective image quality of DLM reconstructions compared to native images (CNR levels; $p < 0.001$). However, the results of subjective image analysis showed no significant differences in image quality between the reconstruction types ($p = 0.055$). Moreover, the assessment of degenerative TMJ lesions was not affected by the type of reconstructions assessed ($p > 0.05$). We concluded that the analyzed DLM reconstruction notably enhanced the objective image quality in TMJ CBCT images, but did not significantly affect the subjective image quality or DJD lesion diagnosis. Our studies provide new insights into the efficacy of the selected DLM in this specific context, separate from its general approval and usage. Therefore, we caution against the generalization of our results beyond this specific context. However, our findings indicate that the use of AI denoising algorithms designed for CT imaging may improve the objective image quality parameters of CBCT images. Further studies, including a larger number of examinations performed using various devices and different diagnostic protocols, could demonstrate greater differences in the results of qualitative and quantitative image assessments. It is likely that the results would be similar to those published on qualitative analyses of studies performed using low-dose protocols in standard CT examinations [22,31,35–39]. Compared with standard and iterative reconstructions (IRs), deep learning reconstructions have already proven to have the potential for radiation dose reductions between 30% and 71% while maintaining diagnostic image quality owing to improved noise reduction [40]. Nevertheless, the trend toward improved image quality with the use of DLM algorithms in CBCT is promising.

Recent studies [41–43] have assessed the effectiveness of generative AI in reducing noise and metal artifacts in dental CT images. Hegazy et al. (2020) [41] evaluated the image quality of low-dose dental CT images reconstructed with a generative adversarial network using the Wasserstein loss function (WGAN). The authors achieved both quantitative and qualitative improvements in image quality; however, interestingly, they encountered the problem of over-smoothing small image details. In a 2021 study [43], Hegazy et al. evaluated the impact of variations in the WGAN and U-WGAN on the image quality of half-scan dental CTs. Both the noise levels and qualitative image parameters were significantly improved in the AI-reconstructed images. Another notable study by Hu et al. [42] proposed a WGAN to decrease the level of noise and metal artifacts in low-dose dental CT images. The results of the study showed that the proposed WGAN algorithm effectively removed artifacts and noise from low-dose dental CT images and outperformed other methods, such as general GANs and convolutional neural networks, in terms of image quality and artifact correction.

The literature concerning noise optimization in dental CBCT examinations, as opposed to conventional CT, is limited. In a recent study by Ramage (2023) [18], the authors assessed the effect of standard filtered back projection (FBP) and iterative reconstruction (IR) on CBCT image noise. They found that compared with FBP, IR significantly reduced image noise (99.84 $\pm$ 16.28 and 198.65 $\pm$ 55.58, respectively). The authors concluded that the additional processing time for IR reconstruction was clinically acceptable. A study by Choi et al. [44] investigated the efficacy of a novel, self-supervised convolutional neural network in projection noise reduction. The phantom study revealed that the peak signal-to-noise ratio (PSNR) and structural similarity index measure (SSIM) significantly improved compared to those of uncorrected images—27.08 and 0.839 vs. 15.68 and 0.103, respectively. A similar phantom study by Han and Yu evaluated the efficacy of a novel self-supervising denoising method based on Bernoulli sampling [45]. The results showed that the proposed method outperforms conventional denoising methods by at least 4.47 dB in PSNR. Brendlin et al. [46] investigated the efficacy of deep-learning denoising (DLD) techniques in mitigating the trade-offs related to the radiation dose and noise of CBCT during interventional procedures. The results showed that the application of DLD enabled significant radiation dose reduction combined with enhanced objective image quality parameters (higher CNR and lower noise). Two studies evaluated the effectiveness of DLD techniques in maxillofacial CBCT [33,47]. Kim et al. confirmed that the use of DLD techniques improved the diagnostic accuracy of readers in diagnosing sinus fungal balls and chronic rhinosinusitis [47]. Ylisiura et al. [33] compared iterative and DLD techniques for effective noise reduction in dentomaxillofacial applications. Their study demonstrated that the proposed method enabled image enhancement comparable to that of the iterative method, but with faster processing time. However, despite promising results, the readers preferred iterative reconstruction over DLD images in hard tissue evaluation. However, none of these studies evaluated commercially available noise reduction methods, and the evaluated techniques were available only to narrow groups of scientists. Therefore, the possibility of comparing different DLD techniques is an exciting topic for further research.

The findings of this study suggest that the application of a DLM to dental CBCT images can improve the CNR without compromising diagnostic quality. These findings are supported by the objective measurements of the CNR, which showed a statistically significant improvement in the DLM-reconstructed images compared with the native reconstructions. It is important to note that while confidence intervals provide an estimate of the range within which the true parameter lies, they do not preclude the possibility of statistically significant differences between groups. Our findings of significant differences in CNR, despite overlapping confidence intervals, underscore the importance of hypothesis testing in statistical analysis. Compared to commercial software such as TrueFidelity™ by GE Healthcare and AiCE by Canon Medical Systems, our vendor-agnostic DLM offers several advantages. Unlike vendor-specific solutions, the vendor-agnostic DLM can be applied to scans from various manufacturers, enhancing its versatility in clinical settings. Although some studies have revealed that while the noise reduction capabilities of our DLM are comparable to those of commercial software, it excels in maintaining image quality across different imaging systems [48]. This flexibility could streamline workflows and reduce the costs associated with acquiring multiple software licenses.

However, this study has several limitations. The sample size, although adequate for a pilot study, was relatively small. Larger studies with more diverse patient populations are needed to generalize these findings. Moreover, the subjective nature of image quality assessment, even for experienced readers, can be influenced by individual biases. Although the study used predefined scales and illustrations to aid in the assessments, these evaluations are inherently subjective and should be interpreted with caution. Notably, this study focused on a specific DLM algorithm and CBCT scanner. Further research is required to evaluate the generalizability of these findings to other DLM algorithms and CBCT scanners. Additionally, we evaluated images acquired only with a "regular quality" preset; therefore, our findings cannot be extrapolated to other protocols, especially low-dose protocols.

5. Conclusions

Overall, the results of this study support the potential of DLMs to objectively improve CBCT image quality by increasing CNR and reducing image noise. However, some issues with the delineation of small bony structures were noted, although no statistically significant differences in subjective image quality ratings were found. Our results could have significant implications for patient care by reducing the radiation dose required for diagnostic-quality images and potentially improving the diagnostic accuracy of dentomaxillofacial pathology. Further research is warranted to fully understand the clinical impact of DLMs on CBCT and to explore their integration into standard practice.

Author Contributions: Conceptualization, W.K. and R.W.; methodology, W.K. and R.W.; software, W.K. and N.K.; validation, W.K., Z.S. and J.J.-O.; formal analysis, W.K. and R.W.; investigation, W.K., R.W., A.W., O.K. and M.D.-K.; resources, W.K.; data curation, W.K. and R.W.; writing—original draft preparation, W.K. and R.W.; writing—review and editing, W.K., R.W., O.K. and N.K.; visualization, W.K. and R.W.; supervision, W.K.; project administration, W.K. and R.W.; funding acquisition, Z.S. and W.K. All authors have read and agreed to the published version of the manuscript.

Funding: This research received no external funding.

Institutional Review Board Statement: This study was conducted in accordance with the Declaration of Helsinki and approved by the Ethics Committee of Collegium Medicum, Nicolaus Copernicus University in Torun, Poland (protocol no. KB 227/2023, 10.04.20223), for studies involving humans.

Informed Consent Statement: Patient consent was waived due to the retrospective nature of the study and the anonymization of patient data.

Data Availability Statement: Data are available upon request.

Conflicts of Interest: The authors declare no conflicts of interest.

References

1. Kaasalainen, T.; Ekholm, M.; Siiskonen, T.; Kortesniemi, M. Dental Cone Beam CT: An Updated Review. *Phys. Medica* **2021**, *88*, 193–217. [CrossRef] [PubMed]
2. Fokas, G.; Vaughn, V.M.; Scarfe, W.C.; Bornstein, M.M. Accuracy of Linear Measurements on CBCT Images Related to Presurgical Implant Treatment Planning: A Systematic Review. *Clin. Oral Implant. Res.* **2018**, *29*, 393–415. [CrossRef] [PubMed]
3. Wikner, J.; Hanken, H.; Eulenburg, C.; Heiland, M.; Gröbe, A.; Assaf, A.T.; Riecke, B.; Friedrich, R.E. Linear Accuracy and Reliability of Volume Data Sets Acquired by Two CBCT-Devices and an MSCT Using Virtual Models: A Comparative In-Vitro Study. *Acta Odontol. Scand.* **2016**, *74*, 51–59. [CrossRef] [PubMed]
4. Gaêta-Araujo, H.; Leite, A.F.; de Faria Vasconcelos, K.; Jacobs, R. Two Decades of Research on CBCT Imaging in DMFR—An Appraisal of Scientific Evidence. *Dentomaxillofac. Radiol.* **2021**, *50*, 20200367. [CrossRef]
5. Abesi, F.; Jamali, A.S.; Zamani, M. Accuracy of Artificial Intelligence in the Detection and Segmentation of Oral and Maxillofacial Structures Using Cone-Beam Computed Tomography Images: A Systematic Review and Meta-Analysis. *Pol. J. Radiol.* **2023**, *88*, 256–263. [CrossRef]
6. Oenning, A.C.; Jacobs, R.; Pauwels, R.; Stratis, A.; Hedesiu, M.; Salmon, B. Cone-Beam CT in Paediatric Dentistry: DIMITRA Project Position Statement. *Pediatr. Radiol.* **2018**, *48*, 308–316. [CrossRef]
7. Widmann, G.; Bischel, A.; Stratis, A.; Bosmans, H.; Jacobs, R.; Gassner, E.-M.; Puelacher, W.; Pauwels, R. Spatial and Contrast Resolution of Ultralow Dose Dentomaxillofacial CT Imaging Using Iterative Reconstruction Technology. *Dentomaxillofac. Radiol.* **2017**, *46*, 20160452. [CrossRef]
8. Schulze, R.; Heil, U.; Groß, D.; Bruellmann, D.D.; Dranischnikow, E.; Schwanecke, U.; Schoemer, E. Artefacts in CBCT: A Review. *Dentomaxillofac. Radiol.* **2011**, *40*, 265–773. [CrossRef]
9. Bechara, B.; McMahan, C.A.; Moore, W.S.; Noujeim, M.; Geha, H.; Teixeira, F.B. Contrast-to-Noise Ratio Difference in Small Field of View Cone Beam Computed Tomography Machines. *J. Oral Sci.* **2012**, *54*, 227–232. [CrossRef]
10. Nagarajappa, A.; Dwivedi, N.; Tiwari, R. Artifacts: The Downturn of CBCT Image. *J. Int. Soc. Prev. Community Dent.* **2015**, *5*, 440–445. [CrossRef]
11. Kocasarac, H.D.; Yigit, D.H.; Bechara, B.; Sinanoglu, A.; Noujeim, M. Contrast-to-Noise Ratio with Different Settings in a CBCT Machine in Presence of Different Root-End Filling Materials: An In Vitro Study. *Dentomaxillofac. Radiol.* **2016**, *45*, 20160012. [CrossRef] [PubMed]
12. Geyer, L.L.; Schoepf, U.J.; Meinel, F.G.; Nance, J.W., Jr.; Bastarrika, G.; Leipsic, J.A.; Paul, N.S.; Rengo, M.; Laghi, A.; De Cecco, C.N. State of the Art: Iterative CT Reconstruction Techniques. *Radiology* **2015**, *276*, 339–357. [CrossRef] [PubMed]
13. Van Gompel, G.; Van Slambrouck, K.; Defrise, M.; Batenburg, K.J.; de Mey, J.; Sijbers, J.; Nuyts, J.; Schafer, A.L.; Kazakia, G.J.; Vittinghoff, E.; et al. Iterative Correction of Beam Hardening Artifacts in CT. *Med. Phys.* **2011**, *38*, S36–S49. [CrossRef] [PubMed]
14. Schmidt, A.M.A.; Grunz, J.-P.; Petritsch, B.; Gruschwitz, P.; Knarr, J.; Huflage, H.; Bley, T.A.; Kosmala, A. Combination of Iterative Metal Artifact Reduction and Virtual Monoenergetic Reconstruction Using Split-Filter Dual-Energy CT in Patients with Dental Artifact on Head and Neck CT. *Am. J. Roentgenol.* **2022**, *218*, 716–727. [CrossRef]
15. Gardner, S.J.; Mao, W.; Liu, C.; Aref, I.; Elshaikh, M.; Lee, J.K.; Pradhan, D.; Movsas, B.; Chetty, I.J.; Siddiqui, F. Improvements in CBCT Image Quality Using a Novel Iterative Reconstruction Algorithm: A Clinical Evaluation. *Adv. Radiat. Oncol.* **2019**, *4*, 390–400. [CrossRef]
16. Chen, B.; Xiang, K.; Gong, Z.; Wang, J.; Tan, S. Statistical Iterative CBCT Reconstruction Based on Neural Network. *IEEE Trans. Med. Imaging* **2018**, *37*, 1511–1521. [CrossRef]
17. Washio, H.; Ohira, S.; Funama, Y.; Morimoto, M.; Wada, K.; Yagi, M.; Shimamoto, H.; Koike, Y.; Ueda, Y.; Karino, T.; et al. Metal Artifact Reduction Using Iterative CBCT Reconstruction Algorithm for Head and Neck Radiation Therapy: A Phantom and Clinical Study. *Eur. J. Radiol.* **2020**, *132*, 109293. [CrossRef]
18. Ramage, A.; Lopez Gutierrez, B.; Fischer, K.; Sekula, M.; Santaella, G.M.; Scarfe, W.; Brasil, D.M.; de Oliveira-Santos, C. Filtered Back Projection vs. Iterative Reconstruction for CBCT: Effects on Image Noise and Processing Time. *Dentomaxillofac. Radiol.* **2023**, *52*, 20230109. [CrossRef]
19. Kim, J.H.; Yoon, H.J.; Lee, E.; Kim, I.; Cha, Y.K.; Bak, S.H. Validation of Deep-Learning Image Reconstruction for Low-Dose Chest Computed Tomography Scan: Emphasis on Image Quality and Noise. *Korean J. Radiol.* **2021**, *22*, 131–138. [CrossRef]
20. Tatsugami, F.; Higaki, T.; Nakamura, Y.; Yu, Z.; Zhou, J.; Lu, Y.; Fujioka, C.; Kitagawa, T.; Kihara, Y.; Iida, M.; et al. Deep Learning–Based Image Restoration Algorithm for Coronary CT Angiography. *Eur. Radiol.* **2019**, *29*, 5322–5329. [CrossRef]
21. Greffier, J.; Hamard, A.; Pereira, F.; Barrau, C.; Pasquier, H.; Beregi, J.P.; Frandon, J. Image Quality and Dose Reduction Opportunity of Deep Learning Image Reconstruction Algorithm for CT: A Phantom Study. *Eur. Radiol.* **2020**, *30*, 3951–3959. [CrossRef] [PubMed]
22. Nam, J.G.; Ahn, C.; Choi, H.; Hong, W.; Park, J.; Kim, J.H.; Goo, J.M. Image Quality of Ultralow-Dose Chest CT Using Deep Learning Techniques: Potential Superiority of Vendor-Agnostic Post-Processing over Vendor-Specific Techniques. *Eur Radiol* **2021**, *31*. [CrossRef] [PubMed]

23. Lim, W.H.; Choi, Y.H.; Park, J.E.; Cho, Y.J.; Lee, S.; Cheon, J.-E.; Kim, W.S.; Kim, I.-O.; Kim, J.H. Application of Vendor-Neutral Iterative Reconstruction Technique to Pediatric Abdominal Computed Tomography. *Korean J. Radiol.* **2019**, *20*, 1358–1367. [CrossRef] [PubMed]
24. Choi, H.; Chang, W.; Kim, J.H.; Ahn, C.; Lee, H.; Kim, H.Y.; Cho, J.; Lee, Y.J.; Kim, Y.H. Dose Reduction Potential of Vendor-Agnostic Deep Learning Model in Comparison with Deep Learning–Based Image Reconstruction Algorithm on CT: A Phantom Study. *Eur. Radiol.* **2022**, *32*, 1247–1255. [CrossRef]
25. Hong, J.H.; Park, E.-A.; Lee, W.; Ahn, C.; Kim, J.-H. Incremental Image Noise Reduction in Coronary CT Angiography Using a Deep Learning-Based Technique with Iterative Reconstruction. *Korean J. Radiol.* **2020**, *21*, 1165–1177. [CrossRef]
26. Shin, Y.J.; Chang, W.; Ye, J.C.; Kang, E.; Oh, D.Y.; Lee, Y.J.; Park, J.H.; Kim, Y.H. Low-Dose Abdominal CT Using a Deep Learning-Based Denoising Algorithm: A Comparison with CT Reconstructed with Filtered Back Projection or Iterative Reconstruction Algorithm. *Korean J. Radiol.* **2020**, *21*, 356–364. [CrossRef]
27. Koivisto, J.; van Eijnatten, M.; Ärnstedt, J.J.; Holli-Helenius, K.; Dastidar, P.; Wolff, J. Impact of Prone, Supine and Oblique Patient Positioning on CBCT Image Quality, Contrast-to-Noise Ratio and Figure of Merit Value in the Maxillofacial Region. *Dentomaxillofac. Radiol.* **2017**, *46*, 20160418. [CrossRef]
28. Zou, G.Y. Sample Size Formulas for Estimating Intraclass Correlation Coefficients with Precision and Assurance. *Stat. Med.* **2012**, *31*, 3972–3981. [CrossRef] [PubMed]
29. R Core Team. *R: A Language and Environment for Statistical Computing*; R Core Team: Vienna, Austria, 2021.
30. Martins, J.N.R.; Versiani, M.A. CBCT and Micro-CT on the Study of Root Canal Anatomy. In *The Root Canal Anatomy in Permanent Dentition*; Springer: Berlin/Heidelberg, Germany, 2018.
31. Brady, S.L.; Trout, A.T.; Somasundaram, E.; Anton, C.G.; Li, Y.; Dillman, J.R. Improving Image Quality and Reducing Radiation Dose for Pediatric CT by Using Deep Learning Reconstruction. *Radiology* **2021**, *298*, 180–188. [CrossRef]
32. AlJehani, Y.A. Diagnostic Applications of Cone-Beam CT for Periodontal Diseases. *Int. J. Dent.* **2014**, *2014*, 865079. [CrossRef]
33. Ylisiurua, S.; Sipola, A.; Nieminen, M.T.; Brix, M.A.K. Deep Learning Enables Time-Efficient Soft Tissue Enhancement in CBCT: Proof-of-Concept Study for Dentomaxillofacial Applications. *Phys. Medica* **2024**, *117*, 103184. [CrossRef] [PubMed]
34. Kazimierczak, W.; Kędziora, K.; Janiszewska-Olszowska, J.; Kazimierczak, N.; Serafin, Z. Noise-Optimized CBCT Imaging of Temporomandibular Joints—The Impact of AI on Image Quality. *J. Clin. Med.* **2024**, *13*, 1502. [CrossRef] [PubMed]
35. Nam, J.G.; Hong, J.H.; Kim, D.S.; Oh, J.; Goo, J.M. Deep Learning Reconstruction for Contrast-Enhanced CT of the Upper Abdomen: Similar Image Quality with Lower Radiation Dose in Direct Comparison with Iterative Reconstruction. *Eur. Radiol.* **2021**, *31*, 5533–5543. [CrossRef] [PubMed]
36. Cheng, Y.; Han, Y.; Li, J.; Fan, G.; Cao, L.; Li, J.; Jia, X.; Yang, J.; Guo, J. Low-Dose CT Urography Using Deep Learning Image Reconstruction: A Prospective Study for Comparison with Conventional CT Urography. *Br. J. Radiol.* **2021**, *94*, 20201291. [CrossRef]
37. Benz, D.C.; Ersözlü, S.; Mojon, F.L.A.; Messerli, M.; Mitulla, A.K.; Ciancone, D.; Kenkel, D.; Schaab, J.A.; Gebhard, C.; Pazhenkottil, A.P.; et al. Radiation Dose Reduction with Deep-Learning Image Reconstruction for Coronary Computed Tomography Angiography. *Eur. Radiol.* **2022**, *32*, 2620–2628. [CrossRef]
38. Racine, D.; Brat, H.G.; Dufour, B.; Steity, J.M.; Hussenot, M.; Rizk, B.; Fournier, D.; Zanca, F. Image Texture, Low Contrast Liver Lesion Detectability and Impact on Dose: Deep Learning Algorithm Compared to Partial Model-Based Iterative Reconstruction. *Eur. J. Radiol.* **2021**, *141*, 109808. [CrossRef]
39. Hata, A.; Yanagawa, M.; Yoshida, Y.; Miyata, T.; Tsubamoto, M.; Honda, O.; Tomiyama, N. Combination of Deep Learning-Based Denoising and Iterative Reconstruction for Ultra-Low-Dose CT of the Chest: Image Quality and Lung-RADS Evaluation. *Am. J. Roentgenol.* **2020**, *215*, 1321–1328. [CrossRef]
40. Koetzier, L.R.; Mastrodicasa, D.; Szczykutowicz, T.P.; van der Werf, N.R.; Wang, A.S.; Sandfort, V.; van der Molen, A.J.; Fleischmann, D.; Willemink, M.J. Deep Learning Image Reconstruction for CT: Technical Principles and Clinical Prospects. *Radiology* **2023**, *306*, e221257. [CrossRef]
41. Hegazy, M.A.A.; Cho, M.H.; Lee, S.Y. Image Denoising by Transfer Learning of Generative Adversarial Network for Dental CT. *Biomed. Phys. Eng. Express* **2020**, *6*, 055024. [CrossRef]
42. Hu, Z.; Jiang, C.; Sun, F.; Zhang, Q.; Ge, Y.; Yang, Y.; Liu, X.; Zheng, H.; Liang, D. Artifact Correction in Low-Dose Dental CT Imaging Using Wasserstein Generative Adversarial Networks. *Med. Phys.* **2019**, *46*, 1686–1696. [CrossRef]
43. Hegazy, M.A.A.; Cho, M.H.; Lee, S.Y. Half-Scan Artifact Correction Using Generative Adversarial Network for Dental CT. *Comput. Biol. Med.* **2021**, *132*, 104313. [CrossRef] [PubMed]
44. Choi, K.; Kim, S.H.; Kim, S. Self-Supervised Denoising of Projection Data for Low-Dose Cone-Beam CT. *Med. Phys.* **2023**, *50*, 6319–6333. [CrossRef] [PubMed]
45. Han, Y.-J.; Yu, H.-J. Self-Supervised Noise Reduction in Low-Dose Cone Beam Computed Tomography (CBCT) Using the Randomly Dropped Projection Strategy. *Appl. Sci.* **2022**, *12*, 1714. [CrossRef]
46. Brendlin, A.S.; Dehdab, R.; Stenzl, B.; Mueck, J.; Ghibes, P.; Groezinger, G.; Kim, J.; Afat, S.; Artzner, C. Novel Deep Learning Denoising Enhances Image Quality and Lowers Radiation Exposure in Interventional Bronchial Artery Embolization Cone Beam CT. *Acad. Radiol.* **2024**, *31*, 2144–2155. [CrossRef]

47. Kim, K.; Lim, C.Y.; Shin, J.; Chung, M.J.; Jung, Y.G. Enhanced Artificial Intelligence-Based Diagnosis Using CBCT with Internal Denoising: Clinical Validation for Discrimination of Fungal Ball, Sinusitis, and Normal Cases in the Maxillary Sinus. *Comput. Methods Programs Biomed.* **2023**, *240*, 107708. [CrossRef]
48. Kim, C.; Kwack, T.; Kim, W.; Cha, J.; Yang, Z.; Yong, H.S. Accuracy of Two Deep Learning–Based Reconstruction Methods Compared with an Adaptive Statistical Iterative Reconstruction Method for Solid and Ground-Glass Nodule Volumetry on Low-Dose and Ultra–Low-Dose Chest Computed Tomography: A Phantom Study. *PLoS ONE* **2022**, *17*, e0270122. [CrossRef]

Disclaimer/Publisher's Note: The statements, opinions and data contained in all publications are solely those of the individual author(s) and contributor(s) and not of MDPI and/or the editor(s). MDPI and/or the editor(s) disclaim responsibility for any injury to people or property resulting from any ideas, methods, instructions or products referred to in the content.

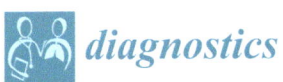

Article

Evaluation of a Decision Support System Developed with Deep Learning Approach for Detecting Dental Caries with Cone-Beam Computed Tomography Imaging

Hakan Amasya [1,2,3], Mustafa Alkhader [4], Gözde Serindere [5], Karolina Futyma-Gąbka [6], Ceren Aktuna Belgin [5], Maxim Gusarev [7], Matvey Ezhov [7], Ingrid Różyło-Kalinowska [6], Merve Önder [8], Alex Sanders [7], Andre Luiz Ferreira Costa [9], Sérgio Lúcio Pereira de Castro Lopes [10] and Kaan Orhan [8,11,12,*]

[1] Department of Oral and Maxillofacial Radiology, Faculty of Dentistry, Istanbul University-Cerrahpaşa, Istanbul 34320, Türkiye; h-amasya@hotmail.com or hakanamasya@iuc.edu.tr
[2] CAST (Cerrahpasa Research, Simulation and Design Laboratory), Istanbul University-Cerrahpaşa, Istanbul 34320, Türkiye
[3] Health Biotechnology Joint Research and Application Center of Excellence, Istanbul 34220, Türkiye
[4] Department of Oral Medicine and Oral Surgery, Faculty of Dentistry, Jordan University of Science and Technology, Irbid 22110, Jordan; mmalkhader@just.edu.jo
[5] Department of Oral and Maxillofacial Radiology, Faculty of Dentistry, Mustafa Kemal University, Hatay 31060, Türkiye; dt.gozde@hotmail.com (G.S.); dtcaktuna@gmail.com (C.A.B.)
[6] Department of Dental and Maxillofacial Radiodiagnostics, Medical University of Lublin, 20-093 Lublin, Poland; lek.dent.karolina.futyma@gmail.com (K.F.-G.); ingrozyl@wp.pl or rozylo.kalinowska@umlub.pl (I.R.-K.)
[7] Diagnocat, Inc., San Francisco, CA 94102, USA; m.gusarev@diagnocat.com (M.G.); matvey@diagnocat.com (M.E.); alex@diagnocat.com (A.S.)
[8] Department of Oral and Maxillofacial Radiology, Faculty of Dentistry, Ankara University, Ankara 0600, Türkiye; merveonder_16@hotmail.com
[9] Postgraduate Program in Dentistry, Cruzeiro do Sul University (UNICSUL), São Paulo 08060-070, SP, Brazil; alfcosta@gmail.com
[10] Science and Technology Institute, Department of Diagnosis and Surgery, São Paulo State University (UNESP), São José dos Campos 01049-010, SP, Brazil; sergio.lopes@unesp.br
[11] Research Center (MEDITAM), Ankara University Medical Design Application, Ankara 06560, Türkiye
[12] Department of Oral Diagnostics, Faculty of Dentistry, Semmelweis University, 1088 Budapest, Hungary
* Correspondence: knorhan@dentistry.ankara.edu.tr or call53@yahoo.com

Abstract: This study aims to investigate the effect of using an artificial intelligence (AI) system (Diagnocat, Inc., San Francisco, CA, USA) for caries detection by comparing cone-beam computed tomography (CBCT) evaluation results with and without the software. 500 CBCT volumes are scored by three dentomaxillofacial radiologists for the presence of caries separately on a five-point confidence scale without and with the aid of the AI system. After visual evaluation, the deep convolutional neural network (CNN) model generated a radiological report and observers scored again using AI interface. The ground truth was determined by a hybrid approach. Intra- and inter-observer agreements are evaluated with sensitivity, specificity, accuracy, and kappa statistics. A total of 6008 surfaces are determined as 'presence of caries' and 13,928 surfaces are determined as 'absence of caries' for ground truth. The area under the ROC curve of observer 1, 2, and 3 are found to be 0.855/0.920, 0.863/0.917, and 0.747/0.903, respectively (unaided/aided). Fleiss Kappa coefficients are changed from 0.325 to 0.468, and the best accuracy (0.939) is achieved with the aided results. The radiographic evaluations performed with aid of the AI system are found to be more compatible and accurate than unaided evaluations in the detection of dental caries with CBCT images.

Keywords: dental caries; cone-beam computed tomography; machine learning; decision support systems

1. Introduction

Dental caries is a multifactorial chronic disease that causes mineral loss in tooth hard tissues. The disease, which has evidence in fossil samples, has a high prevalence today [1–3]. Symptoms such as pain, swelling, and abscess may be seen depending on the stage of the disease [4–8]. Caries diagnosis is a clinical decision regarding the presence of caries, while the detection of caries is a result of the clinical and radiographic evaluation of caries signs. Dental probes used for tactile feedback during visual inspection may damage weakened tooth tissues. Although bitewing radiographs are successful in showing the posterior approximal surfaces, they require attention to the rules of projection geometry in the production of images [1,7–9]. Cone-beam computed tomography (CBCT) is a volumetric imaging tool which require less patient dose than the medical CTs but more when compared to other plain imaging methods in dentistry. The SEDENTEXCT Panel in 2011 concluded that evaluating dental caries is not an indication for CBCT. However, dental caries findings in volumetric data taken for other reasons should be evaluated [10–12].

Digital radiology provides number-based images, paving the way for the development of a clinical decision support system (CDSS) to be integrated into clinical workflows [13–16]. Moreover, such systems can be developed using artificial intelligence (AI) techniques on subjects such as acute care management, drug ordering, clinical oncology, and many more [17–23]. AI tools can be developed using a machine learning approach, mainly based on supervised learning, unsupervised learning, semi-supervised learning, and reinforced learning. In supervised learning, data are labeled by experts, while in unsupervised learning, features are extracted by algorithms. In semi-supervised learning, a combination of these two approaches is applied, while in reinforcement learning, the model is developed by giving reward or punishment according to its outputs [24–26]. Deep learning, generally combined with the transfer learning approach, is a popular technique used in the automation of tasks such as lesion detection, segmentation, and classification in radiographic data [27–29].

The potential of using CBCT volumes for caries detection has been evaluated in several studies [11,30–32]. Some researchers proposed AI models for the detection of dental caries with different imaging modalities such as periapical, panoramic, or bitewings [33–35]. Lee et al. developed a convolutional neural network (CNN) for dental caries detection and diagnosis using periapical images. A total of 3000 periapical radiographs were labeled as dental caries and non-caries based on medical records and expert evaluation (equal in numbers), then the images were cropped to show one tooth per image and resized to 299×299 pixels. The dataset was split into training and testing subsets with the ratio of 4:1, randomly, and the training dataset was augmented 10 times using rotation, width and height shifting, zooming, shearing, and horizontal flipping. The model was based on a pre-trained GoogLeNet Inception v3 CNN network and trained using transfer learning. The model had 9 inception modules, including an auxiliary classifier, two fully connected layers, and softmax functions. The data were given in batches of 32, and 1000 epochs were run at a learning rate of 0.01; the model was fine-tuned by optimizing the weights. The diagnostic performance of the developed model was reported between 82.0–89.0% according to anatomical regions, while AUC values varied between 845 (95% CI 0.790–0.901) and 0.917 (95% CI 0.860–0.975) [33]. Bui et al. proposed a computer-aided diagnosis (CAD) system to detect dental caries in panoramic radiographs. The dataset consisted of a total of 533 single-tooth images (229 caries and 304 non-caries) which was manually segmented from panoramic radiographs. The system was based on two modules: feature extraction and classification. In the first module, the pre-trained CNN models such as Alexnet, Googlenet, VGG16, VGG19, Resnet18, Resnet50, Resnet101, and Xception were used to extract the deep activated features. The extracted features were optimized using mathematical descriptors, such as mean and STD, and texture features such as Haralick's features; the results of the deep networks and geometric features were optimized mainly based on a Support Vector Machine (SVM) model, prior to being fed into the second module. The fusion features were tested using SVM, Naïve Bayes, k-nearest neighbor, decision tree, and random forest classifier models, and the authors reported that the proposed method achieved 91.70%,

90.43%, and 92.67% accuracy, sensitivity, and specificity, respectively [34]. Devito et al. proposed an artificial multilayer perceptron neural network for the diagnosis of proximal dental caries using bitewing radiographs. The tooth surfaces were divided as sound and dental caries (non-cavitated) by visual evaluation, and a total of 40 pre-molar and 40 molar-extracted teeth were embedded in silicone models to develop 20 tooth models, including canines for proximal contact. The neural network was based on a one-hidden layer perceptron model with a back-propagation algorithm and had 25 neurons in the input and the hidden layer, and 1 in the output layer. Samples were divided into training, testing and cross-validation subsets with the ratio of 2:1:1, and the initial weights of each "synapse" was determined using the Nguyen–Windrow algorithm. A total number of 160 tooth surfaces were scored by 25 examiners (from 1 to 5), each with over 20 years' experience, and each result was given as inputs. The training was optimized by analyzing the reduction in the mean square error. The golden standard was obtained by histopathological evaluation of the samples after the radiographic acquisition. The area under the ROC curve was reported to be 0.884, and the developed model performed 23.3% better than the best examiner and 39.4% better than the mean human performance [35]. Cantu et at. developed a fully CNN model based on U-Net architecture to detect caries lesions with varying radiographic stages on bitewing radiographs. A total of 3686 bitewings were labeled by three expert dentists in a pixel-wise fashion, and a fourth expert dentist reviewed and revised the process. Each annotation was further classified into four categories by two independent dentists according to the radiographic stage. All images were resized to 512 × 416 pixels, and the data were divided into a training (3293), validation (252), and test dataset (141). Researchers initialized the current model's weights using the data obtained in a previously developed model for caries segmentation on panoramic radiographs (unpublished) and then applied data augmentation techniques based on geometric level (image flipping, center cropping, xy-translation, and rotations) and pixel level (gaussian-blur, sharpening, contrast, and brightness) random transformation techniques to improve the generalization of the previous model. Several models were trained with different training strategies, loss functions, and combinations of the parameters to improve the performance. First, they started with 10 epochs with a constant encoder weight and a learning rate value of $5e^{-3}$. Then, the training was further improved for 190 epochs by allowing the optimization of weights in all layers, with a batch size of two and an initial learning rate of $5e^{-4}$. The results of each epoch were saved and improvements in the mean Intersection-over-Union (IoU) were analyzed. After adjusting the optimal weights, the outputs were converted into binary results by determining a cutoff threshold using Adam optimizer. Further, the system's results were compared with a cohort of seven dentists with 3–14 years of experience. The authors reported a higher accuracy (0.80) in results of the model when compared to the dentists (0.71) and significantly more sensitivity when compared to the dentists (0.75 versus 0.36). The specificity of the model (0.83) was found to be lower than the dentists (0.91); however, the results were not significant [36].

This study aims to investigate the effect of using a CDSS (Diagnocat, Inc., San Francisco, CA, USA) with caries detection function to enhance CBCT evaluations in terms of detecting dental caries by comparing the results of the observers with and without the aid of the software. For this purpose, volumetric data that met the criteria such as absence of gross artifacts and presence of sufficient teeth were collected among CBCT volumes obtained for other clinical reasons; this study does not support the justification of the use of CBCT only for caries diagnosis. According to the literature review conducted on Pubmed and Google Scholar using the keywords of "caries" or "dental caries" and "cbct" or "cone beam computed tomography" or "cone-beam computed tomography" and "artificial intelligence" or "AI" or "machine learning" or "ML", no other study was found on this subject other than the Diagnocat system. Hence, this study contributes to the literature in terms of evaluating the performance of an AI model developed for the evaluation of secondary diagnoses using CBCT images obtained in real clinical conditions.

2. Materials and Methods

Using retrospective data from our faculty, a power analysis (Power and Precision software, Biostat, Englewood, NJ, USA) was conducted which indicated that detection of differences between the observers with and without the aid of the software could be obtained with 432 CBCT volumes and at least 1098 caries at a power of 0.8 (alpha = 0.05). Thus, this study conducted 500 CBCT volumes retrospectively and all caries lesions were included in the CBCT volumes of the patients between 18 and 64 years of age selected from a Jordan Technological University Hospital's database.

Patients with fixed prosthetics, implants, caries lesions, missing, or restored teeth were included, while edentulous patients and volumes with exceeding artifacts were excluded. This study was approved by the Institutional Research Board of Jordan Institute of Technology with the protocol number of 792-2019. Informed consent was obtained from all individual participants included in the study. CBCT volumes of the patients were acquired by CS 8100 3D (Carestream Health, NY, USA) CBCT machine in a standing position during imaging. The scanner offers multiple fields of view (FOVs), allowing the dentist to select the optimum scan on a case-by-case basis. Digital radiographs were acquired with the imaging parameters of 80 kVp, 6 mA (6300 µA), 15 s of imaging time, and 8 × 9 FOV (0.150 mm^3 voxel size) with isotropic voxels. All cases were selected from the database to be examined by the decision of a dentomaxillofacial radiology consultant with more than 10 years of experience. The radiographic data were anonymized (except gender and age) and CBCT volumes were exported in DICOM format. The dataset was split into encrypted compressed files and distributed to independent observers for radiographic evaluation using the cloud service.

Three observers in dentomaxillofacial radiology evaluated CBCT volumes for dental caries signs, without and with the Diagnocat system. An online conference was conducted prior to evaluations for the calibration of the observers with different levels of experience. The results of aided and unaided evaluations were collected in a template document to ensure standardization among observers. The template with dedicated columns for 'tooth condition', 'mesial surface', and 'distal surface' for each tooth was prepared to collect the responses in an organized manner. Tooth conditions were saved as 'intact', 'missing', 'restored', 'support' and 'excluded'. Mesial and distal surfaces of the tooth were scored by independent observers separately for the presence of caries on a five-point confidence scale: (1) caries definitely absent, (2) caries probably absent, (3) unsure, (4) caries probably present, and (5) caries definitely present. Primarily, the dataset was imported to Sante DICOM Viewer Pro (Santesoft Ltd., Nicosia, Cyprus) by each observer independently (version 11.6.2 for Windows, 2.0.1 for macOS), and unaided evaluations were performed without any restriction and saved (Figure 1). After a month-long time interval, the dataset was uploaded to the Diagnocat system, and CBCT volumes were analyzed to generate a radiological report. Observers were granted access to the web-based system (Figure 2) to re-evaluate the samples with the aid of the Diagnocat system, and the results were saved using new duplicates of the template.

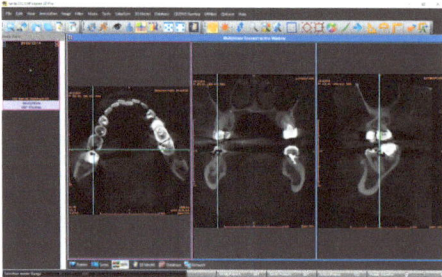

Figure 1. Interface for unaided evaluations in the multiplanar reconstruction view (Sante DICOM Viewer Pro for macOS). In multiplanar (MPR) reconstruction mode, the purple frame indicates the active

plane (axial in this case), while the blue frames represent other dimensions which follow the actions in the active plane. The green lines represent the intersection point in all three planes, which demonstrate an approximal dental caries in the distal surface of the tooth number 36. Thus, findings in the active frame are evaluated together with other axes.

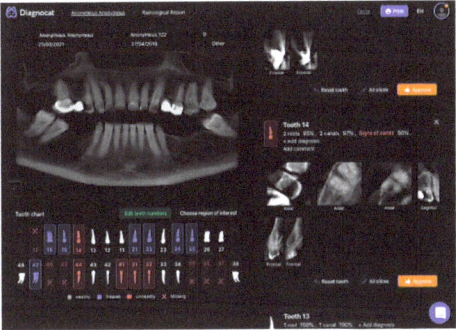

Figure 2. Interface for aided evaluation (Diagnocat). On the left side, at the top, the synthetic–panoramic image produced from the CBCT volume is provided for an overall view, while underneath, there is a dental chart that provides information about the condition of each tooth. The colors of white and purple represent a healthy and treated tooth, while the red means an unhealthy or missing tooth. On the right, the predictions of the system for the relevant tooth are provided by image slices in different axes.

2.1. Model Pipeline

The Diagnocat system generates a radiological report based on a pipeline of multiple pre-trained fully CNN and algorithmic slice extraction. A radiological report includes a panoramic reformat of a CBCT and a section with slices and evaluations for each tooth (Figure 3). Predictions crucial for signs of caries evaluation include only voxel-perfect segmentations of teeth, although segmentations of different anatomy elements are also used for other evaluations (e.g., orthodontic aid).

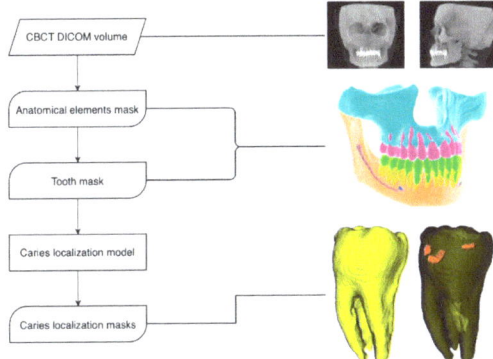

Figure 3. Diagnocat system model pipeline.

The tooth volume was cropped from a CBCT using a boundary box of a tooth segmentation mask extended by 3 mm from each side of the box. It was rescaled to have isotropic voxels and a 0.25 mm voxel size and resized to a fixed shape of $96 \times 64 \times 64$. The tooth volume was fed to a caries localization model, and the model prediction was rescaled to the original voxel size and resized to an initial tooth volume shape. During the first step of post-processing of the caries localization model, the predicted caries lesion mask was labeled by connected components, resulting in a set of separate predicted lesions situated inside the tooth. Lesions with a volume less than 0.3 cm^3 were ignored. The magnitude of volume threshold was derived from the training dataset lesion volume distribution. During the second step, predicted probability from the classification head of the model was rescaled in a way that a probability value of 0.5 corresponded to the maximum score based on sensitivity and specificity. The last step of post-processing the caries localization model was an intersection of a segmentation mask of the tooth of interest with a predicted caries lesion mask. This step was used to eliminate from final prediction caries lesion predictions situated inside neighboring teeth. The intersection was conducted with a morphological operation of binary dilation of a tooth segmentation mask and a multiplication of boolean masks of a tooth and caries lesions. The final prediction masks were used as visualizations of caries lesion locations via imposition of lesion masks on the tooth volume in axial, mesiodistal, and frontal views (Figure 4).

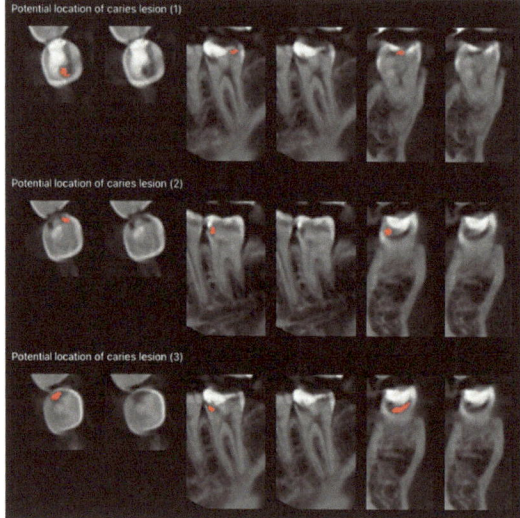

Figure 4. Extended slice section of aided evaluations (Diagnocat) showing separate predicted caries lesion masks (red) in axial, mesiodistal, and buccolingual views of tooth 37.

2.2. The Architecture of the Deep CNNs

The Diagnocat system exploits a set of pre-trained semantic segmentation networks based on internally modified fully convolutional 3D U-Net architecture from Isensee et al. [37] to obtain voxel-perfect segmentation masks of teeth, caries lesions, and anatomical elements. As well as the original U-Net, the modified architecture consists of a contraction path (the encoder) that encodes abstract representations of the input, followed by a symmetric expanding path (the decoder) that takes into consideration these features with high dimensional feature representations to precisely localize regions of interest. Blocks of the encoder were connected by $3 \times 3 \times 3$ convolutions with stride 2 to reduce the resolution of the feature maps. Nearest neighbor interpolation was used to up-sample the low-resolution feature maps. Blocks of the decoder consisted of $3 \times 3 \times 3$ convolution followed by $1 \times 1 \times 1$ convolution which halves the number of feature maps. Features at each up-sampling level were concatenated with the features from the corresponding level of the encoder. Additionally, in the localization pathway, we integrated segmentation layers at different levels of the network and combined them via element-wise summation to form the final network output.

Additive attention gates were used at each up-sampling level to highlight salient image regions and preserve only the activations relevant to the main task. In such a gate, a single scalar attention coefficient (in range from 0 to 1) was obtained for each pixel vector which corresponds to the number of feature maps at the current layer of the model. Finally, after the last step of the up-sampling pathway, the classification block was added to predict the probability of the input being pathological in conventional classification fashion.

Leaky ReLU non-linearities were used as an activation function throughout the architecture. Additionally, traditional batch normalization was replaced with instance normalization due to small batch sizes of 3D volumes.

All networks were not initialized with any pre-trained weights and were trained from scratch. The combination of Jaccard loss and cross-entropy loss was utilized for segmentation tasks. The anatomical elements were labeled separately, while all signs of caries were labeled as a single class and further assigned to specific teeth.

2.3. Statistical Analysis

The results of the observers on the five-point confidence scale were transformed into binary categories (score 1, 2, and 3 as 'absence of caries', score 4 and 5 as 'presence of caries'), and the ground truth was determined by calculating the consensus of the observers. After cleaning the data, in case three observers scored the same, the result was considered ground truth, and conflicting surfaces were identified in online sessions under the supervision of senior dentomaxillofacial radiologists.

After a two-month-long time interval, 50 randomly chosen samples were evaluated again to calculate the intra-observer agreement for both aided and unaided evaluations. Consistency between the aided and the unaided results of the observers were evaluated by kappa statistics (95% CI) for the assessment of intra- and inter-observer agreement. In addition, Fleiss kappa was used to demonstrate the agreement among all observers in their aided and unaided evaluations, regardless of the ground truth. Consistency between the binary results and the ground truth was analyzed with sensitivity, specificity, accuracy, and kappa statistics. Sensitivity, specificity, and accuracy values were calculated using Equation (1):

$$\text{Sensitivity} = TP/(TP + FN)$$
$$\text{Specificity} = TN/(TN + FP) \qquad (1)$$
$$\text{Accuracy} = (TP + TN)/(TP + FP + TN + FP)$$

(TP: True positive, FP: False positive, TN: True negative, FP: False positive)

Statistics were calculated using SPSS (Version 25). A p-value of less than 0.05 was determined as the threshold for statistical significance.

3. Results

The kappa and weighted kappa coefficients are interpreted as described by Viera et al. [38] in Table 1.

Table 1. Interpretation of Kappa statistics [38].

Kappa	Agreement
<0	Less than change agreement
0.01–0.20	Slight agreement
0.21–0.40	Fair agreement
0.41–0.60	Moderate agreement
0.61–0.80	Substantial agreement
0.81–0.99	Almost perfect agreement
1	Perfect agreement

Intra-observer agreements of each observer are demonstrated by kappa coefficients in Table 2. For Cohen's kappa coefficient values, Observer 3's repeatability for the five-point scale scoring increased from substantial agreement to almost perfect agreement with software support.

Table 2. Intra-observer agreement for unaided and aided evaluations.

	Cohen's Kappa				Weighted Kappa			
	Five-Point Scale		Binary Scale		Five-Point Scale		Binary Scale	
	Unaided	Aided	Unaided	Aided	Unaided	Aided	Unaided	Aided
Observer 1	0.820	0.903	0.926	0.939	0.938	0.958	0.926	0.939
Observer 2	0.903	0.923	0.932	0.945	0.962	0.968	0.932	0.945
Observer 3	0.735	0.911	0.865	0.939	0.849	0.937	0.865	0.939

Consistency between the observer's aided and unaided evaluations is shown in Table 3. For binary results, Cohen's kappa coefficients were found to be almost perfect agreement, substantial agreement, and moderate agreement for Observer 1, Observer 2, and Observer 3, respectively.

Table 3. Consistency between each observer's aided and unaided results.

Score	Kappa	Observer 1	Observer 2	Observer 3
Multiple	Weighted	0.749	0.713	0.607
	Cohen's	0.438	0.349	0.308
Binary	Cohen's	0.816	0.683	0.410

The distribution of absence or presence of caries in binary scores is demonstrated in Table 4. The ratio of absence/presence of caries in ground truth was found to be approximately 2.32.

Table 4. Distribution of absence or presence of caries for binary scores.

n		Absence	Presence
Observer 1	Unaided	15,302	4634
	Aided	14,225	5711
Observer 2	Unaided	14,756	5180
	Aided	14,253	5683
Observer 3	Unaided	11,604	8332
	Aided	13,584	6352
Ground Truth		13,928	6008

The areas under the ROC curve of Observers 1, 2, and 3 were found to be 0.855, 0.863, and 0.747 for unaided and 0.920, 0.917, and 0.903 for aided (Figure 5) evaluations, respectively.

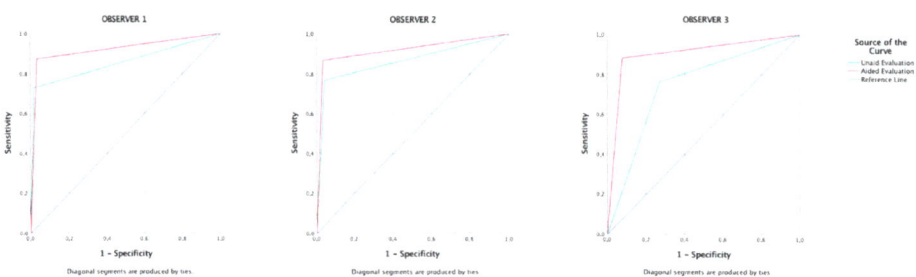

Figure 5. The ROC curves of aided and unaided evaluation of each observer.

The general consensus among all observers in binary scores is shown in Table 5. Agreement among the three observers for the presence of caries changed from substantial agreement (Fleiss Kappa: 0.612) to almost perfect agreement (Fleiss Kappa: 0.829) in the aided results. Overall agreement changed from moderate agreement (Fleiss Kappa: 0.443) to substantial agreement (Fleiss Kappa: 0.757) in the binary results.

Table 5. General consensus among all observers in binary scores.

Fleiss Kappa Coefficient	Binary	
Tooth Condition	Unaided	Aided
1. Absence of caries	0.831	0.928
2. Presence of caries	0.612	0.829
Overall Consensus	0.443	0.757

The general consensus among all observers on the five-point confidence scale is shown in Table 6. Overall agreement changed from fair agreement (Fleiss Kappa: 0.325) to moderate agreement (Fleiss Kappa: 0.468) on the five-point confidence scale.

Table 6. General consensus among all observers in multiple scores.

Fleiss Kappa Coefficient	Multiple	
Tooth Condition	Unaided	Aided
1. Definitely not	0.534	0.581
2. Probably not	0.494	0.628
3. Not sure	0.420	0.330
4. Probably yes	0.305	0.709
5. Definitely yes	0.561	0.668
Overall Consensus	0.325	0.468

The accuracy of the observers' aided and unaided responses in determining the presence or absence of caries according to the ground truth along with kappa coefficients is shown in Table 7. The difference in accuracy between aided and unaided responses of the Observer 3 were found to be the highest, while Observer 1 achieved the best accuracy (0.939) in the aided results.

Table 7. The sensitivity and specificity of unaided and aided evaluations of each observer.

		TP	TN	FP	FN	Sensitivity	Specificity	Accuracy	Kappa
Observer 1	Unaided	4377	13,671	257	1631	0.729	0.982	0.905	0.759
	Aided	5248	13,465	463	760	0.874	0.967	0.939	0.852
Observer 2	Unaided	4609	13,357	571	1399	0.767	0.959	0.901	0.756
	Aided	5210	13,455	473	798	0.867	0.966	0.936	0.846
Observer 3	Unaided	4588	10,184	3744	1420	0.764	0.731	0.741	0.446
	Aided	5299	12,875	1053	709	0.882	0.924	0.912	0.793

FN: False negative, FP: False positive, TN: True negative, TP: True positive.

The agreement between the observers is shown in Table 8. The highest agreement was found between the aided results of Observer 1 and Observer 2, with substantial to almost perfect agreement for different types of kappa coefficients (five-point confidence scale quadratic results, weighted kappa: 0.859 and kappa: 0.664; binary results, kappa: 0.810).

Table 8. Pairwise agreement among observers.

Observer			Five-Point Confidence Scale				Binary Score	
			Weighted Kappa		Cohen's Kappa			
1	2	3	Unaided	Aided	Unaided	Aided	Unaided	Aided
X	X		0.557	0.859	0.332	0.664	0.583	0.810
X		X	0.406	0.578	0.355	0.420	0.388	0.740
	X	X	0.435	0.574	0.317	0.373	0.408	0.724

4. Discussion

CBCT has become a very important radiographic technique in dentistry. The use of CBCT in dental procedures has gained popularity in recent years due to its low cost, fast image production rate, and lower radiation dose in comparison to medical CT [39]. However, CBCT machines are operated at milliamperes that are roughly one order of magnitude below the medical CT machines. Noise is defined as an unwanted disturbance of a signal that tends to obscure the signal's information. Despite the reduction in the radiation dose, a high noise level or lower signal-to-noise ratio is expected in CBCT images. Noise reduces contrast resolution and affects the ability to segment low-density tissues effectively [40,41]. Artifact is any distortion or error in the image that is unrelated to the subject. Image artifacts are one of the drawbacks of the clinical use of CBCT. Artifacts may obscure or simulate the pathology of the head and neck region, including dental caries [39,41].

Scatter is caused by those photons that are diffracted from their original path after interaction with matter. The scattered photons are captured by the sensor and simply added to the primary intensity. The geometry of the detector is an important factor for this image-degrading effect of scattered radiation; as the sensor gets larger, the probability of catching a scattered photon is raised. Scatters reduce soft-tissue contrast and affect the density of all tissues [40]. The streak artifacts caused by scatter are very similar to those of beam hardening [40,41]. Beam hardening is one of the most common sources of artifacts. As the beam passes through the object, a highly absorbing material in the object, such as metal, can function as a filter to absorb the lower energetic photons more rapidly than the higher energetic photons. Hence, the beam spectrum becomes rich in high-energy photons and the mean energy increases. When the spectrum of the captured beam contains relatively more higher energetic photons than the emitted ray, the beam becomes 'hardened' and an artifact is induced, resulting in dark streaks [39,40]. Artifacts are related to several factors such as the object, material type, FOV, imaging device, and parameters [42,43]. The effectiveness of metal artifact reduction algorithm has been investigated by several authors [44–46]. Xie et al. proposed a deep CNN to reduce scatter artifacts for CBCT in an image-guided radiation therapy system [47].

Several authors investigated the potential of using CBCT instead of plain radiographs in detecting dental caries. Studies on this issue have reported varying results, perhaps due to differences in methodology. Young et al. evaluated the CBCT images in detecting proximal and occlusal caries by mounting 146 non-restored extracted human teeth in plaster. Caries lesions are categorized according to location and depth, and practicing dentists are found to be more successful in CBCT images with the average sensitivity of 0.61 when compared to plain radiographs but with not occlusal caries [48]. Kayipmaz et al. investigated the use of CBCT in detecting occlusal and approximal caries using 72 extracted human teeth. In their study, CBCT was reported to be superior in detecting not the approximal but the occlusal caries, when compared to plain radiographs [49]. Krzyzostaniak et al. conducted a study using 135 extracted human posterior teeth, and the accuracy of detecting non-cavitated proximal caries with CBCT unit was reported to be (0.629) inferior to other intra-oral radiography techniques. However, the CBCT system is reported to be slightly better for detecting occlusal carious lesions [50].

Unlike researchers that included occlusal caries, some studies excluded this location, as we have, and focused on approximal caries detection. Zhang ZL et al. evaluated 39 non-cavitated and unrestored human permanent teeth for approximal caries. The mean ROC values for two different CBCT devices were reported to be 0.528 and 0.525 ($p = 0.763$). The performance of CBCT was reported to be a little better than chance when compared to plain radiography [51]. Valizadeh et al. embedded 84 extracted human teeth in blocks, and the area under the ROC curve, sensitivity, specificity, accuracy, and positive and negative predictive values of CBCT images were reported to be 0.568, 0.835, 0.637, 0.714, 0.598, and 0.856, respectively. Afterall, CBCT images did not enhance the detection of proximal caries in comparison with plain radiography [52]. Wenzel et al. mounted 257 non-filled human teeth in plaster to be evaluated and found that CBCT was more accurate than intra-oral radiography in detecting approximal caries [53].

Several studies are performed with the motivation that the artifacts caused by restorative materials may affect the diagnosis of caries. Charuakkra et al. compared CBCT and bitewing radiographs in detecting secondary caries using 120 cavity slots with different restorative materials. The mean ROC values for the CBCT system were reported to be 0.995, and 0.978, making CBCT superior to bitewing radiographs [54]. Melo et al. evaluated the use of CBCT in detecting recurrent caries-like lesions by creating artificial caries lesions under restorative materials. In their study, CBCT and intra-oral radiography were found to be similar in detecting demineralization under restorations [55]. In addition, not all CBCT machines are duplicates due to the adoption of different production technologies. Considering that differences in production technology may affect the diagnosis of dental caries, Qu et al. investigated the effect of two different detector types employed in five CBCT systems on the diagnostic accuracy of approximal carious lesions by evaluating 78 approximal surfaces. According to the results of this study, the differences between five different CBCT devices and two different detector types were not found to be statistically significant [56].

In this study, the areas under ROC curves (0.747–0.863 for unaided, and 0.903–0.920 for the aided evaluations) were found to be better than those in Zhang ZL et al. (0.525–0.528) and Valizadeh et al. (0.568) and close to the Charuakkra et al. (0.978–0.995) [51,52,54]. Sensitivities (0.729–0.767 for unaided, 0.874–0.882 for aided evaluations) were found to be better than the research of Young et al. (0.61) and similar to the study of Valizadeh et al. (0.835) [48,52]. Higher coefficients in Table 2 can provide evidence to the higher repeatability of observers for evaluations without the CDSS support (Sante DICOM Viewer Pro) and with the software support (Diagnocat), separately. Repeatability values for all observers were found to be almost perfect, except for one variable. Unaided results of Observer 3 on the five-point scale evaluation were found to be in substantial agreement (0735) with Cohen's kappa coefficient; however, the same observer reached almost perfect agreement (0.911) in the observations made with DiagnoCat system. The results of Table 3 may represent the magnitude of the decision changes before and after using the Diagnocat system, inversely. Kappa coefficients of Cohen's and weighted were calculated in the range of fair agreement (0.438) and almost perfect agreement (0.816) for Observer 1, fair agreement (0.349) and substantial agreement (0.713) for Observer 2, and fair agreement (0.308) and substantial agreement (0.607) for Observer 3. Accordingly, the decision changes made with the use of the Diagnocat system were found to be minimal in Observer 1, while the magnitude of the decision changes in Observer 3 was found to be slightly greater than in Observer 2. According to Table 7, in unaided evaluations, Observer 1 achieved the lowest sensitivity (0.729) and highest specificity (0.982). While sensitivity values were calculated similarly for Observer 2 (0.767) and Observer 3 (0.764), the lowest specificity value was found in Observer 3 (0.731). In aided evaluations, sensitivity values were increased to 0.874, 0.867, and 0.882 for Observer 1, Observer 2, and Observer 3, respectively. Specificity values were improved in both Observer 2 (0.966) and Observer 3 (0.924), while there was some loss in Observer 1 (0.967). Afterall, accuracies of all observers were improved when using the Diagnocat system. Kappa coefficients for Observer 1 were changed from substantial agreement (0.759) to almost perfect agreement (0.852) for Observer 2, they were changed from substantial agreement (0.756) to almost perfect agreement (0.846); and for Observer

3, they were changed from moderate agreement (0.446) to substantial agreement (0.793) before and after using the Diagnocat system. According to the results, it can be thought that Observer 1 was more cautious in caries scoring than Observer 3. This difference may be due to the difference in approach in distinguishing artifacts from caries findings. The results of our research show that the impact of the Diagnocat system on clinicians' decisions varies in magnitude and nature. Based on the findings, it can be suggested that Observer 3 is the one most affected by software support. The general consensus was improved from moderate agreement (0.443) to substantial agreement (0.757) using the software (Table 5), and the pair-wise agreements were improved (Table 8). While the findings of our research show that there is a general improvement in the evaluations made with Diagnocat, the slight decrease in the specificity of Observer 1 reminds us that these systems are not mistake-free and are auxiliary tools, and the importance of the final decision remains with the clinician.

Cardoso et al. defined gold standard data or methods as something that has already been checked (histologically, microscopically, chemically, etc.) and presents the best accuracy (sensitivity and specificity). Ground truth was reported as data and/or methods related to a consensus or more reliable values/aspects that can be used as references but were not or cannot be checked [57]. Experiments with extracted teeth allow for histopathological evaluation, and the lack of histopathological inspection can be considered as the limitations of this study. In our study, not the golden standard but ground truth was obtained and not for caries diagnosis but for radiographic caries detection. To address this point, a consensus was obtained among observers, similar to previous studies [58–61]. Thus, by using real patient images, there was no need to simulate conditions such as artifacts in translating the experimental results to clinical environment. Artifacts seen in CBCT imaging, especially those associated with metallic restorations, may affect the effectiveness of caries detection [32]. The lack of a distinction for restorations in our study can be considered as a limitation. In the meantime, samples with gross artifacts were not included in our study, and we aimed to overcome this situation by keeping the number of samples surplus. Thus, we aimed to reflect a realistic clinical situation by avoiding the bias caused by the distinction between images with and without artifacts. Evaluating the effect of artifacts due to restorations may be the subject of future studies. Caries identification by CBCT is a controversial topic and beyond the scope of this study. The developed system analyzes the volumetric data already saved and presents the dental caries signs to the operator. Further clinical review and final decision rests with the clinician. We suggest that machine learning tools, such as the system in our study, may be useful in detecting secondary findings, rather than for the primary imaging purpose, for better diagnosis and treatment planning.

5. Conclusions

In this study, radiographic evaluations performed by three observers were found to be more compatible and accurate with the aid of the AI system, when compared to the evaluations without the AI system, in detecting dental caries on CBCT images. Our study does not recommend justifying the use of CBCT imaging for caries diagnosis but suggests that once the volumetric data are acquired, machine learning tools can be helpful in detecting the caries signs. As technology advances, the integration of similar tools into the digital radiology workflow can assist clinicians in evaluating radiographic data.

Author Contributions: Conceptualization, M.A., I.R.-K., and K.O.; methodology, H.A., I.R.-K., A.L.F.C., S.L.P.d.C.L., and K.O.; software, M.G., M.E., and A.S.; validation, H.A. and K.O.; formal analysis, H.A., M.G., M.E., and A.S.; investigation, G.S., K.F.-G., C.A.B., and K.O.; resources, M.A.; data curation, H.A., M.A., and K.O.; writing—original draft preparation, H.A. and M.Ö.; writing—review and editing, G.S., K.F.-G., C.A.B., M.G., M.E., A.S., A.L.F.C., and S.L.P.d.C.L.; visualization, M.Ö.; supervision, I.R.-K. and K.O.; project administration, K.O. All authors have read and agreed to the published version of the manuscript.

Funding: This research received no external funding.

Institutional Review Board Statement: This study was conducted in accordance with the Declaration of Helsinki and approved by the Institutional Review Board (or Ethics Committee) of the Institutional Research Board of Jordan Institute of Technology (protocol code 792-2019).

Informed Consent Statement: Informed consent was obtained from all subjects involved in the study. The CBCT volume of the patients are anonymized (except gender and age) prior to exporting in DICOM format.

Data Availability Statement: The data presented in this study are available on request from the corresponding author.

Conflicts of Interest: Maxim Gusarev, Matvey Ezhov, and Alex Sanders are employees of Diagnocat Co., Ltd. Kaan Orhan is a scientific research advisor for Diagnocat Co., Ltd., San Francisco CA. Hakan Amasya, Mustafa Alkhader, Gözde Serindere, Karolina Futyma-Gąbka, Ceren Aktuna Belgin, Ingrid Różyło-Kalinowska, Merve Önder, Andre Luiz Ferreira Costa, and Sérgio Lúcio Pereira de Castro Lopes have no potential competing interests.

References

1. Machiulskiene, V.; Campus, G.; Carvalho, J.C.; Dige, I.; Ekstrand, K.R.; Jablonski-Momeni, A.; Maltz, M.; Manton, D.J.; Martignon, S.; Martinez-Mier, E.A.; et al. Terminology of Dental Caries and Dental Caries Management: Consensus Report of a Workshop Organized by ORCA and Cariology Research Group of IADR. *Caries Res.* **2020**, *54*, 7–14. [CrossRef]
2. Towle, I.; Irish, J.D.; De Groote, I.; Fernee, C.; Loch, C. Dental caries in South African fossil hominins. *S. Afr. J. Sci.* **2021**, *117*, 3–4. [CrossRef]
3. Selwitz, R.H.; Ismail, A.I.; Pitts, N.B. Dental caries. *Lancet* **2007**, *369*, 51–59. [CrossRef]
4. Vachirarojpisan, T.; Shinada, K.; Kawaguchi, Y.; Laungwechakan, P.; Somkote, T.; Detsomboonrat, P. Early childhood caries in children aged 6-19 months. *Community Dent. Oral Epidemiol.* **2004**, *32*, 133–142. [CrossRef]
5. Jiang, Q.; Liu, J.; Chen, L.; Gan, N.; Yang, D. The Oral Microbiome in the Elderly With Dental Caries and Health. *Front. Cell. Infect. Microbiol.* **2019**, *8*, 442. [CrossRef]
6. Usha, C.; Sathyanarayanan, R. Dental caries-A complete changeover (Part I). *JCD* **2009**, *12*, 46–54. [CrossRef]
7. Mathur, V.P.; Dhillon, J.K. Dental Caries: A Disease Which Needs Attention. *Indian J. Pediatr.* **2018**, *85*, 202–206. [CrossRef]
8. Pitts, N.B.; Zero, D.T.; Marsh, P.D.; Ekstrand, K.; Weintraub, J.A.; Ramos-Gomez, F.; Tagami, J.; Twetman, S.; Tsakos, G.; Ismail, A. Dental caries. *Nat. Rev. Dis. Primers* **2017**, *3*, 17030. [CrossRef]
9. Yılmaz, H.; Keleş, S. Recent methods for diagnosis of dental caries in dentistry. *Meandros Med. Dent. J.* **2018**, *19*, 1–8. [CrossRef]
10. Sukovic, P. Cone beam computed tomography in craniofacial imaging. *Orthod. Craniofac. Res.* **2003**, *6*, 31–36. [CrossRef]
11. Price, J.B. Caries Detection with Dental Cone Beam Computed Tomography. In *Detection and Assesment of Dental Caries: A Clinical Guide*; Zandona, A.F., Longbottom, C., Eds.; Springer: Cham, Switzerland, 2019; pp. 127–138.
12. Radiation Protection No 172. Cone beam CT for dental and maxillofacial radiology (Evidence-based guidelines). Available online: https://www.sedentexct.eu/files/radiation_protection_172.pdf (accessed on 10 October 2023).
13. Bansal, G.J. Digital radiography. A comparison with modern conventional imaging. *Postgrad. Med. J.* **2006**, *82*, 425–428. [CrossRef] [PubMed]
14. Jayachandran, S. Digital Imaging in Dentistry: A Review. *Contemp. Clin. Dent.* **2017**, *8*, 193–194. [CrossRef] [PubMed]
15. Mendonça, E.A. Clinical decision support systems: Perspectives in dentistry. *J. Dent. Educ.* **2004**, *68*, 589–597. [CrossRef]
16. Musen, M.A.; Shahar, Y.; Shortliffe, E.H. Clinical Decision-Support Systems. In *Medical Informatics*; Health Informatics; Shortliffe, E.H., Perreault, L.E., Eds.; Springer: New York, NY, USA, 2001; pp. 573–609. [CrossRef]
17. Sahota, N.; Lloyd, R.; Ramakrishna, A.; Mackay, J.A.; Prorok, J.C.; Weise-Kelly, L.; Navarro, T.; Wilczynski, N.L.; Haynes, R.B.; CCDSS Systematic Review Team. Computerized clinical decision support systems for acute care management: A decision-maker-researcher partnership systematic review of effects on process of care and patient outcomes. *Implement. Sci.* **2011**, *6*, 91. [CrossRef]
18. Jaspers, M.W.; Smeulers, M.; Vermeulen, H.; Peute, L.W. Effects of clinical decision-support systems on practitioner performance and patient outcomes: A synthesis of high-quality systematic review findings. *J. Am. Med. Inform. Assoc.* **2011**, *18*, 327–334. [CrossRef] [PubMed]
19. Ali, S.M.; Giordano, R.; Lakhani, S.; Walker, D.M. A review of randomized controlled trials of medical record powered clinical decision support system to improve quality of diabetes care. *Int. J. Med. Inform.* **2016**, *87*, 91–100. [CrossRef]
20. Pawloski, P.A.; Brooks, G.A.; Nielsen, M.E.; Olson-Bullis, B.A. A Systematic Review of Clinical Decision Support Systems for Clinical Oncology Practice. *J. Natl. Compr. Canc. Netw.* **2019**, *17*, 331–338. [CrossRef]
21. Kahn, C.E., Jr. Artificial intelligence in radiology: Decision support systems. *Radiographics* **1994**, *14*, 849–861. [CrossRef]
22. Syeda-Mahmood, T. Role of Big Data and Machine Learning in Diagnostic Decision Support in Radiology. *J. Am. Coll. Radiol.* **2018**, *15*, 569–576. [CrossRef]
23. Kök, H.; İzgi, M.S.; Acılar, A.M. Evaluation of the Artificial Neural Network and Naive Bayes Models Trained with Vertebra Ratios for Growth and Development Determination. *Turk. J. Orthod.* **2020**, *34*, 2–9. [CrossRef] [PubMed]

24. Goh, G.; Sing, S.; Yeong, W. A review on machine learning in 3D printing: Applications, potential, and challenges. *Artif. Intell. Rev.* **2021**, *54*, 63–94. [CrossRef]
25. Burkov, A. *The Hundred-Page Machine Learning Book*; Andriy Burkov: Quebec City, QC, Canada, 2019; pp. 3–7.
26. Zhu, X.; Goldberg, A.B. *Introduction to Semi-Supervised Learning*; Synthesis Lectures on Artificial Intelligence and Machine Learning (SLAIML); Springer: Berlin/Heidelberg, Germany, 2009; Volume 3, pp. 1–130.
27. Montagnon, E.; Cerny, M.; Cadrin-Chênevert, A.; Hamilton, V.; Derennes, T.; Ilinca, A.; Vandenbroucke-Menu, F.; Turcotte, S.; Kadoury, S.; Tang, A. Deep learning workflow in radiology: A primer. *Insights Imaging* **2020**, *11*, 22. [CrossRef]
28. Erickson, B.J.; Korfiatis, P.; Kline, T.L.; Akkus, Z.; Philbrick, K.; Weston, A.D. Deep Learning in Radiology: Does One Size Fit All? *J. Am. Coll. Radiol.* **2018**, *15*, 521–526. [CrossRef] [PubMed]
29. Sin, Ç.; Akkaya, N.; Aksoy, S.; Orhan, K.; Öz, U. A deep learning algorithm proposal to automatic pharyngeal airway detection and segmentation on CBCT images. *Orthod. Craniofac. Res.* **2021**, *24*, 117–123. [CrossRef] [PubMed]
30. Isman, O.; Aktan, A.M.; Ertas, E.T. Evaluating the effects of orthodontic materials, field of view, and artifact reduction mode on accuracy of CBCT-based caries detection. *Clin. Oral Investig.* **2020**, *24*, 2487–2496. [CrossRef]
31. Kumar, T.P.; Sujatha, S.; Rakesh, N.; Shwetha, V. Applications of CBCT in Caries Detection and Endodontics-A Review. *J. Dent. Res.* **2019**, *15*, 71–76.
32. Cebe, F.; Aktan, A.M.; Ozsevik, A.S.; Ciftci, M.E.; Surmelioglu, H.D. The effects of different restorative materials on the detection of approximal caries in cone-beam computed tomography scans with and without metal artifact reduction mode. *Oral Surg. Oral Med. Oral Pathol. Oral Radiol.* **2017**, *123*, 392–400. [CrossRef]
33. Lee, J.H.; Kim, D.H.; Jeong, S.N.; Choi, S.H. Detection and diagnosis of dental caries using a deep learning-based convolutional neural network algorithm. *J. Dent.* **2018**, *77*, 106–111. [CrossRef] [PubMed]
34. Bui, T.H.; Hamamoto, K.; Paing, M.P. Deep Fusion Feature Extraction for Caries Detection on Dental Panoramic Radiographs. *Appl. Sci.* **2021**, *11*, 2005. [CrossRef]
35. Devito, K.L.; de Souza Barbosa, F.; Felippe Filho, W.N. An artificial multilayer perceptron neural network for diagnosis of proximal dental caries. *Oral Surg. Oral Med. Oral Pathol. Oral Radiol. Endod.* **2008**, *106*, 879–884. [CrossRef]
36. Cantu, A.G.; Gehrung, S.; Krois, J.; Chaurasia, A.; Rossi, J.G.; Gaudin, R.; Elhennawy, K.; Schwendicke, F. Detecting caries lesions of different radiographic extension on bitewings using deep learning. *J. Dent.* **2020**, *100*, 103425. [CrossRef] [PubMed]
37. Isensee, F.; Kickingereder, P.; Wick, W.; Bendszus, M.; Maier-Hein, K. Brain tumor segmentation and radiomics survival prediction: Contribution to the brats 2017 challenge. In Proceedings of the International MICCAI Brainlesion Workshop, BrainLes 2017, Quebec City, QC, Canada, 14 September 2017; pp. 287–297.
38. Viera, A.J.; Garrett, J.M. Understanding interobserver agreement: The kappa statistic. *Fam. Med.* **2005**, *37*, 360–363.
39. Esmaeili, F.; Johari, M.; Haddadi, P.; Vatankhah, M. Beam Hardening Artifacts: Comparison between Two Cone Beam Computed Tomography Scanners. *J. Dent. Res. Dent. Clin. Dent. Prospects* **2012**, *6*, 49–53. [CrossRef] [PubMed]
40. Schulze, R.; Heil, U.; Gross, D.; Bruellmann, D.D.; Dranischnikow, E.; Schwanecke, U.; Schoemer, E. Artefacts in CBCT: A review. *Dentomaxillofac. Radiol.* **2011**, *40*, 265–273. [CrossRef]
41. Nagarajappa, A.K.; Dwivedi, N.; Tiwari, R. Artifacts: The downturn of CBCT image. *J. Int. Soc. Prev. Community Dent.* **2015**, *5*, 440–445. [CrossRef]
42. Codari, M.; de Faria Vasconcelos, K.; Ferreira Pinheiro Nicolielo, L.; Haiter Neto, F.; Jacobs, R. Quantitative evaluation of metal artifacts using different CBCT devices, high-density materials and field of views. *Clin. Oral Implants Res.* **2017**, *28*, 1509–1514. [CrossRef]
43. Panjnoush, M.; Kheirandish, Y.; Kashani, P.M.; Fakhar, H.B.; Younesi, F.; Mallahi, M. Effect of Exposure Parameters on Metal Artifacts in Cone Beam Computed Tomography. *J. Dent.* **2016**, *13*, 143–150.
44. Candemil, A.P.; Salmon, B.; Freitas, D.Q.; Ambrosano, G.M.B.; Haiter-Neto, F.; Oliveira, M.L. Are metal artefact reduction algorithms effective to correct cone beam CT artefacts arising from the exomass? *Dentomaxillofac. Radiol.* **2019**, *48*, 20180290. [CrossRef] [PubMed]
45. Queiroz, P.M.; Oliveira, M.L.; Groppo, F.C.; Haiter-Neto, F.; Freitas, D.Q. Evaluation of metal artefact reduction in cone-beam computed tomography images of different dental materials. *Clin. Oral Investig.* **2018**, *22*, 419–423. [CrossRef]
46. Vasconcelos, T.V.; Bechara, B.B.; McMahan, C.A.; Freitas, D.Q.; Noujeim, M. Evaluation of artifacts generated by zirconium implants in cone-beam computed tomography images. *Oral Surg. Oral Med. Oral Pathol. Oral Radiol.* **2017**, *123*, 265–272. [CrossRef] [PubMed]
47. Xie, S.; Yang, C.; Zhang, Z.; Li, H. Scatter artifacts removal using learning-based method for CBCT in IGRT system. *IEEE Access* **2018**, *6*, 78031–78037. [CrossRef]
48. Young, S.M.; Lee, J.T.; Hodges, R.J.; Chang, T.L.; Elashoff, D.A.; White, S.C. A comparative study of high-resolution cone beam computed tomography and charge-coupled device sensors for detecting caries. *Dentomaxillofac. Radiol.* **2009**, *38*, 445–451. [CrossRef] [PubMed]
49. Kayipmaz, S.; Sezgin, Ö.S.; Saricaoǧlu, S.T.; Çan, G. An in vitro comparison of diagnostic abilities of conventional radiography, storage phosphor, and cone beam computed tomography to determine occlusal and approximal caries. *Eur. J. Radiol.* **2011**, *80*, 478–482. [CrossRef]
50. Krzyżostaniak, J.; Kulczyk, T.; Czarnecka, B.; Surdacka, A. A comparative study of the diagnostic accuracy of cone beam computed tomography and intraoral radiographic modalities for the detection of noncavitated caries. *Clin. Oral Investig.* **2015**, *19*, 667–672. [CrossRef] [PubMed]
51. Zhang, Z.L.; Qu, X.M.; Li, G.; Zhang, Z.Y.; Ma, X.C. The detection accuracies for proximal caries by cone-beam computerized tomography, film, and phosphor plates. *Oral Surg. Oral Med. Oral Pathol. Oral Radiol. Endod.* **2011**, *111*, 103–108. [CrossRef] [PubMed]

52. Valizadeh, S.; Tavakkoli, M.A.; Karimi Vasigh, H.; Azizi, Z.; Zarrabian, T. Evaluation of Cone Beam Computed Tomography (CBCT) System: Comparison with Intraoral Periapical Radiography in Proximal Caries Detection. *J. Dent. Res. Dent. Clin. Dent. Prospects.* **2012**, *6*, 1–5. [CrossRef]
53. Wenzel, A.; Hirsch, E.; Christensen, J.; Matzen, L.H.; Scaf, G.; Frydenberg, M. Detection of cavitated approximal surfaces using cone beam CT and intraoral receptors. *Dentomaxillofac. Radiol.* **2013**, *42*, 39458105. [CrossRef]
54. Charuakkra, A.; Prapayasatok, S.; Janhom, A.; Pongsiriwet, S.; Verochana, K.; Mahasantipiya, P. Diagnostic performance of cone-beam computed tomography on detection of mechanically-created artificial secondary caries. *Imaging Sci. Dent.* **2011**, *41*, 143–150. [CrossRef]
55. Sousa Melo, S.L.; Belem, M.D.F.; Prieto, L.T.; Tabchoury, C.P.M.; Haiter-Neto, F. Comparison of cone beam computed tomography and digital intraoral radiography performance in the detection of artificially induced recurrent caries-like lesions. *Oral Surg. Oral Med. Oral Pathol. Oral Radiol.* **2017**, *124*, 306–314. [CrossRef] [PubMed]
56. Qu, X.; Li, G.; Zhang, Z.; Ma, X. Detection accuracy of in vitro approximal caries by cone beam computed tomography images. *Eur. J. Radiol.* **2011**, *79*, e24–e27. [CrossRef]
57. Cardoso, J.R.; Pereira, L.M.; Iversen, M.D.; Ramos, A.L. What is gold standard and what is ground truth? *Dental Press J. Orthod.* **2014**, *19*, 27–30. [CrossRef] [PubMed]
58. Lin, X.; Hong, D.; Zhang, D.; Huang, M.; Yu, H. Detecting Proximal Caries on Periapical Radiographs Using Convolutional Neural Networks with Different Training Strategies on Small Datasets. *Diagnostics* **2022**, *12*, 1047. [CrossRef] [PubMed]
59. Takahashi, N.; Lee, C.; Da Silva, J.D.; Ohyama, H.; Roppongi, M.; Kihara, H.; Hatakeyama, W.; Ishikawa-Nagai, S.; Izumisawa, M. A comparison of diagnosis of early stage interproximal caries with bitewing radiographs and periapical images using consensus reference. *Dentomaxillofac. Radiol.* **2019**, *48*, 20170450. [CrossRef]
60. Kallio-Pulkkinen, S.; Huumonen, S.; Haapea, M.; Liukkonen, E.; Sipola, A.; Tervonen, O.; Nieminen, M.T. Effect of display type, DICOM calibration and room illuminance in bitewing radiographs. *Dentomaxillofac. Radiol.* **2016**, *45*, 20150129. [CrossRef] [PubMed]
61. Jeon, K.J.; Han, S.S.; Lee, C.; Choi, Y.J.; Jung, H.I.; Kim, Y.H. Application of panoramic radiography with a multilayer imaging program for detecting proximal caries: A preliminary clinical study. *Dentomaxillofac. Radiol.* **2020**, *49*, 20190467. [CrossRef] [PubMed]

Disclaimer/Publisher's Note: The statements, opinions and data contained in all publications are solely those of the individual author(s) and contributor(s) and not of MDPI and/or the editor(s). MDPI and/or the editor(s) disclaim responsibility for any injury to people or property resulting from any ideas, methods, instructions or products referred to in the content.

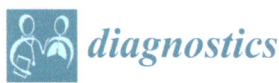 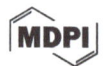

Systematic Review

Accuracy of Artificial Intelligence Models in Dental Implant Fixture Identification and Classification from Radiographs: A Systematic Review

Wael I. Ibraheem

Department of Preventive Dental Sciences, College of Dentistry, Jazan University, Jazan 45142, Saudi Arabia; wibraheem@jazanu.edu.sa or dr.wael007@yahoo.com

Abstract: *Background and Objectives*: The availability of multiple dental implant systems makes it difficult for the treating dentist to identify and classify the implant in case of inaccessibility or loss of previous records. Artificial intelligence (AI) is reported to have a high success rate in medical image classification and is effectively used in this area. Studies have reported improved implant classification and identification accuracy when AI is used with trained dental professionals. This systematic review aims to analyze various studies discussing the accuracy of AI tools in implant identification and classification. *Methods*: The Preferred Reporting Items for Systematic Reviews and Meta-Analyses (PRISMA) guidelines were followed, and the study was registered with the International Prospective Register of Systematic Reviews (PROSPERO). The focused PICO question for the current study was "What is the accuracy (outcome) of artificial intelligence tools (Intervention) in detecting and/or classifying the type of dental implant (Participant/population) using X-ray images?" Web of Science, Scopus, MEDLINE-PubMed, and Cochrane were searched systematically to collect the relevant published literature. The search strings were based on the formulated PICO question. The article search was conducted in January 2024 using the Boolean operators and truncation. The search was limited to articles published in English in the last 15 years (January 2008 to December 2023). The quality of all the selected articles was critically analyzed using the Quality Assessment and Diagnostic Accuracy Tool (QUADAS-2). *Results*: Twenty-one articles were selected for qualitative analysis based on predetermined selection criteria. Study characteristics were tabulated in a self-designed table. Out of the 21 studies evaluated, 14 were found to be at risk of bias, with high or unclear risk in one or more domains. The remaining seven studies, however, had a low risk of bias. The overall accuracy of AI models in implant detection and identification ranged from a low of 67% to as high as 98.5%. Most included studies reported mean accuracy levels above 90%. *Conclusions*: The articles in the present review provide considerable evidence to validate that AI tools have high accuracy in identifying and classifying dental implant systems using 2-dimensional X-ray images. These outcomes are vital for clinical diagnosis and treatment planning by trained dental professionals to enhance patient treatment outcomes.

Keywords: artificial intelligence; deep learning; dental implant; convolutional neural network; machine learning; implant classification; implant identification; implant fixture

1. Introduction

Advancements in science and technology have influenced people's lives in various fields, including dentistry. With the introduction of precise digital machines, dentists can provide high-quality treatment to their patients [1,2]. Various studies have shown that these computer-aided machines help dentists in various ways, from the fabrication of prostheses using CAD/CAM [2–5] to the use of robots in the treatment of patients [6–8]. The introduction of AI has taken dentistry to the next level. These tools help/act as supplementary aids to guide dentists' diagnosis and treatment planning. Artificial intelligence involves developing and training machines through a set of data so that they are capable of decision making and problem solving, mimicking the human brain [9–11]. Machine learning (ML), a segment of AI, involves using algorithms to perform tasks without human intervention. Deep learning (DL), e.g., convolutional neural network (CNN), is an element of ML that creates a neural network capable of identifying patterns by itself, which enhances feature identification [11–13].

AI functions on two levels. The first level involves training, in which data are used to train and set the parameters. The second level is the testing level, in which AI performs its designated task of problem solving or decision making based on the training data. The training data are generally from the pool of collected data of interest [14–17]. Currently, AI is widely used in dentistry, which involves caries detection [18,19], periapical lesion detection [20], oral cancer diagnosis [21,22], screening of osteoporosis [23], working length determination during endodontic treatment [24,25], determination of root morphology [26,27], forensic odontology [28], pediatric dentistry [29], and implant dentistry for identification [30–32], diagnosis, and treatment planning [33,34]. Studies have shown that, in general, AI helps dentists in diagnosis and treatment planning, as it provides logical reasons that aid in scientific assessment.

Dental implants are commonly used for replacing missing teeth. Studies have reported a high long-term success rate with a ten-year survival rate above 95% [35–38]. With constantly increasing demands, dental implant manufacturers are developing different implant systems to increase the success rate [39]. With the increase in the use of dental implants, an increase in complications has also been reported. These complications may be related to prosthetic or fixture components or may be biological in nature [40–43]. To manage these complications, the treating dentist should know the type of implant system used so that he or she can provide the best possible treatment outcome [44]. The data related to the implant system can be retrieved easily from the patient's previous records. However, in case of inaccessibility or loss of previous records due to any reason, it becomes difficult for the dentist to identify and classify the implant system using the available X-rays and clinical observation [45]. Dentists with vast experience in implantology may also find this task challenging. AI is reported to have a high success rate in medical image classification and is effectively used in this area. AI has been used to manage the problem of implant system identification and classification [30–32,46–63]. The AI tool is trained using a database of implant images and is later used to identify and classify the implants. Studies have reported improved implant classification and identification accuracy when AI is used with trained dental professionals [51,53,60,62]. This systematic review aims to analyze various studies discussing the accuracy of AI tools in implant identification and classification.

2. Materials and Methods

2.1. Registration

The Preferred Reporting Items for Systematic Reviews and Meta-Analyses (PRISMA) guidelines [64] were followed to systematize and compile this systematic review. The study was registered with the International Prospective Register of Systematic Reviews (PROSPERO registration No.: CRD42024500347).

2.2. Inclusion and Exclusion Criterias

The details of inclusion and exclusion criteria are given in Table 1.

2.3. Exposure and Outcome

In the current study, the exposure was the identification of the type and classification of an implant system using an artificial intelligence tool. The outcome was the accuracy of identification. The focused PICO (Population (P), Intervention (I), Comparison (C), and Outcome (O)) question for the current study was "What is the accuracy (outcome) of artificial intelligence tools (Intervention) in detecting and/or classifying the type of dental implant (Participant/population) using X-ray images?"

P: Human X-rays with dental implants.
I: Artificial intelligence tools.
C: Expert opinions and reference standards.
O: Accuracy of detection of the dental implant.

Table 1. Selection criteria.

Inclusion Criteria	Exclusion Criteria
Literature in English language	Literature in a language other than English
Human clinical studies	Animal studies, cadaver studies, technical reports, case reports, posters, case series, reports, commentaries, reviews, unpublished abstracts and dissertations, incomplete trials, and non-peer reviewed articles
Articles published between January 2008 and December 2023	Articles published prior to January 2008
Studies evaluating the diagnostic accuracy of artificial intelligence tools in the identification and classification of dental implants	Studies evaluating the accuracy of artificial intelligence tools in identification of other dental/oral structures
Studies in which three or more implant models were identified	Studies having only the abstract and not the full text
	Studies in which less than three implant models were identified
	Studies discussing artificial intelligence tools under trial

2.4. Information Sources and Search Strategy

Four electronic databases (Web of Science, Scopus, MEDLINE-PubMed, and Cochrane) were searched systematically to collect the relevant published literature. The search strings were based on the formulated PICO question. The article search was conducted in January 2024 using the Boolean operators and truncation. The search was limited to articles published in English in the last 15 years (January 2008 to December 2023). Studies performed on animals were not included. Details about the search strategy are mentioned in Table 2. Minor changes were made in the search strings based on the requirements of the database. Grey literature was searched, and bibliographies of selected studies and other review articles were checked manually to ensure that no relevant articles were left.

2.5. Screening, Selection of Studies, and Data Extraction

Two reviewers, M.S.A. and M.N.A., independently reviewed the titles and abstracts obtained by the electronic search. Duplicate titles were eliminated. The remaining titles were assessed based on the preset selection criteria and the PICO question. Full texts of the selected studies were reviewed independently by two reviewers, R.S.P. and W.I.I., and relevant articles were shortlisted. Any disagreements were resolved by discussion between them and with the third reviewer, M.N.A. Articles that did not meet the selection criteria were discarded, and the reason for exclusion was noted. The inter-examiner agreement was calculated using kappa statistics. W.I.I. created a data extraction chart and collected information related to the author, year of publication, country where the research was conducted, type and name of the algorithm network architecture, architecture depth, number of training epochs, learning rate, type of radiographic image, patient data collection duration, number of implant images evaluated, number and names of implant brands and models evaluated, comparator, test group, and training/validation number and ratio. Accuracy reported by the studies, author's suggestions, and conclusions were also extracted. These data were checked and verified by a second reviewer (M.S.A.).

Table 2. Strategy and search terms for the electronic databases.

Database	Combination of Search Terms and Strategy	Number of Titles
MEDLINE-PubMed	(((((((dental implants[MeSH Terms]) OR (dental implantation[MeSH Terms])) OR (dental implant*)) OR (dental implant system*)) OR (Dental Implant System Classification)) OR (dental implant fixture)) OR (dental implant fixture classification)) AND (((((((((((((dental diagnostic imaging) OR (dental digital radiography[MeSH Terms])) OR (dental radiography[MeSH Terms])) OR (oral digital radiography) OR (dental Digital radiograph))) OR (Panoramic image*)) OR (panoramic radiography[MeSH Terms])) OR (Periapical images)) OR (dental radiology)) OR (periapical radiograph*)) OR (dental X-ray image)) OR (synthetic dental X-ray image)) OR (OPG)) OR (Orthopantomogram)) OR (Intro oral radiograph) AND ((((((((((((((artificial intelligence[MeSH Terms]) OR (machine learning[MeSH Terms])) OR (neural networks computer[MeSH Terms])) OR (algorithms[MeSH Terms])) OR (deep learning)) OR (supervised machine learning)) OR (Automated deep learning)) OR (Object detection)) OR (Yolov3)) OR (object detection algorithm)) OR (convolutional neural network*)) OR (Deep Neural Network*)) OR (multi-task learning)) OR (deep convolutional neural network)) OR (Transfer Learning)) OR (attention branch network)) OR (Ensemble Deep Learning) AND ((((((((sensitivity and specificity[MeSH Terms]) OR (Accuracy)) OR (sensitivity)) OR (specificity)) OR (Positive Predictive Value*)) OR (Negative Predictive Value*)) OR (Precision)) OR (Recall)) OR (F1 score)) OR (Area under receiver operating characteristics curve) Filters: Humans, English, from 1 January 2008 to 31 December 2023	119
Scopus	("dental implants" OR "dental implantation" OR "dental implant*" OR "dental implant system*" OR "Dental Implant System Classification" OR "dental implant fixture" OR "dental implant fixture classification") AND ("dental diagnostic imaging" OR "dental digital radiography" OR "dental radiography" OR "oral digital radiography" OR "dental Digital radiograph" OR "Panoramic image*" OR "panoramic radiography" OR "Periapical images" OR "dental radiology" OR "periapical radiograph*" OR "dental X-ray image" OR "synthetic dental X-ray image" OR "OPG" OR "Orthopantomogram" OR "Intro oral radiograph") AND ("artificial intelligence" OR "machine learning" OR "neural networks computer" OR "algorithms" OR "deep learning" OR "supervised machine learning" OR "Automated deep learning" OR "Object detection" OR "Yolov3" OR "object detection algorithm" OR "convolutional neural network*" OR "Deep Neural Network*" OR "multi-task learning" OR "deep convolutional neural network" OR "Transfer Learning" OR "attention branch network" OR "Ensemble Deep Learning") AND ("sensitivity and specificity" OR "Accuracy" OR "sensitivity" OR "specificity" OR "Positive Predictive Value*" OR "Negative Predictive Value*" OR "Precision" OR "Recall" OR "F1 score" OR "Area under receiver operating characteristics curve") AND PUBYEAR > 2008 AND PUBYEAR <2023 AND (LIMIT-TO (SUBJAREA, "DENT")) AND (LIMIT-TO (DOCTYPE, "ar")) AND (LIMIT-TO (LANGUAGE, "English")) AND (LIMIT-TO(SRCTYPE, "j"))	205
Web of Science	#1 (P) TS = ('dental implants' OR 'dental implantation' OR 'dental implant*'OR 'dental implant system*' OR 'Dental Implant System Classification' OR 'dental implant fixture' OR 'dental implant fixture classification' OR 'dental diagnostic imaging' OR 'dental digital radiography' OR 'dental radiography' OR 'oral digital radiography' OR 'dental Digital radiograph' OR 'Panoramic image*' OR 'panoramic radiography' OR 'Periapical images' OR 'dental radiology' OR 'periapical radiograph*' OR 'dental X-ray image' OR 'synthetic dental X-ray image' OR 'OPG' OR Orthopantomogram OR 'Intro oral radiograph') #2 (I) TS = ('artificial intelligence' OR 'machine learning' OR 'neural networks computer' OR algorithms OR 'deep learning' OR 'supervised machine learning' OR 'Automated deep learning' OR 'Object detection' OR 'Yolov3' OR 'object detection algorithm' OR 'convolutional neural network*' OR 'Deep Neural Network*' OR 'multi-task learning' OR 'deep convolutional neural network' OR 'Transfer Learning' OR 'attention branch network' OR 'Ensemble Deep Learning') #3 (O) TS = ('sensitivity and specificity' OR Accuracy OR sensitivity OR specificity OR 'Positive Predictive Value*' OR 'Negative Predictive Value*' OR Precision OR Recall OR 'F1 score' OR 'Area under receiver operating characteristics curve') #3 AND #2 AND #1 Indexes = SCI-EXPANDED, SSCI, A&HCI, CPCI-S, CPCI-SSH, ESCI, CCR-EXPANDED, IC Timespan = January 2008 to December 2023 and English (Languages)	8

Table 2. Cont.

Database	Combination of Search Terms and Strategy	Number of Titles
Cochrane Library	#1 MeSH descriptor: [Dental Implants] explode all trees #2 MeSH descriptor: [Dental Implantation] explode all trees #3 dental implant* #4 dental implant system* #5 Dental Implant System Classification #6 dental implant fixture #7 dental implant fixture classification #8 dental diagnostic imaging #9 MeSH descriptor: [Radiography, Dental, Digital] explode all trees #10 MeSH descriptor: [Radiography, Dental] explode all trees #11 oral digital radiography #12 dental Digital radiograph #13 Panoramic image* #14 panoramic radiography #15 Periapical images #16 dental radiology #17 periapical radiograph* #18 dental X-ray image #19 synthetic dental X-ray image #20 OPG #21 Orthopantomogram #22 Intro oral radiograph #23 MeSH descriptor: [Artificial Intelligence] explode all trees #24 MeSH descriptor: [Machine Learning] explode all trees #25 MeSH descriptor: [Neural Networks, Computer] explode all trees #26 MeSH descriptor: [Algorithms] explode all trees #27 deep learning #28 supervised machine learning #29 Automated deep learning #30 Object detection #31 Yolov3 #32 object detection algorithm #33 convolutional neural network* #34 Deep Neural Network* #35 multi-task learning #36 deep convolutional neural network #37 Transfer Learning #38 attention branch network #39 Ensemble Deep Learning #40 MeSH descriptor: [Sensitivity and Specificity] explode all trees #41 Accuracy #42 sensitivity #43 specificity #44 Positive Predictive Value* #45 Negative Predictive Value* #46 Precision #47 Recall #48 F1 score #49 Area under receiver operating characteristics curve #50 #1 OR #2 OR #3 OR #4 OR #5 OR #6 OR #7 #51 #8 OR #9 OR #10 OR #11 OR #12 OR #13 OR #14 OR #15 OR #16 OR #17 OR #18 OR #19 OR #20 OR #21 OR #22 #52 #23 OR #24 OR #25 OR #26 OR #27 OR #28 OR #29 OR #30 OR #31 OR #32 OR #33 OR #34 OR #35 OR #36 OR #37 OR #38 OR #39 #53 #40 OR #41 OR #42 OR #43 OR #44 OR #45 OR #46 OR #47 OR #48 OR #49 #54 #50 AND #51 AND #52 AND #53	6

* truncation. P, population; I, intervention; O, outcome.

2.6. Quality Assessment of Included Studies

The quality of all the selected articles was critically analyzed using the Quality Assessment and Diagnostic Accuracy Tool (QUADAS-2) [65]. This tool is used for studies evaluating diagnostic accuracy (Table S1). This tool assesses the risk of bias and applicability concerns. The risk of bias arm has four domains that primarily focus on patient selection, index test, reference standard, and flow and timing. Meanwhile, the applicability concern arm has three domains focusing on patient selection, index test, and reference standards.

3. Results

3.1. Identification and Screening

After an electronic search of the databases, 561 hits were displayed. A total of 36 articles were found to be duplicates and were removed, and the titles and abstracts of 525 articles were reviewed and checked for eligibility based on inclusion and exclusion criteria. Twenty-eight articles were selected for full-text review. Out of these twenty-eight articles, six were rejected, as they discussed the use of AI in diagnosis and treatment planning of dental implants, and one was rejected because it discussed the diagnostic accuracy of AI in evaluating the misfit of abutment and implant. Eventually, twenty-one articles were included in the study. No relevant articles meeting the selection criteria were found during the manual search of the bibliographies of the selected studies and other review articles (Figure 1). During the full-text review phase, Cohen's kappa value was found to be 0.89 for two reviewers (R.S.P. and W.I.I.), which is an excellent agreement.

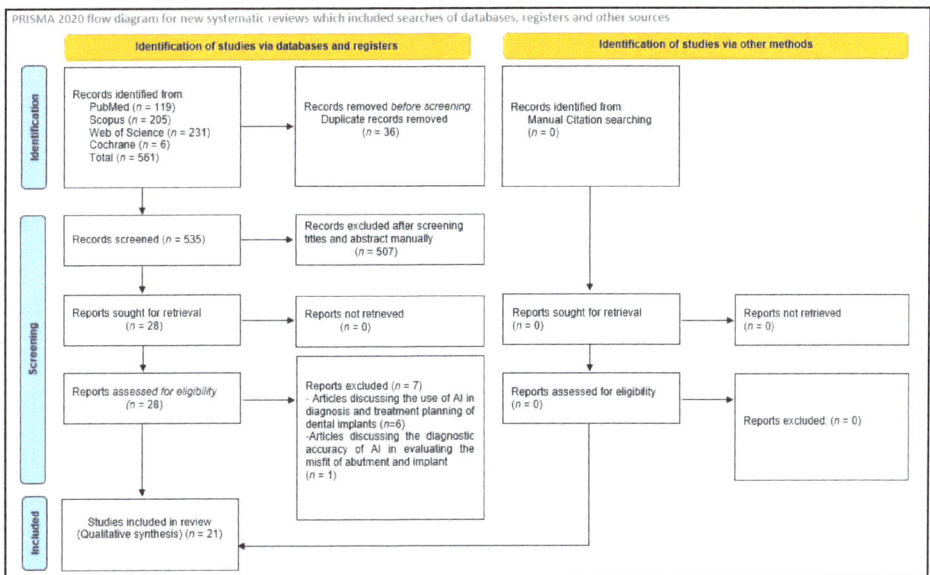

Figure 1. Flow chart illustrating the search strategy.

3.2. Study Characteristics

Table 3 displays the characteristics of studies involved in the review. All the involved studies were published in the last four years (2020: six; 2021: four; 2022: five; 2023: six) (Figure 2). Out of selected 21 studies, 12 were conducted in the Republic of Korea [31,48,51,53–55,57–62], four in Japan [30,47,50,52], and one each in Brazil [49], India [56], France [46], South Africa [32], and the United States [63] (Figure 3). Some of the included studies were conducted by the same research groups (Kong et al. [31,61],

Park et al. [48,62], Sukegawa et al. [30,50,52], and Lee et al. [51,53,54]). Each of them shared common funding sources and grant numbers, respectively, but the studies by Kong et al. [31,61] also shared a common research registration number. The number of algorithm networks evaluated for accuracy varied in the selected studies. Ten studies [46–49,51,53,57,58,60,62] evaluated the accuracy of one algorithm network; three evaluated two algorithm networks [32,59,61]; two tested three algorithm networks [31,54]; one tested four algorithm networks [56]; three tested five algorithm networks [50,52,55]; one study each tested six [30] and ten [63] algorithm networks. All the included studies evaluated the accuracy of tested AI tools in implant detection and classification, whereas four studies [51,53,60,62] also compared this to trained dental professionals.

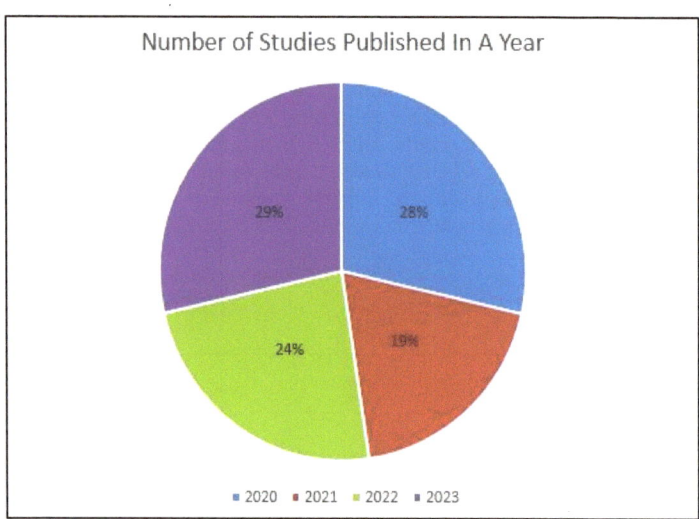

Figure 2. Year-wise distribution of published studies.

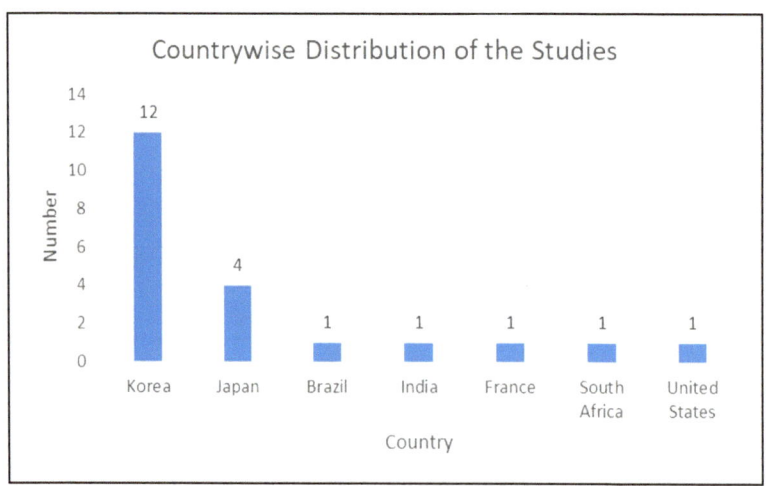

Figure 3. Country-wise distribution of published studies.

Table 3. Study characteristics and accuracy results of the included studies.

Author, Year Country	Algorithm Network Architecture and Name	Architecture Depth (Number of Layers), Number of Training Epochs, and Learning Rate	Type of Radiographic Image	Patient Data Collection/X-ray Collection Duration	Number of X-rays/Implant Images Evaluated (N)	Number and Names of Implant Brands and Models Evaluated	Comparator	Test Group and Training/Validation Number and Ratio	Accuracy Reported	Authors Suggestions/Conclusions
Kong, et al., 2023, Republic of Korea [61]	- 2 DL - YOLOv5 - YOLOv7	Training Epochs: YOLOv5: 146, 184, 200 YOLOv7: 200	Pano	2001 to 2021	N = 14,037	Implant models: N = 130 * Implant design classification: 1. Coronal one-third 2. Middle one-third 3. Apical part	EORS	Test Group: 20% Training Group: 80%	mAP (area under the precision–recall curve): YOLOv5: Implant-dataset-1:0.929 Implant-dataset-2: 0.940 Implant-dataset-3:0.873 YOLOv7: Implant-dataset-1: 0.931 Implant-dataset-2: 0.984 Implant-dataset-3: 0.884 YOLOv7 Implant-dataset-1: IPA: 0.986 IPA + Magnification ×2: 0.988 IPA + Magnification ×4: 0.986	mAP: YOLOv7 > YOLOv5 The tested DL has a high accuracy
Kong, 2023, Republic of Korea [58]	- Fine-tuned CNN - Google automated machine learning (AutoML) Vision	Training: 32 node hours	PA	January 2005 to December 2019	N = 4800	Implant Brands: N = 3 (A) Osstem Implant (B) Biomet 3i LLC (C) Dentsply Sirona Implant models: N = 4 (1) Osstem TSIII (25%) (2) Osstem USII (25%) (3) Biomet 3i Osseotite External (25%) (4) Dentsply Sirona Xive (25%)	EORS	Test Group: 10% Training Group: 80% Fine-tuning Group:10%	Overall Accuracy: 0.981 Precision: 0.963 Recall: 0.961 Specificity: 0.985 F1 score: 0.962	Tested fine-tuned CNN showed high accuracy in the classification of DISs
Park, et al., 2023, Republic of Korea [62]	- Fine-tuned and pretrained DL - ResNet-50	- Depth: 50 layers	PA and Pano	NM	N = 150,733 PA (24.8%) and Pano (75.2%)	Implant Brands: N = 10 (A) Neobiotech (n = 14.1%) (B) NB (n = 2.41%) (C) Dentsply (n = 10.14%) (D) Dentium (n = 27.26%) (E) Dio (n = 1.01%) (F) Megagen (n = 5.17%) (G) ST (n = 3.30%) (H) Shinhung (n = 2.23%) (I) Osstem (n = 28.47%) (J) Warantec (n = 5.86%) Implant Models: N = 25 (A) Neobiotech: (1) IS I 1, (2) IS II, (3) IS III, (4) EB; (B) NB: (1) Branemark; (C) Dentsply: (1) Astra, (2) Xive; (D) Dentium: (1) Implantium, (2) Superline; (E) Dio: (1) UF, (2) UF II, (F) Megagen: (1) Any ridge, (2) Anyone internal, (3) Anyone external, (4) Esteel external; (G) ST: (1) TS standard, (2) TS standard plus, (3) Bone level; (H) Shinhung: (1) Luna; (I) Osstem: (1) GS II, (2) SS II, (3) TS III, (4) US II, (5) US III; (J) Warantec: (1) Hexplant	DL vs. 28 dental professionals (9 dentists specialized in implantology and 19 dentists not specialized in implantology)	Training Group: 80% Validation Group: 10% Test Group: 10%	Accuracy (1) DL: (a) Both Pano and PA: 82.3% (95% CI, 78.0–85.9%) (b) PA: 83.8% (95% CI, 79.6–87.2%) (c) Pano: 73.3% (95% CI, 68.5–77.6%) (2) All dental professionals: (a) Both Pano and PA: 23.5% ± 18.5 (b) PA: 26.2% ± 18.2 (c) Pano: 24.5% ± 19.0 (3) Dentist specialized in Implantology: (a) Both Pano and PA: 43.3% ± 20.4 (b) PA: 43.3% ± 19.7 (c) Pano: 43.2% ± 21.2 (4) Dentist not specialized in implantology: (a) Both Pano and PA: 16.8% ± 9 (b) PA: 18.1% ± 9.9 (c) Pano: 15.6% ± 8.5 Deep learning (For both Pano and PA) AUC: 0.823 Sensitivity: 80.0% Specificity: 84.5% PPV: 83.8% NPV: 80.9%	Classification accuracy performance of DL was significantly superior

121

Table 3. Cont.

Author, Year Country	Algorithm Network Architecture and Name	Architecture Depth (Number of Layers), Number of Training Epochs, and Learning Rate	Type of Radiographic Image	Patient Data Collection/X-ray Collection Duration	Number of X-ray/Implant Images Evaluated (N)	Number and Names of Implant Brands and Models Evaluated	Comparator	Test Group and Training/Validation Number and Ratio	Accuracy Reported	Authors Suggestions/Conclusions
Hsiao et al., 2023, USA [63]	- 10 CNN architectures (1) MnasNet (2) ShuffleNet7 (3) MobileNet8 (4) AlexNet9 (5) VGG10 (6) ResNet11 (7) DenseNet12 (8) SqueezeNet13 (9) ResNeXt14 (10) Wide ResNet15	- Learning rate: 0.001 - For training accuracy, the CNN assessed data 90 times per image	PA	January 2011 to January 2019	N = 788	Implant Brands: N = 3 (A) BioHorizons (22.84%) (B) ST (34.51%) (C) NB (42.63%) Implant Models (A) BioHorizons: (1) Legacy implant Tapered Pro; (B) ST: (1) Bone Level, Bone Level Tapered, Standard Straumann, Tapered Effect; (C) NB: (1) Active, (2) Parallel, (3) Replace, (4) Replace Select Straight, (5) Replace Select Tapered, (6) Speedy Groovy, (7) Speedy Replace	EORS	Training Group: 75% Test Group: 25%	Overall implant-identification Accuracy: >90% Test accuracy (1) MnasNet6: 81.89% (2) ShuffleNet7: 96.85% (3) MobileNet8: 92.68% (4) AlexNet9: 94.35% (5) VGG10: 92.94% (6) ResNet11: 96.43% (7) DenseNet12: 96.41% (8) SqueezeNet13: 91.55% (9) ResNeXt14: 93.90% (10) Wide ResNet15: 92.01%	Tested CNN has high accuracy and speed
Park et al., 2023, Republic of Korea [48]	- Customized automatic DL - Neuro-T version 3.0.1	- Training epochs: 500	PA and Pano	NM	N = 156,965 (Pano: 116,756; PA: 40,209)	Implant Brands: N = 10 (A) Neobiotech, (B) NB, (C) Dentsply, (D) Dentium, (E) Dioimplant, (F) Megagen, (G) ST, (H) Shinhung, (I) Osstem, (J) Warrantec Implant models: N = 27 1. IS I (Neobiotech) (5%); 2. IS II (Neobiotech) (1.83%); 3. IS III (Neobiotech) (5.18%); 4. EB (Neobiotech) (1.53%); 5. Branemark (NB) (2.32%); 6. Astra (Dentsply) (8.90%); 7. Xive (Dentsply) (0.84%); 8. Implantium (Dentium) (12.20%); 9. Superline (Dentium) (13.98%); 10. UF Any ridge (Megagen) (0.22%); 13. Anyone international (Megagen) (2.43%); 14. Anyone external (Megagen) (1.63%); 15. Esset external (Megagen) (0.69%); 16. TS standard (Straumann) (0.85%); 17. TS standard plus (Straumann) (0.66%); 18. Bone level (Straumann) (1.66%); 19. Luna (Shinhung) (2.15%); 20. GS II (Osstem) (1.10%); 21. SS II (Osstem) (0.53%); 22. TS III (Osstem) (18.96%); 23. US II (Osstem) (6.15%); 24. US III (Osstem) (0.60%); 25. Hexplant (Warrantec) (5.63%); 26. Internal (Warrantec) (3.68%); 27. IT (Warrantec) (0.28%)	EORS	Training Group: 80% Validation Group: 10% Test Group: 10%	Overall 1. Accuracy: 88.53% 2. Precision: 85.70% 3. Recall: 82.30% 4. F1 score: 84.00% Using Pano: 1. Accuracy: 87.89% 2. Precision: 85.20% 3. Recall: 81.10% 4. F1 score: 83.10% Using PA: 1. Accuracy: 86.87% 2. Precision: 84.40% 3. Recall: 81.70% 4. F1 score: 83.00%	- DL has reliable classification accuracy - No statistically significant difference in accuracy performance between the Pano and PA - Suggestion: Additional dataset needed for confirming clinical feasibility of DL
Kong et al., 2023, Republic of Korea [31]	3 DLs (1) EfficientNet (2) Res2Next (3) Ensemble model	NM	Pano	March 2001 and April 2021	N = 45,909	Implant Brands: N = 20 (A) Bicon; (B) BioHorizons; (C) BIOMET 3i; (D) Biotem; (E) Dental Ratio; (F) Dentis; (G) Dentium; (H) Dentsply Sirona; (I) Dio Implant; (J) Hi-ossen implant; (K) IBS Implant; (L) Keystone Dental; (M) MegaGen Implant; (N) Neobiotech; (O) NB; (P) Osstem Implant; (Q) Point Implant; (R) ST; (S) Thommen Medical; (T) Zimmer Dental Implant models: N = 130*	EORS	Training Group: 80% Test Group:20%	Top-1 accuracy (ratio that the nearest class was predicted, and the answer was correct) (a) EfficientNet: 73.83 (b) Res2Next: 73.09 (c) Ensemble model: 75.27 Top-5 accuracy (ratio in which the five nearest classes were predicted, and the answer was among them) (a) EfficientNet: 93.84 (b) Res2Next: 93.60 (c) Ensemble model: 95.02 Precision: (a) EfficientNet: 74.61 (b) Res2Next: 77.79 (c) Ensemble model: 78.84 Recall: (a) EfficientNet: 73.83 (b) Res2Next: 73.08 (c) Ensemble model: 75.27 F1 score: (a) EfficientNet: 72.02 (b) Res2Next: 73.55 (c) Ensemble model: 74.89	Accuracy: Ensemble model > EfficientNet > Res2Next

Table 3. Cont.

Author, Year Country	Algorithm Network Architecture and Name	Architecture Depth (Number of Layers), Number of Training Epochs, and Learning Rate	Type of Radiographic Image	Patient Data Collection/X-ray Collection Duration	Number of X-rays/Implant Images Evaluated (N)	Number and Names of Implant Brands and Models Evaluated	Comparator	Test Group and Training/Validation Number and Ratio	Accuracy Reported	Authors Suggestions/Conclusions
Jang et al., 2022, Republic of Korea [57]	Faster R-CNN Resnet 101	- Training epochs: 1000	PA	January 2016 to June 2020	N = 300	NM	EORS	Test Group: 20% Training Group: 80%	Classification: Precision: 0.977 Recall: 0.992 F1 score: 0.984	Faster R-CNN model provided high-quality object detection for dental implants and peri-implant tissues
Kohlakala et al., 2022, South Africa [32]	DL (1) FCN-1 (2) FCN-2	- Training epochs: 1000	Artificially generated (simulated) X-ray images	NM	NM	Implant brands: N = 1 MIS Dental implant Implant models: N = 9 (1) Conical narrow platform V3 (2) Conical narrow platform C1 (3) Conical standard platform V3 (4) Conical wide platform C1 Internal diameter 4.00 mm (5) Internal hex narrow platform SEVEN (6) Internal hex standard platform SEVEN (7) Internal hex wide platform SEVEN (8) External hex standard platform LANCE (9) External hex wide platform	EORS	Test Group: 17–18% Training Group: 82–83% Validation: 12–13%	Semi-automated system (human jaws) Full precision: 70.52% Recall: 69.76% Accuracy: 69.76% F1 score: 69.70% Fully automated system (human jaws) Full precision: 70.55% Recall: 68.67% Accuracy: 68.67% F1 score: 67.60%	Proposed fully automated system displayed promising results for implant classification
Sukegawa et al., 2022, Japan [30]	CNN and CNN + ABN (1) ResNet18 (2) ResNet18 + ABN (3) ResNet50 (4) ResNet50 + ABN (5) ResNet152 (6) ResNet152 + ABN	- Depth: (1 and 2) 18 layers (3 and 4) 50 layers (5 and 6) 152 layers - Training epochs: 100 - Learning rate: 0.001	Pano	NM	N = 10,191	Implant brands: N = 5 (A) ZB (4.19%) (B) NB (25.25%) (C) Kyocera Co. (7.07%) (D) ST (8.94%) (E) Dentsply IH AB (54.16%) Implant models: N = 13 1. Full OSSEOTITE 4.0 (4.19%) 2. Astra EV 4.2 (8.29%) 3. Astra TX 4.0 (24.73%) 4. Astra TX 4.5 (10.93%) 5. Astra Micro Thread 4.0 (6.91%) 6. Astra Micro Thread 4.5 (3.73%) 7. Branemark Mk III 4.0 (3.48%) 8. FINESIA 4.2 (3.33%) 9. POI EX 4.2 (3.74%) 10. Replace Select Tapered 4.3 (6.04%) 11. Nobel Replace CC 4.3 (15.69%) 12. Straumann Tissue 4.1 (6.43%) 13. Straumann Bone Level 4.1 (2.51%)	EORS	Test dataset split Training: validation: 8:2.	Test accuracy (95% CI): (a) ResNet18: 0.9486 (b) ResNet18 + ABN: 0.9719 (c) ResNet50: 0.9578 (d) ResNet50 + ABN: 0.9511 (e) ResNet152: 0.9624 (f) ResNet152 + ABN: 0.9564 Precision: (a) ResNet18: 0.9441 (b) ResNet18 + ABN: 0.9686 (c) ResNet50: 0.9546 (d) ResNet50 + ABN: 0.9477 (e) ResNet152: 0.9575 (f) ResNet152 + ABN: 0.9514 Recall: (a) ResNet18: 0.9333 (b) ResNet18 + ABN: 0.9627 (c) ResNet50: 0.9471 (d) ResNet50 + ABN: 0.9382 (e) ResNet152: 0.9509 (f) ResNet152 + ABN: 0.9450 F1 score: (a) ResNet18: 0.9382 (b) ResNet18 + ABN: 0.9652 (c) ResNet50: 0.9508 (d) ResNet50 + ABN: 0.9416 (e) ResNet152: 0.9530 (f) ResNet152 + ABN: 0.9470 AUC: (a) ResNet18: 0.9979 (b) ResNet18 + ABN: 0.9993 (c) ResNet50: 0.9983 (d) ResNet50 + ABN: 0.9975 (e) ResNet152: 0.9985 (f) ResNet152 + ABN: 0.9955	ResNet 18 showed very high compatibility in the ABN model Accuracy: ResNet18 + ABN > ResNet152 > ResNet50 > 0.9578 > ABN > ResNet50 + ABN > ResNet18

123

Table 3. Cont.

Author, Year Country	Algorithm Network Architecture and Name	Architecture Depth (Number of Layers), Number of Training Epochs, and Learning Rate	Type of Radiographic Image	Patient Data Collection/X-ray Collection Duration	Number of X-rays/Implant Images Evaluated (N)	Number and Names of Implant Brands and Models Evaluated	Comparator	Test Group and Training/Validation Number and Ratio	Accuracy Reported	Authors Suggestions/Conclusions
Kim et al., 2022, Republic of Korea [59]	- DCNN - YOLOv3 (Darknet-53)	- Depth: 53 layers - Training epochs: 100, 200, and 300	PA	April 2020 to July 2021	N = 355	Implant models: N = 3 (1) Superline (Dentium Implant Co. Ltd., Seoul, Republic of Korea) (34.08%) (2) TS III (Osstem Implant Co. Ltd., Seoul, Republic of Korea) (32.39%) (3) Bone Level Implant (Institut ST AG, Basel, Switzerland) (33.52%)	EORS	Test Group: 20% Training Group: 80% (10% used for validation)	At 200 epochs training: Accuracy: 96.7% Sensitivity: 94.4% Specificity: 97.9% Confidence score: 0.75	High performance could be achieved with YOLOv3 DCNN
Lee et al., 2022, Republic of Korea [60]	- Automated DL - Neuro-T version 2.0.1, Neurocle Inc., Seoul, Republic of Korea	NM	Pano	NM	N = 180	Implant models: N = 6 (1) Astra OsseoSpeed® TX (16.66%) (2) Dentium Implantium® (16.66%) (3) Dentium Superline® (16.66%) (4) Osstem TSIII® (16.66%) (5) Straumann SLActive® BL (16.66%) (6) Straumann SLActive® BLT (16.66%).	DL vs. 44 dental professionals (3 board-certified periodontists, 8 periodontology residents, 17 conservative and pediatric dentistry residents, and 14 interns)	Training Group: 80% Validation Group: 20%	Mean Accuracy: - Automated DL algorithm: 80.56% - All participants (without DL assistance): 63.13% - All participants (with DL assistance): 78.88%	The DL algorithm significantly helps improve the classification accuracy of dental professionals. Average accuracy: board-certified periodontists with DL > Automated DL
Benakatti et al., 2021, India [56]	4 machine learning algorithms: (1) Support vector machine (SVM) (2) Logistic regression (3) K-nearest neighbor (KNN) (4) X boost classifiers	NM	Pano	January 2021 to April 2021	NM	Implant models: N = 3 1. Osstem TS III SA Regular, 2. Osstem TS III SA Medium, 3. Norris Medical Tuff.	EORS	Test Group: 20% Training Group: 80%	Average accuracy overall: 0.67 Accuracy based on Hu moments (a) SVM:0.47 (b) Logistic regression: 0.33 (c) KNN: 0.50 (d) X boost classifiers: 0.33 Accuracy based on eigenvalues (a) SVM: 0.67 (b) Logistic regression: 0.17 (c) KNN: 0.67 (d) X boost classifiers: 0.67	The machine learning models tested are proficient enough to identify DISs Accuracy: logistic regression > SVM > KNN > X boost
Santos et al., 2021, Brazil [49]	- DCNN - Stochastic Gradient Descent optimization algorithm	- Depth: 5 convolutional layers + 5 dense layers - Training epochs: 25 - Learning rate: 0.005	PA	2018–2020	N = 1800	Implant Brands and Model: N = 3 (A) ST (internal-connection) (33.33%) (B) Neodent (Neodent) (33.33%) (C) SIN Implante (SIN Morse taper with prosthetic platform) (33.33%)	EORS	Test Group: 20% Training Group: 80%	1. Accuracy = 85.29% (78.4% to 90.5%) 2. Sensitivity = 89.9% (81.1% to 95.6%) 3. Specificity = 82.4% (73.7% to 87.3%) 4. PPV = 82.6% (74.1% to 86.6%) 5. NPV = 88.5% (79.8% to 93.9%	- DCNN has high degree of accuracy for implant identification Suggestion: Need for more comprehensive database

124

Table 3. Cont.

Author, Year Country	Algorithm Network Architecture and Name	Architecture Depth (Number of Layers), Number of Training Epochs, and Learning Rate	Type of Radiographic Image	Patient Data Collection/X-ray Collection Duration	Number of X-rays/Implant Images Evaluated (N)	Number and Names of Implant Brands and Models Evaluated	Comparator	Test Group and Training/Validation Number and Ratio	Accuracy Reported	Authors Suggestions/Conclusions
Sugegawa et al., 2021, Japan [52]	5 CNNs 1. ResNet18 2. ResNet34 3. ResNet50 4. ResNet101 5. ResNet152	- Depth: 1. 18 layers 2. 34 layers 3. 50 layers 4. 101 layers 5. 152 layers - Training epochs: 50 - Learning rate: 0.001	Pano	January 2005 to December 2020	N = 9767	Implant brands: N = 5 (A) ZB, (B) Dentsply, (C) NB, (D) Kyocera, (E) ST Implant models: N = 12 1. Full OSSEOTITE 4.0 (ZB) (4.37%); 2. Astra EV 4.2 (Dentsply) (8.65%); 3. Astra TX 4.0 (Dentsply) (25.80%); 4. Astra MicroThread 4.0 (Dentsply) (7.20%); 5. Astra MicroThread 4.5 (Dentsply) (3.89%); 6. Astra TX 4.5 (Dentsply) (11.40%); 7. Brånemark Mk III 4.0 (NB) (3.63%); 8. FINESIA 4.2 (Kyocera) (3.39%); 9. Replace Select Tapered 4.3 (NB) (6.30%); 10. Nobel CC 4.3 (NB) (16.37%); 11. Straumann Tissue 4.1 (ST) (6.70%); 12. Straumann Bone Level 4.1 (ST) (2.25%)	EORS	Validation Group: 20% Training Group: 80%	Single task: accuracy: (a) ResNet18: 0.9787 (b) ResNet34: 0.9800 (c) ResNet50: 0.9800 (d) ResNet101: 0.9841 (e) ResNet152: 0.9851 Precision: (a) ResNet18: 0.9737 (b) ResNet34: 0.9790 (c) ResNet50: 0.9816 (d) ResNet101: 0.9822 (e) ResNet152: 0.9839 Recall: (a) ResNet18: 0.9726 (b) ResNet34: 0.9743 (c) ResNet50: 0.9746 (d) ResNet101: 0.9789 (e) ResNet152: 0.9809 F1 score: (a) ResNet18: 0.9724 (b) ResNet34: 0.9762 (c) ResNet50: 0.9776 (d) ResNet101: 0.9805 (e) ResNet152: 0.9820 AUC: (a) ResNet18: 0.9996 (b) ResNet34: 0.9997 (c) ResNet50: 0.9996 (d) ResNet101: 0.9997 (e) ResNet152: 0.9998	- CNNs conferred high validity in the classification of DIs - The larger the number of parameters and the deeper the network, the better the performance for classifications
Lee et al., 2021, Republic of Korea [54]	- 3 DCNN (1) VGGNet-19 (2) GoogLeNet Inception-v3 (3) Automated DCNN (Neuro-T version 2.1.1.)	- Depth: (1) 19 layers (2) 22 layers (3) 18 layers - Training epochs: 2000 - Learning rate: 0.0001	PA and Pano	January 2006 to December 2019	251 intact and 198 fractured dental implants images (Pano: 45.2%, PA: 54.8%)	Not mentioned Intact and fractured dental implants were identified and classified	EORS	Test Group: 20% Training Group: 60% Validation Group: 20%	Overall: AUC: - VGGNet-19: 0.929 (95% CI: 0.854–0.972) - GoogLeNet Inception-v3: 0.967 (95% CI: 0.906–0.993) - Automated DCNN: 0.972 (95% CI: 0.913–0.995) Sensitivity: - VGGNet-19: 0.933 - GoogLeNet Inception-v3: 1.00 - Automated DCNN: 0.866 Specificity: - VGGNet-19: 0.933 - GoogLeNet Inception-v3: 0.866 - Automated DCNN: 0.966 Youden index: - VGGNet-19: 0.866 - GoogLeNet Inception-v3: 0.866 - Automated DCNN: 0.833	- All tested DCNNs showed acceptable accuracy in the detection and classification of fractured dental implants - Best accuracy: Automated DCNN architecture using only PA images

Table 3. Cont.

Author, Year Country	Algorithm Network Architecture and Name	Architecture Depth (Number of Layers), Number of Training Epochs, and Learning Rate	Type of Radiographic Image	Patient Data Collection/X-ray Collection Duration	Number of X-rays/Implant Images Evaluated (N)	Number and Names of Implant Brands and Models Evaluated	Comparator	Test Group and Training/Validation Number and Ratio	Accuracy Reported	Authors Suggestions/Conclusions
Hadj Said et al., 2020, France [46]	- DCNN - Pretrained GoogLeNet Inception v3	- Depth: 22 layers deep (27 including the pooling layers) - Training epochs: 1000 - Learning rate: 0.02	PA and Pano	NM	N = 1206	Implant brands: N = 3 (A) NB (49.4%), (B) ST (25.5%), (C) ZB (25%) Implant models: N = 6 1. NobelActive (21.64%);2. Brånemark system (21.77%); 3. Straumann Bone Level (12.43%); 4. Straumann Tissue Level (13.1%); 5. Zimmer Biomet Dental Tapered Screw-Vent (12.6%); 6. SwissPlus (Zimmer) (12.43%)	EORS	Test Group: 19.9% Training and Validation Group: 80%	1. Diagnostic accuracy = 93.8% (87.2% to 99.4%) 2. Sensitivity = 93.5% (84.2% to 99.3%) 3. Specificity = 94.2% (83.5% to 99.4%) 4. PPV = 92% (83.9% to 97.2%) 5. NPV = 91.5% (80.2% to 97.1%)	- Good performance of DCNN in implant identification - Suggestion: Creation of a giant database of implant radiographs
Lee et al., 2020, Republic of Korea [53]	- Automated DCNN - Neuro-T version 2.0.1 (Neurocle Inc., Republic of Korea)	- Depth: 18 layers	PA and Pano	January 2006 to May 2019	N = 11,980 (Pano: 59.6% and PA: 40.4%)	Implant brands: N = 4 (A) Osstem implant system (46.9%) (B) Dentium implant system (40.7%) (C) Institut ST implant system (9.2%) (D) Dentsply implant system (3.2%) Implant models: N = 6 1. Astra Osseo Speed TX (Dentsply) (3.2%) 2. Implantium (Dentium) (21%) 3. Superline (Dentium) (19.7%) 4. TSIII® (Osstem) (46.9%) 5. SLActive BL (Institut ST) (4.5%) 6. SLActive BLT (Institut ST) (4.7%)	DCNN vs. 25 dental professionals (board-certified periodontist, periodontology residents, other specialty residents)	Test Group: 20% Training Group: 80%	DCNN overall (based on 180 images): Accuracy (AUC): 0.954 Youden index: 0.808 Sensitivity: 0.955 Specificity: 0.853 Using Pano images: AUC: 0.929 Youden index: 0.804 Sensitivity: 0.922 Specificity: 0.882 Using PA images: AUC: 0.961 Youden index: 0.802 Sensitivity: 0.955 Specificity: 0.846 AUC Dental Professionals: i. Board-certified periodontist: 0.501–0.968 ii. Periodontology residents: 0.503–0.915 iii. Other specialty residents: 0.544–0.915	Accuracy: DCNN > Dental professionals
Takahashi et al., 2020, Japan [47]	- DL - Fine-tuned Yolo v3	- Training epochs: 1000 - Learning rate: 0.01	Pano	Feb. 2000–2020	N = 1282	Implant brands: N = 3 (A) NB, (B) ST, (C) GC Implant models: N = 6 1. MK III (NB); 2. MK III Groovy (NB); 3. Bone level implant (ST); 4. Genesio Plus ST (Genesio) (GC); 5. MK IV (NB); 6. Speedy Groovy (NB)	EORS	Test Group: 20% Training Group: 80%	1. True-positive ratio: 0.50 to 0.82 2. Average precision: 0.51 to 0.85 3. Mean average precision: 0.71 4. Mean intersection over union: 0.72	- Implants can be identified by using DL - Suggestion: More images of other implant systems will be necessary to increase the learning performance

126

Table 3. Cont.

Author, Year Country	Algorithm Network Architecture and Name	Architecture Depth (Number of Layers), Number of Training Epochs, and Learning Rate	Type of Radiographic Image	Patient Data Collection/X-ray Collection Duration	Number of X-rays/Implant Images Evaluated (N)	Number and Names of Implant Brands and Models Evaluated	Comparator	Test Group and Training/Validation Number and Ratio	Accuracy Reported	Authors Suggestions/Conclusions
Sukegawa et al., 2020, Japan [50]	- 5 DCNNs 1. Basic CNN 2. VGG16 transfer-learning model 3. Finely tuned VGG16 4. VGG19 transfer-learning model 5. Finely tuned VGG19	- Depth: 1: 3 convolution layers, 2 and 3: 16 layers (13 convolutional layers + 3 fully connected layers), 4 and 5: 19 layers (16 convolutional layers + 3 fully connected layers) - Training epochs: 700 - Learning rate: 0.0001	Pano	January 2005 to December 2019	N = 8859	Implant brands: N = 5 (A) ZB, (B) Dentsply, (C) NB, (D) Kyocera, (E) ST Implant models: N = 11 1. Full OSSEOTITE 4.0 (ZB) (4.81%); 2. Astra EV 4.2 (Dentsply) (4.7%); 3. Astra TX 4.0 (Dentsply) (28.45%); 4. Astra MicroThread 4.0 (Dentsply) (12.28%); 5. Astra MicroThread 4.5 (Dentsply) (7.87%); 6. Astra TX 4.5 (Dentsply) (4.36%); 7. Brånemark Mk III 4.0 (NB) (4.77%); 8. FINESIA 4.2 (Kyocera) (2.63%); 9. Replace Select Tapered 4.3 (NB) (5.48%); 10. Nobel CC 4.3 (NB) (18.97%); 11. Straumann Tissue 4.1 (ST) (5.53%)	EORS	Test Group: 25% Training Group: 75%	1. Basic CNN: i. Accuracy: 0.860 ii. Precision: 0.842 iii. Recall: 0.802 iv. F1 score: 0.819 2. VGG16-transfer learning: i. Accuracy: 0.899 ii. Precision: 0.888 iii. Recall: 0.864 iv. F1 score: 0.874 3. Finely tuned VGG16: i. Accuracy: 0.935 ii. Precision: 0.928 iii. Recall: 0.907 iv. F1 score: 0.916 4. VGG19 transfer-learning: i. Accuracy: 0.880 ii. Precision: 0.873 iii. Recall: 0.840 iv. F1 score: 0.853 5. Finely tuned VGG19: i. Accuracy: 0.927 ii. Precision: 0.913 iii. Recall: 0.894 iv. F1 score: 0.902	High accuracy demonstrated by all tested DCNNs Accuracy: Finely tuned VGG16 > Finely tuned VGG19 > VGG16-transfer learning > VGG19 transfer-learning > Basic CNN
Lee and Jong, 2020, Republic of Korea [51]	- DCNN - GoogLeNet Inception v3	- Depth: 22 layers deep, 2 fully connected layers - Training epochs: 1000	PA and Pano	January 2010 to December 2019	N = 10,770 (Pano: 5390, PA: 5380)	Implant brands: N = 3 (A) Osstem TSIII implant system (42.71%) (B) Dentium Superline implant system (40.57%) (C) Straumann BLT implant system (16.71%)	DCNN vs. board-certified periodontist	Test Group: 20% Training Group: 60% Validation Group: 20%	i. AUC: 1. Overall: - DCNN: 0.971 (95% CI: 0.963–0.978) - Periodontist: 0.925 (95% CI: 0.913–0.935) 2. Pano: - DCNN: 0.956 (95% CI: 0.942–0.967) - Periodontist: 0.891 (95% CI: 0.871–0.909) 3. PA: - DCNN: 0.979 (95% CI: 0.969–0.987) - Periodontist: 0.959 (95% CI: 0.945–0.970) ii. Sensitivity and specificity 1. Overall: - DCNN: 95.3% and 97.6% - Periodontist: 88.7% and 87.1% 2. Pano: - DCNN: 93.6% and 95.7% - Periodontist: 82.9% and 90.3% 3. PA: - DCNN: 97.1% and 99.5% - Periodontist: 94.2% and 95.8%	DCNN is useful for the identification and classification of DISs Accuracy: DCNN > Periodontist (both are reliable)

Table 3. Cont.

Author, Year Country	Algorithm Network Architecture and Name	Architecture Depth (Number of Layers), Number of Training Epochs, and Learning Rate	Type of Radiographic Image	Patient Data Collection/X-ray Collection Duration	Number of X-rays/Implant Images Evaluated (N)	Number and Names of Implant Brands and Models Evaluated	Comparator	Test Group and Training/Validation Number and Ratio	Accuracy Reported	Authors Suggestions/Conclusions
Kim et al., 2020, Republic of Korea [55]	5 different CNNs (1) SqueezeNet (2) GoogLeNet (3) ResNet-18 (4) MobileNet-v2 (5) ResNet-50	-Depth: (1) 18 layers (2) 22 layers (3) 18 layers (4) 54 layers (5) 50 layers -Training epochs: 500	PA	2005 to 2019	N = 801	Implant models: N = 4 1. Brånemark Mk TiUnite 2. Dentium Implantium 3. Straumann Bone Level 4. Straumann Tissue Level	EORS	NM	Test accuracy: (a) SqueezeNet: 96% (b) GoogLeNet: 93% (c) ResNet-18: 98% (d) MobileNet-v2: 97% (e) ResNet-50: 98% Precision: (a) SqueezeNet: 0.96 (b) GoogLeNet: 0.92 (c) ResNet-18: 0.98 (d) MobileNet-v2: 0.96 (e) ResNet-50: 0.98 Recall: (a) SqueezeNet: 0.96 (b) GoogLeNet: 0.94 (c) ResNet-18: 0.98 (d) MobileNet-v2: 0.95 (e) ResNet-50: 0.98 F1 score: (a) SqueezeNet: 0.96 (b) GoogLeNet: 0.93 (c) ResNet-18: 0.98 (d) MobileNet-v2: 0.96 (e) ResNet-50: 0.98	CNNs can classify implant fixtures with high accuracy

DCNN, deep convolutional neural network; CNN, convolutional neural network; PA, periapical radiograph; Pano, panoramic radiograph; NM, not mentioned; DL, deep learning; EORS, expert opinions, reference standards; YOLO, you only look once; NB, Nobel Biocare; ST, Straumann; ZB, Zimmer Biomet; AUC, area under the receiver operating characteristic curve; PPV, positive predictive value; NPV, negative predictive value; VGG, Visual Geometry Group, Oxford University; CI, confidence interval; DISs, dental implant systems; ABN, attention branch network; *, details not mentioned due to high number; FCN, fully convolutional neural network; IPA, image processing augmentation; R-CNN, region-based convolutional neural network; mAP, mean average precision.

More than 431,000 implant images were used to train and test the selected AI tools' implant detection and classification accuracy. Eight studies [30,31,47,50,52,56,60,61] used cropped panoramic X-ray images, and six studies [49,55,57–59,63] used cropped periapical X-ray images, whereas another six studies [46,48,51,53,54,62] used both periapical and panoramic implant images. In one study [32], artificially generated X-ray images were used to test AI accuracy. In most of the selected studies, the test group to training group ratio was 1:4. The learning rate of the AI algorithm ranged between 0.0001 and 0.02, the number of training epochs ranged from 50 to 2000, and the architecture depth varied from 3 to 150 layers. Also, the number of implant brands and models identified and classified varied from $N = 3$ to $N = 130$.

3.3. Quality Assessment of Included Studies

The QUADAS-2 tool was used to assess the risk of bias in diagnostic tests. Out of the 21 studies evaluated, 14 were found to be at risk of bias, with high or unclear risk in one or more domains. The remaining seven studies, however, had a low risk of bias. All the included studies utilized photographic data as input to AI, resulting in a low risk of bias in the data selection domain across all studies. The results from the risk-of-bias arm demonstrated that 80.95% of the studies had a low risk, 14.28% had an unclear risk, and 4.76% had a high risk in the index test domain. In contrast, in the reference standard domain, 47.62% of the studies had a low or unclear risk of bias, while 4.76% had a high risk of bias. As the data feeding in AI technology is standardized, the final output will not affect the flow or time frame. Therefore, all studies regarded both aspects as low-risk categories (100%). Based on the risk-of-bias arm of the QUADAS-2 assessment tool, applicability concerns generated similar results. (Table S1 and Figure 4).

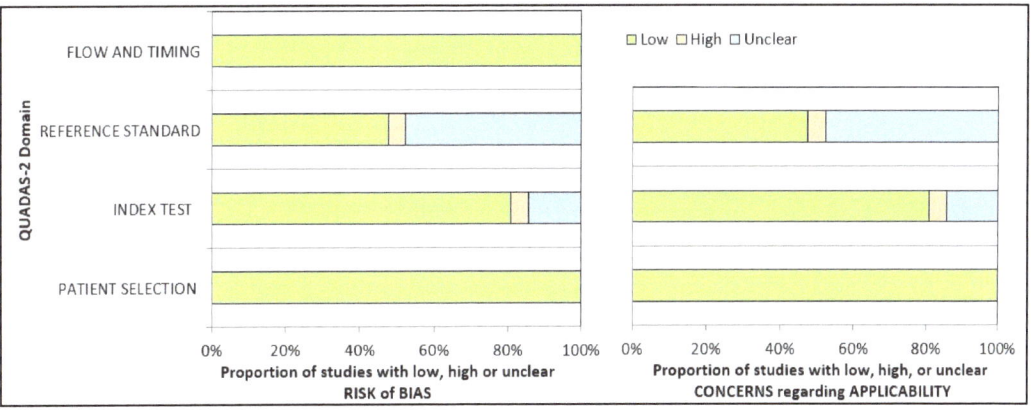

Figure 4. Presentation of the risk of quality assessment summary of risk bias and applicability concerns for included studies according to the QUADAS-2 tool.

3.4. Accuracy Assessment

The overall accuracy of deep learning algorithms (DLA) in implant detection and identification ranged from a low of 67% [56] to as high as 98.5% [52]. Most included studies reported mean accuracy levels above 90% [30,46,50–55,58,59,63]. The accuracy of the latest finely tuned versions of DLAs was reported to be higher when compared to basic DLAs. Six studies [46,48,51,53,54,62] used both periapical and panoramic implant images to test the DLA models. Four studies reported higher accuracy when periapical radiographs were used [46,51,53,54,62]. One study reported higher accuracy with panoramic radiographs [48], whereas one study did not provide these details [46]. Four studies compared the accuracy of DLAs with dental professionals [51,53,60,62]. All four reported higher accuracy for DLAs when compared to dental professionals. A study by Lee et al. [60] reported that the board-certified periodontists with the assistance of DLA reported higher accuracy when compared to automated DL alone.

4. Discussion

The current systematic review involved all the recently published studies evaluating the accuracy of AI in implant detection and classification [30–32,46–63]. Overall, the outcome of this review revealed that the application of AI in implant detection and classification is a reliable and accurate method and can help dentists manage cases with no previous data related to the type of implant. With the advancements in AI, the accuracy levels may improve to a great extent.

However, the outcomes of this review should be inferred with caution because there was a significant variation between the numbers of implant models evaluated for testing the accuracy in the included studies. These ranged from as low as three [49,51,56,59] to as high as one hundred and thirty [61]. In general, the lower the number, the higher the accuracy rate of identification and classification, generally. There was a large variation in the sample size in the selected studies, which varied from 300 [57] to more than 150,000 [62].

The included studies have variations in the annotation process. PA images were used for training and testing the AI tool in six studies [49,55,57–59,63] and panoramic images in eight studies [30,31,47,50,52,56,60,61], whereas both PA and panoramic images were used in six studies [46,48,51,53,54,62]. One study used simulated images generated artificially [32]. In the studies where both PA and panoramic images were used, four studies reported that the accuracy of identification and classification was higher with PA images as compared to panoramic images [51,53,54,62], whereas one study reported that the accuracy was higher with the panoramic images [48].

The dental professionals involved in image selection, cropping, image standardization, training, and validation varied in areas of practice from periodontists and prosthodontists to oral and maxillofacial surgeons [30,48,51,53,54,63]. In contrast, other included studies were lacking in this information. One study validated the collected data with the help of board-certified oral and maxillofacial radiologists [48] and periodontists [53]. To reduce the heterogeneity and standardize the outcomes, the validation of the selected X-ray images should be performed by a trained radiologist. There was variation in training epochs, which varied from 50 to 2000, and the architecture depth varied from 3 to 150 layers. These parameters can affect the accuracy outcomes of the included studies. The accuracy of identification and classification also depends on the generation of Dl architecture used. There was a difference in the tested algorithms in the selected studies.

In their study, Sukegawa et al. [52] trained a CNN algorithm to analyze the implant brand and treatment stage simultaneously. The AI tool was annotated for both parameters. The classification accuracy of the implant treatment stage was reported as 0.996, with a large effect size of 0.818. The accuracy of single-task and multi-task AI tools were found to be comparable. Lee et al. [54] trained and tested the accuracy of AI tools to identify and classify fractured implants. They reported an implant classification accuracy varying from 0.804 to 0.829. They reported higher accuracy levels when DCNN architecture used only PA images for identification.

All the included studies evaluated the accuracy of tested AI tools in implant detection and classification, whereas four studies [51,53,60,62] also compared this to the trained dental professionals. Lee et al. [51,53,60] and Park et al. [62] compared the accuracy of the tested DL algorithm in implant detection and classification with trained dental professionals. All the studies reported that the accuracy performance of the DL algorithm was significantly superior when compared to humans. The accuracy reported by Park et al. [62] for DL was 82.3% and for humans varied from 16.8% (dentist not specialized in implantology) to 43.3% (dentist specialized in implantology). Lee et al. [60] reported mean accuracy of 80.56% for the automated DL algorithm, 63.13% for all participants without DL assistance, and 78.88% for all participants with DL assistance. They reported that the DL algorithm significantly helped in improving the classification accuracy of all dental professionals. Lee et al. [53], in another study, reported an accuracy of 95.4% for DL and between 50.1% to 96.8% for dentists. Another study by Lee et al. [51] reported a similar accuracy rate with DL at 97.1% and periodontists at 92.5%.

Most of the currently reported AI models use two-dimensional X-rays (periapical or panoramic). In contrast, three-dimensional X-rays like cone-beam computed tomography, widely used in implantology, were not evaluated. Also, the studies included have limitations in the type of implant systems evaluated. Thus, there is a need for more studies with a vast database that can include most of the commonly used implant systems and can utilize all forms of radiographic techniques.

The DL algorithm's identification and classification abilities in all the selected studies were limited to the implant models the authors trained. There is a need to include more implant systems and models and create a vast database to help identify a wider variety of implant models and their characteristics. A comprehensive search strategy and rigorous selection strategy are the strong points of this systematic review. All articles mentioning AI and dental implants were assessed based on pre-set selection criteria, thus ensuring that every relevant article was reviewed.

4.1. Inferences and Future Directions

The field of AI is growing exponentially. There is vast literature discussing the advancements of AI in the healthcare field. Most of these AI tools focus on identification, diagnosis, and treatment planning and ways to improve them to help healthcare professionals provide the best possible treatment to their patients. All the included studies used two-dimensional images (periapical or panoramic) to identify and classify the implant systems. Three-dimensional imaging techniques like CBCT are considered a gold-standard imaging technique in dental implant planning and treatment. Thus, there is a need to develop AI tools that can use these 3D images to identify and classify the implant systems. Additionally, with the availability of newer generations of AI tools, there is a need for constant up-gradation to increase the accuracy levels of these tools.

4.2. Limitations

The current systematic review has a few limitations. This review included studies published only in English. The search period was limited to the last 25 years only (2008–2023). As AI is a recent and advancing field, the authors believed that conducting a search before this time may provide studies in which the technology is in an immature stage. Lastly, a meta-analysis was not feasible due to the lack of heterogeneity among the selected studies.

5. Conclusions

To conclude, it can be stated that the articles in the present review provide considerable evidence to validate AI tools as having high accuracy in identifying and classifying dental implant systems using 2-dimensional X-ray images. These outcomes are vital for clinical diagnosis and treatment planning by trained dental professionals to enhance patient treatment outcomes.

Supplementary Materials: The following supporting information can be downloaded at: https://www.mdpi.com/article/10.3390/diagnostics14080806/s1, Table S1: Quality Assessment (QUADAS-2) Summary of Risk Bias and Applicability Concerns.

Funding: This research received no external funding.

Institutional Review Board Statement: Not applicable.

Informed Consent Statement: Not applicable.

Data Availability Statement: The data that support the findings of this study are available from the corresponding author upon reasonable request.

Acknowledgments: Author would like to thank Mohammed Sultan Al-Ak'hali (M.S.A.), Mohammad N. Alam (M.N.A.), and Reghunathan S. Preethanath (R.S.P.) for their help in the screening and selection of the reviewed articles.

Conflicts of Interest: The author declares no conflicts of interest.

References

1. Abad-Coronel, C.; Bravo, M.; Tello, S.; Cornejo, E.; Paredes, Y.; Paltan, C.A.; Fajardo, J.I. Fracture Resistance Comparative Analysis of Milled-Derived vs. 3D-Printed CAD/CAM Materials for Single-Unit Restorations. *Polymers* **2023**, *15*, 3773. [CrossRef] [PubMed]
2. Martín-Ortega, N.; Sallorenzo, A.; Casajús, J.; Cervera, A.; Revilla-León, M.; Gómez-Polo, M. Fracture resistance of additive manufactured and milled implant-supported interim crowns. *J. Prosthet. Dent.* **2022**, *127*, 267–274. [CrossRef] [PubMed]
3. Jain, S.; Sayed, M.E.; Shetty, M.; Alqahtani, S.M.; Al Wadei, M.H.D.; Gupta, S.G.; Othman, A.A.A.; Alshehri, A.H.; Alqarni, H.; Mobarki, A.H.; et al. Physical and mechanical properties of 3D-printed provisional crowns and fixed dental prosthesis resins compared to CAD/CAM milled and conventional provisional resins: A systematic review and meta-analysis. *Polymers* **2022**, *14*, 2691. [CrossRef] [PubMed]
4. Gad, M.M.; Fouda, S.M.; Abualsaud, R.; Alshahrani, F.A.; Al-Thobity, A.M.; Khan, S.Q.; Akhtar, S.; Ateeq, I.S.; Helal, M.A.; Al-Harbi, F.A.; et al. Strength and surface properties of a 3D-printed denture base polymer. *J. Prosthodont.* **2021**, *31*, 412–418. [CrossRef]
5. Al Wadei, M.H.D.; Sayed, M.E.; Jain, S.; Aggarwal, A.; Alqarni, H.; Gupta, S.G.; Alqahtani, S.M.; Alahmari, N.M.; Alshehri, A.H.; Jain, M.; et al. Marginal Adaptation and Internal Fit of 3D-Printed Provisional Crowns and Fixed Dental Prosthesis Resins Compared to CAD/CAM-Milled and Conventional Provisional Resins: A Systematic Review and Meta-Analysis. *Coatings* **2022**, *12*, 1777. [CrossRef]
6. Wang, D.; Wang, L.; Zhang, Y.; Lv, P.; Sun, Y.; Xiao, J. Preliminary study on a miniature laser manipulation robotic device for tooth crown preparation. *Int. J. Med. Robot. Comput. Assist. Surg.* **2014**, *10*, 482–494. [CrossRef] [PubMed]
7. Toosi, A.; Arbabtafti, M.; Richardson, B. Virtual reality haptic simulation of root canal therapy. *Appl. Mech. Mater.* **2014**, *666*, 388–392. [CrossRef]
8. Jain, S.; Sayed, M.E.; Ibraheem, W.I.; Ageeli, A.A.; Gandhi, S.; Jokhadar, H.F.; AlResayes, S.S.; Alqarni, H.; Alshehri, A.H.; Huthan, H.M.; et al. Accuracy Comparison between Robot-Assisted Dental Implant Placement and Static/Dynamic Computer-Assisted Implant Surgery: A Systematic Review and Meta-Analysis of In Vitro Studies. *Medicina* **2024**, *60*, 11. [CrossRef] [PubMed]
9. Bellman, R. *Artificial Intelligence: Can Computers Think? Thomson Course Technology*; Boyd & Fraser: Boston, MA, USA, 1978; 146p.
10. Akst, J. A primer: Artificial intelligence versus neural networks. Inspiring Innovation. *The Scientist Exploring Life*, 1 May 2019; p. 65802.
11. Kozan, N.M.; Kotsyubynska, Y.Z.; Zelenchuk, G.M. Using the artificial neural networks for identification unknown person. *IOSR J. Dent. Med. Sci.* **2017**, *1*, 107–113.
12. Khanagar, S.B.; Al-ehaideb, A.; Maganur, P.C.; Vishwanathaiah, S.; Patil, S.; Baeshen, H.A.; Sarode, S.C.; Bhandi, S. Developments, application, and performance of artificial intelligence in dentistry—A systematic review. *J. Dent. Sci.* **2021**, *16*, 508–522. [CrossRef] [PubMed]
13. Sikka, A.; Jain, A. Sex determination of mandible: A morphological and morphometric analysis. *Int. J. Contemp. Med. Res.* **2016**, *3*, 1869–1872.
14. Kaladhar, D.; Chandana, B.; Kumar, P. Predicting Cancer Survivability Using Classification Algorithms. Books 1 View project Protein Interaction Networks in Metallo Proteins and Docking Approaches of Metallic Compounds with TIMP and MMP in Control of MAPK Pathway View project Predicting Cancer. *Int. J. Res. Rev. Comput. Sci.* **2011**, *2*, 340–343.
15. Kalappanavar, A.; Sneha, S.; Annigeri, R.G. Artificial intelligence: A dentist's perspective. *Pathol. Surg.* **2018**, *5*, 2–4. [CrossRef]
16. Krishna, A.B.; Tanveer, A.; Bhagirath, P.V.; Gannepalli, A. Role of artificial intelligence in diagnostic oral pathology-A modern approach. *J. Oral Maxillofac. Pathol.* **2020**, *24*, 152–156. [CrossRef] [PubMed]
17. Katne, T.; Kanaparthi, A.; Gotoor, S.; Muppirala, S.; Devaraju, R.; Gantala, R. Artificial intelligence: Demystifying dentistry—The future and beyond artificial intelligence: Demystifying dentistry—The future and beyond. *Int. J. Contemp. Med. Surg. Radiol.* **2019**, *4*, 4. [CrossRef]
18. Tuzoff, D.V.; Tuzova, L.N.; Bornstein, M.M.; Krasnov, A.S.; Kharchenko, M.A.; Nikolenko, S.I.; Sveshnikov, M.M.; Bednenko, G.B. Tooth detection and numbering in panoramic radiographs using convolutional neural networks. *Dentomaxillofac. Radiol.* **2019**, *48*, 20180051. [CrossRef]
19. Murata, M.; Ariji, Y.; Ohashi, Y.; Kawai, T.; Fukuda, M.; Funakoshi, T.; Kise, Y.; Nozawa, M.; Katsumata, A.; Fujita, H.; et al. Deep-learning classification using convolutional neural network for evaluation of maxillary sinusitis on panoramic radiography. *Oral Radiol.* **2019**, *35*, 301–307. [CrossRef] [PubMed]
20. Ekert, T.; Krois, J.; Meinhold, L.; Elhennawy, K.; Emara, R.; Golla, T.; Schwendicke, F. Deep Learning for the Radiographic Detection of Apical Lesions. *J. Endod.* **2019**, *45*, 917–922.e5. [CrossRef]

21. Deif, M.A.; Attar, H.; Amer, A.; Elhaty, I.A.; Khosravi, M.R.; Solyman, A.A.A. Diagnosis of Oral Squamous Cell Carcinoma Using Deep Neural Networks and Binary Particle Swarm Optimization on Histopathological Images: An AIoMT Approach. *Comput. Intell. Neurosci.* 2022, *2022*, 6364102. [CrossRef]
22. Yang, S.Y.; Li, S.H.; Liu, J.L.; Sun, X.Q.; Cen, Y.Y.; Ren, R.Y.; Ying, S.C.; Chen, Y.; Zhao, Z.H.; Liao, W. Histopathology-Based Diagnosis of Oral Squamous Cell Carcinoma Using Deep Learning. *J. Dent. Res.* 2022, *101*, 1321–1327. [CrossRef]
23. Lee, K.S.; Jung, S.K.; Ryu, J.J.; Shin, S.W.; Choi, J. Evaluation of transfer learning with deep convolutional neural networks for screening osteoporosis in dental panoramic radiographs. *J. Clin. Med.* 2020, *9*, 392. [CrossRef]
24. Saghiri, M.A.; Garcia-Godoy, F.; Gutmann, J.L.; Lotfi, M.; Asgar, K. The reliability of artificial neural network in locating minor apical foramen: A cadaver study. *J. Endod.* 2012, *38*, 1130–1134. [CrossRef] [PubMed]
25. Saghiri, M.A.; Asgar, K.; Boukani, K.K.; Lotfi, M.; Aghili, H.; Delvarani, A.; Karamifar, K.; Saghiri, A.M.; Mehrvarzfar, P.; Garcia-Godoy, F. A new approach for locating the minor apical foramen using an artificial neural network. *Int. Endod. J.* 2012, *45*, 257–265. [CrossRef] [PubMed]
26. Hatvani, J.; Horváth, A.; Michetti, J.; Basarab, A.; Kouamé, D.; Gyöngy, M. Deep learning-based super-resolution applied to dental computed tomography. *IEEE Trans. Rad. Plasma Med. Sci.* 2019, *3*, 120–128. [CrossRef]
27. Hiraiwa, T.; Ariji, Y.; Fukuda, M.; Kise, Y.; Nakata, K.; Katsumata, A.; Fujita, H.; Ariji, E. A deep-learning artificial intelligence system for assessment of root morphology of the mandibular first molar on panoramic radiography. *Dentomaxillofac. Radiol.* 2019, *48*, 20180218. [CrossRef]
28. Vila-Blanco, N.; Carreira, M.J.; Varas-Quintana, P.; Balsa-Castro, C.; Tomas, I. Deep neural networks for chronological age estimation from OPG images. *IEEE Trans. Med. Imaging* 2020, *39*, 2374–2384. [CrossRef]
29. Vishwanathaiah, S.; Fageeh, H.N.; Khanagar, S.B.; Maganur, P.C. Artificial Intelligence Its Uses and Application in Pediatric Dentistry: A Review. *Biomedicines* 2023, *11*, 788. [CrossRef]
30. Sukegawa, S.; Yoshii, K.; Hara, T.; Tanaka, F.; Yamashita, K.; Kagaya, T.; Nakano, K.; Takabatake, K.; Kawai, H.; Nagatsuka, H.; et al. Is attention branch network effective in classifying dental implants from panoramic radiograph images by deep learning? *PLoS ONE* 2022, *17*, e0269016. [CrossRef]
31. Kong, H.J.; Eom, S.H.; Yoo, J.Y.; Lee, J.H. Identification of 130 Dental Implant Types Using Ensemble Deep Learning. *Int. J. Oral Maxillofac. Implants* 2023, *38*, 150–156. [CrossRef] [PubMed]
32. Kohlakala, A.; Coetzer, J.; Bertels, J.; Vandermeulen, D. Deep learning-based dental implant recognition using synthetic X-ray images. *Med. Biol. Eng. Comput.* 2022, *60*, 2951–2968. [CrossRef]
33. Kurt Bayrakdar, S.; Orhan, K.; Bayrakdar, I.S.; Bilgir, E.; Ezhov, M.; Gusarev, M.; Shumilov, E. A deep learning approach for dental implant planning in cone-beam computed tomography images. *BMC Med. Imaging* 2021, *21*, 86. [CrossRef] [PubMed]
34. Moufti, M.A.; Trabulsi, N.; Ghousheh, M.; Fattal, T.; Ashira, A.; Danishvar, S. Developing an artificial intelligence solution to autosegment the edentulous mandibular bone for implant planning. *Eur. J. Dent.* 2023, *17*, 1330–1337. [CrossRef] [PubMed]
35. Howe, M.S.; Keys, W.; Richards, D. Long-term (10-year) dental implant survival: A systematic review and sensitivity meta-analysis. *J. Dent.* 2019, *84*, 9–21. [CrossRef] [PubMed]
36. Simonis, P.; Dufour, T.; Tenenbaum, H. Long-term implant survival and success: A 10-16-year follow-up of non-submerged dental implants. *Clin. Oral Implants Res.* 2010, *21*, 772. [CrossRef] [PubMed]
37. Romeo, E.; Lops, D.; Margutti, E.; Ghisolfi, M.; Chiapasco, M.; Vogel, G. Longterm survival and success of oral implants in the treatment of full and partial arches: A 7-year prospective study with the ITI dental implant system. *Int. J. Oral Maxillofac. Implants.* 2004, *19*, 247–249. [PubMed]
38. Papaspyridakos, P.; Mokti, M.; Chen, C.J.; Benic, G.I.; Gallucci, G.O.; Chronopoulos, V. Implant and prosthodontic survival rates with implant fixed complete dental prostheses in the edentulous mandible after at least 5 years: A systematic review. *Clin. Implant. Dent. Relat. Res.* 2014, *16*, 705–717. [CrossRef] [PubMed]
39. Jokstad, A.; Braegger, U.; Brunski, J.B.; Carr, A.B.; Naert, I.; Wennerberg, A. Quality of dental implants. *Int. Dent. J.* 2003, *53*, 409–443. [CrossRef]
40. Sailer, I.; Karasan, A.; Todorovic, A.; Ligoutsikou, M.; Pjetursson, B.E. Prosthetic failures in dental implant therapy. *Periodontol. 2000* 2022, *88*, 130–144. [CrossRef]
41. Lee, D.W.; Kim, N.H.; Lee, Y.; Oh, Y.A.; Lee, J.H.; You, H.K. Implant fracture failure rate and potential associated risk indicators: An up to 12-year retrospective study of implants in 5124 patients. *Clin. Oral Implants Res.* 2019, *30*, 206–217. [CrossRef] [PubMed]
42. Tabrizi, R.; Behnia, H.; Taherian, S.; Hesami, N. What are the incidence and factors associated with implant fracture? *J. Oral Maxillofac. Surg.* 2017, *75*, 1866–1872. [CrossRef] [PubMed]
43. Srinivasan, M.; Meyer, S.; Mombelli, A.; Müller, F. Dental implants in the elderly population: A systematic review and meta-analysis. *Clin. Oral Implants Res.* 2017, *28*, 920–930. [CrossRef]
44. Al-Wahadni, A.; Barakat, M.S.; Abu Afifeh, K.; Khader, Y. Dentists' most common practices when selecting an implant system. *J. Prosthodont.* 2018, *27*, 250–259. [CrossRef] [PubMed]
45. Tyndall, D.A.; Price, J.B.; Tetradis, S.; Ganz, S.D.; Hildebolt, C.; Scarfe, W.C.; American Academy of Oral and Maxillofacial Radiology. Position statement of the American Academy of Oral and Maxillofacial Radiology on selection criteria for the use of radiology in dental implantology with emphasis on cone beam computed tomography. *Oral Surg. Oral Med. Oral Pathol. Oral Radiol.* 2012, *113*, 817–826. [CrossRef] [PubMed]

46. Hadj Saïd, M.; Le Roux, M.K.; Catherine, J.H.; Lan, R. Development of an Artificial Intelligence Model to Identify a Dental Implant from a Radiograph. *Int. J. Oral Maxillofac. Surg.* **2020**, *36*, 1077–1082. [CrossRef]
47. Takahashi, T.; Nozaki, K.; Gonda, T.; Mameno, T.; Wada, M.; Ikebe, K. Identification of dental implants using deep learning-pilot study. *Int. J. Implant. Dent.* **2020**, *6*, 53. [CrossRef]
48. Park, W.; Huh, J.K.; Lee, J.H. Automated deep learning for classification of dental implant radiographs using a large multi-center dataset. *Sci. Rep.* **2023**, *13*, 4862. [CrossRef]
49. Da Mata Santos, R.P.; Vieira Oliveira Prado, H.E.; Soares Aranha Neto, I.; Alves de Oliveira, G.A.; Vespasiano Silva, A.I.; Zenóbio, E.G.; Manzi, F.R. Automated Identification of Dental Implants Using Artificial Intelligence. *Int. J. Oral Maxillofac. Implants* **2021**, *36*, 918–923. [CrossRef] [PubMed]
50. Sukegawa, S.; Yoshii, K.; Hara, T.; Yamashita, K.; Nakano, K.; Yamamoto, N.; Nagatsuka, H.; Furuki, Y. Deep Neural Networks for Dental Implant System Classification. *Biomolecules* **2020**, *10*, 984. [CrossRef] [PubMed]
51. Lee, J.H.; Jeong, S.N. Efficacy of deep convolutional neural network algorithm for the identification and classification of dental implant systems, using panoramic and periapical radiographs: A pilot study. *Medicine* **2020**, *99*, e20787. [CrossRef]
52. Sukegawa, S.; Yoshii, K.; Hara, T.; Matsuyama, T.; Yamashita, K.; Nakano, K.; Takabatake, K.; Kawai, H.; Nagatsuka, H.; Furuki, Y. Multi-Task Deep Learning Model for Classification of Dental Implant Brand and Treatment Stage Using Dental Panoramic Radiograph Images. *Biomolecules* **2021**, *11*, 815. [CrossRef] [PubMed]
53. Lee, J.-H.; Kim, Y.-T.; Lee, J.-B.; Jeong, S.-N. A Performance Comparison between Automated Deep Learning and Dental Professionals in Classification of Dental Implant Systems from Dental Imaging: A Multi-Center Study. *Diagnostics* **2020**, *10*, 910. [CrossRef] [PubMed]
54. Lee, D.-W.; Kim, S.-Y.; Jeong, S.-N.; Lee, J.-H. Artificial Intelligence in Fractured Dental Implant Detection and Classification: Evaluation Using Dataset from Two Dental Hospitals. *Diagnostics* **2021**, *11*, 233. [CrossRef] [PubMed]
55. Kim, J.-E.; Nam, N.-E.; Shim, J.-S.; Jung, Y.-H.; Cho, B.-H.; Hwang, J.J. Transfer Learning via Deep Neural Networks for Implant Fixture System Classification Using Periapical Radiographs. *J. Clin. Med.* **2020**, *9*, 1117. [CrossRef] [PubMed]
56. Benakatti, V.B.; Nayakar, R.P.; Anandhalli, M. Machine learning for identification of dental implant systems based on shape—A descriptive study. *J. Indian Prosthodont. Soc.* **2021**, *21*, 405–411. [CrossRef] [PubMed]
57. Jang, W.S.; Kim, S.; Yun, P.S.; Jang, H.S.; Seong, Y.W.; Yang, H.S.; Chang, J.S. Accurate detection for dental implant and peri-implant tissue by transfer learning of faster R-CNN: A diagnostic accuracy study. *BMC Oral Health* **2020**, *22*, 591. [CrossRef] [PubMed]
58. Kong, H.J. Classification of dental implant systems using cloud-based deep learning algorithm: An experimental study. *J. Yeungnam Med. Sci.* **2023**, *40* (Suppl.), S29–S36. [CrossRef] [PubMed]
59. Kim, H.S.; Ha, E.G.; Kim, Y.H.; Jeon, K.J.; Lee, C.; Han, S.S. Transfer learning in a deep convolutional neural network for implant fixture classification: A pilot study. *Imaging Sci. Dent.* **2022**, *52*, 219–224. [CrossRef] [PubMed]
60. Lee, J.H.; Kim, Y.T.; Lee, J.B.; Jeong, S.N. Deep learning improves implant classification by dental professionals: A multi-center evaluation of accuracy and efficiency. *J. Periodontal Implant Sci.* **2022**, *52*, 220–229. [CrossRef]
61. Kong, H.J.; Yoo, J.Y.; Lee, J.H.; Eom, S.H.; Kim, J.H. Performance evaluation of deep learning models for the classification and identification of dental implants. *J. Prosthet. Dent.* **2023**, in press. [CrossRef] [PubMed]
62. Park, W.; Schwendicke, F.; Krois, J.; Huh, J.K.; Lee, J.H. Identification of Dental Implant Systems Using a Large-Scale Multicenter Data Set. *J. Dent. Res.* **2023**, *102*, 727–733. [CrossRef] [PubMed]
63. Hsiao, C.Y.; Bai, H.; Ling, H.; Yang, J. Artificial Intelligence in Identifying Dental Implant Systems on Radiographs. *Int. J. Periodontics Restor. Dent.* **2023**, *43*, 363–368.
64. Moher, D.; Shamseer, L.; Clarke, M.; Ghersi, D.; Liberati, A.; Petticrew, M.; Shekelle, P.; Stewart, L.A.; PRISMA-P Group. Preferred reporting items for systematic review and meta-analysis protocols (PRISMA-P) 2015 statement. *Syst. Rev.* **2015**, *4*, 1. [CrossRef] [PubMed]
65. Whiting, P.F.; Rutjes, A.W.; Westwood, M.E.; Mallett, S.; Deeks, J.J.; Reitsma, J.B.; Leeflang, M.M.; Sterne, J.A.; Bossuyt, P.M.; QUADAS-2 Group (2011). QUADAS-2: A revised tool for the quality assessment of diagnostic accuracy studies. *Ann. Intern. Med.* **2011**, *155*, 529–536. [CrossRef] [PubMed]

Disclaimer/Publisher's Note: The statements, opinions and data contained in all publications are solely those of the individual author(s) and contributor(s) and not of MDPI and/or the editor(s). MDPI and/or the editor(s) disclaim responsibility for any injury to people or property resulting from any ideas, methods, instructions or products referred to in the content.

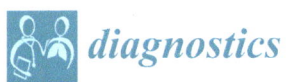

Case Report

The Stresses and Deformations in the Abfraction Lesions of the Lower Premolars Studied by the Finite Element Analyses: Case Report and Review of Literature

Bogdan Constantin Costăchel [1], Anamaria Bechir [2,*], Mihail Târcolea [3,*,†], Lelia Laurenţa Mihai [2,†], Alexandru Burcea [2,†] and Edwin Sever Bechir [4]

[1] Doctoral School in Dental Medicine, "Titu Maiorescu" University of Bucharest, 189 Calea Văcărești, 040056 Bucharest, Romania; costachel.bogdan@gmail.com
[2] Faculty of Dental Medicine, "Titu Maiorescu" University of Bucharest, 67A Gh. Petrascu Street, 031592 Bucharest, Romania; lelia_mihai2000@yahoo.com (L.L.M.); alexandru.burcea@helpdent.ro (A.B.)
[3] Faculty of Materials Science and Engineering, University Politehnica of Bucharest, 313 Splaiul Independenței, 060042 Bucharest, Romania
[4] Faculty of Dental Medicine, "George Emil Palade" University of Medicine, Pharmacy, Science, and Technology of Targu Mures, 38 Gh. Marinescu Street, 540142 Targu Mures, Romania; bechir.edwin@gmail.com
* Correspondence: anamaria.bechir@gmail.com (A.B.); mihai.tarcolea@upb.ro (M.T.)
† These authors contributed equally to this work.

Abstract: Background: The purpose of the study was to investigate the behavior of hard dental structures of the teeth with abfraction lesions when experimental occlusal loads were applied. Methods: A 65-year-old patient came to the dentist because she had painful sensitivity in the temporomandibular joints and the lower right premolars. The patient was examined, and cone-beam computed tomography (CBCT) of the orofacial area was indicated. The data provided from the CBCT were processed with Mimics Innovation Suite 17 software to create the desired anatomical area in 3D format. Then, the structural calculation module was used in order to perform a finite element analysis of the lower right premolar teeth. A focused review of articles published between 2014 and 2023 from specialty literature regarding the FEA of premolars with abfraction lesions was also conducted. Results: The parcel area and the cervical third of the analyzed premolars proved to be the most vulnerable areas under the inclined direction of occlusal loads. The inclined application of experimental loads induced 3–4 times higher maximum shears, stresses, and deformations than the axial application of the same forces. Conclusions: FEA can be used to identify structural deficiencies in teeth with abfractions, a fact that is particularly important during dental treatments to correct occlusal imbalances.

Keywords: mandibular premolars; abfraction lesions; FEA; experimental forces; evaluation

1. Introduction

The complex formed by periodontal tissues (cementum, ligaments, and bone) confers the characteristic flexibility of the tooth root in the alveolar socket, flexibility necessary for dispersing the occlusal forces [1–3]. Irreversible structural defects that are located in the cervical area at the level of the enamel–cement junction on the buccal/labial surface of the teeth are named non-carious cervical lesions (NCCLs) [4]. In the area of the enamel–cementum junction, the enamel prisms have a horizontal orientation [5]. The volume and composition of enamel and dentin contribute to the development of NCCLs [6].

The term "abfraction" nominates stress-induced NCCLs in the cervical region of the dental crowns that determine the progressive damage to mineralized dental tissues because of flexion [7,8]. Micro-fractures of hydroxyapatite (HA) crystals of enamel, cementum, and dentine thus appear in the zone of stress concentration. Abfraction lesions are located at the site of the least resistance in the cervical region, at the enamel–cementum junction [7–9].

The etiology of abfraction lesions remains disputable, and current evidence shows that the apparition of NCCLs is multifactorial, and that the degrees of tooth hard tissue vary and may differ from patient to patient [7,10–13]. Correct diagnosis and treatment decisions require in-depth knowledge regarding the multifactorial etiological conditions of abfraction lesions. The therapeutic possibilities for these lesions currently vary; therefore, clinicians need to be informed regarding the major etiological factors and the clinical particularities that differentiate them [7,14].

Computational modeling is a computer-based method that studies the behavior of complex systems through computer simulations. It can be used to resolve mathematical models that characterize physical phenomena but also to make predictions of the system's behavior under different conditions [15,16]. Finite element analysis (FEA) is a numerical technique that slices the structure of the analyzed object into several elements; later, the elements are reconnected at points called nodes [17]. FEA has reformed scientific modeling in engineering methods and can also be used in the analysis of the components of the orofacial system [18–22].

The detection of non-carious abfraction lesions in the cervical area of dental hard tissues by the clinician is an alarm signal that can predict the patient's need for occlusal balancing therapy in the future. The originality of this study consists in carrying out an experimental FEA study (which is a non-invasive repeatable method that does not require the presence of the patient, realized in accordance with data from the patient's CBCT), and determining how the obtained results can represent a first step in the phasing of the dental treatment applied by the clinician to patients with abfraction lesions. Later, various occlusion analysis systems can be used to record detailed data regarding the existence of excessive occlusal forces (including the use of a T-Scan digital device), but these types of analyses can only be performed in the presence of the patient. The aim of the present study was to assess, using FEA, the behavior of hard dental tissues at the level of the lower premolar with abfraction under perpendicular and 45-degree inclined experimental forces.

2. Case Description

A 65-year-old female patient came to the dental practice for the treatment of dental pain. The patient complained of dental sensitivity to cold, hot, sweet, and sour agents in the lower right premolar area. Anamnesis revealed that the patient was not under treatment for chronic diseases. According to what was stated in the anamnesis, the patient had not previously undergone orthodontic treatments and had no traumatic injury. The patient also complained of the signs and symptoms of bruxism (teeth grinding or clenching loud enough to wake up the sleep partner, jaw and face soreness, tired or tight jaw muscles, and a dull headache in the temporal area). The patient declared that she did not drink fruit juices and other acidic drinks, that she has no digestive diseases (reflux and/or vomiting), that she uses a soft-bristled toothbrush and toothpaste containing fluoride, that her teeth are brushed gently, and that she does not wear a mouth guard or occlusal splint.

During the extraoral examination, it was observed that the masseter muscles presented with hypertonicity, especially on the left side, and painful sensitivity in the temple area.

The intraoral examination revealed that the patient presented with multiple simple odontal lesions that were partially treated, correctly and incorrectly. A simple carious lesion affected the right upper first premolar (1.4) (Figure 1). Wear areas were also observed in the incisal and occlusal regions of the right lower canine and premolars, as well as abfractions, with exposed dentine, located in the buccal cervical zone of the mandibular right premolars. The aspect of abfractions was mixed-shaped (wedge and saucer), located in enamel and dentine, without prepared cavities, and without any bacterial deposits. The abfraction lesions were 1.2 mm in depth. The most commonly used index that categorizes tooth wear in the cervical region is the Tooth Wear Index by Smith and Knight [23]. The abfraction lesions of the lower right premolars were determined to be 3rd class (defects ranging from 1 to 2 mm deep).

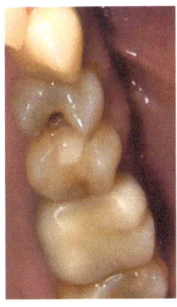 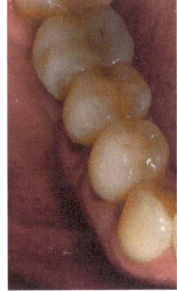 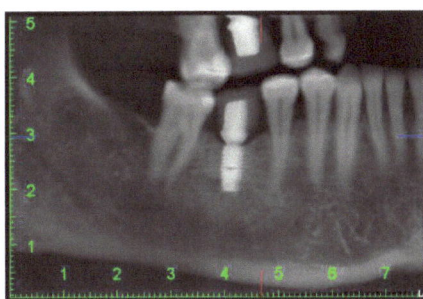

Figure 1. Intraoral aspects and CBCT image of patient.

The cervical margin of the patient's abfraction lesions were located at the level of the free gingival margin. No gingival recessions were detected at the level of the cervical area of the two premolars. During the anamnesis and the clinical examination of the patient as well as later during the treatment and monitoring, no changes of periodontal tissues were detected (e.g., inflammation, gingival bleeding, the apparition of periodontal pockets, or dental mobility).

These mandibular right premolars presented with painful tooth sensitivity. The teeth appeal revealed the absence of 1.8, 1.6, 2.6, 3.5, 3.6, 4.6, and 4.8 teeth (after the FDI two-digit notation system). Cone-beam computed tomography (CBCT) of the orofacial area was indicated as a complementary examination. The patient's missing teeth were already prosthodontically rehabilitated when she came to the dentist, through dental implants. She told us that these were short Bicon dental implants (facts confirmed by analysis of the CBCT images) with the superstructure made of hybrid ceramics.

After the professional prophylactic cleaning of both dental arches, the patient was trained regarding the proper toothbrushing technique in order to abolish any eventual horizontal movements with excessive force during toothbrushing.

The specific dental treatment started with the desensitization of abfraction areas (with GLUMA desensitizer, KulzerGmbH, Mitsui chemical group, Hanau, Germany) and the manufacturing of a thermoformed polyethylene occlusal mouth guard (of Sof-Tray Sheets, Ultradent Products Inc., South Jordan, UT, USA). The mouth guard had a thickness of 1.5 mm and was inserted on the lower dental arch. The patient was instructed on how to use the mouth guard to control the bruxism parafunction.

3. Finite Element Analysis (FEA) of Mandibular Right Premolars

The data provided by the CBCT were also used for performing the finite element analysis (FEA).

The FEM analysis in the presented case represented the first step in clarifying the stages of applied dental treatment in future sessions, especially since these experimental studies did not require the presence of the patient. By performing finite element analysis (FEA), it was possible to identify the harmful direction of forces as well as the actual and future structural deficiencies in the lower right premolar teeth with abfractions.

To carry out the numerical analyses, we selected the clinical case of a 65-year-old patient who presented with abfractions at the level of the lower right premolar group. The patient underwent a CBCT at an imaging center, and the information provided by the computed tomography was processed with dedicated software and subsequently subjected to finite element analysis. The processing of the information provided by CBCT, and the numerical study, were carried out at the University POLITEHNICA of Bucharest.

Tomographic information was imported into the software package Mimics Innovation Suite 17, © Materialise NV. It has two components: Mimics and 3-matic. In Mimics, information from the CBCT was read in axial incidence whereupon the program immediately calculated the other two incidences, coronal and sagittal. The area of interest in the study was selected by applying the filters corresponding to predefined areas of Hounsfield units (grayscale masks). The mask was limited in its expansion by cropping. The desired anatomical area was created in a 3D format (Figure 2).

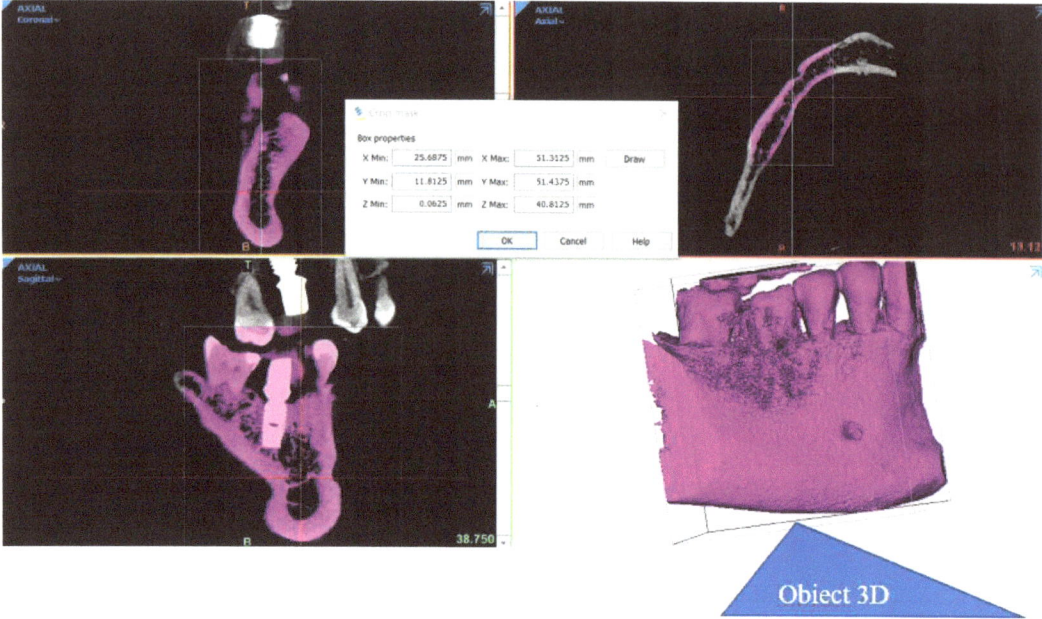

Figure 2. The stages in obtaining the desired anatomical area in 3D format.

From the desired anatomical zone, the area of interest for the study was delimited through specific sectioning operations in order to be able to analyze the region of the two premolars affected by abfraction (Figure 3a,b).

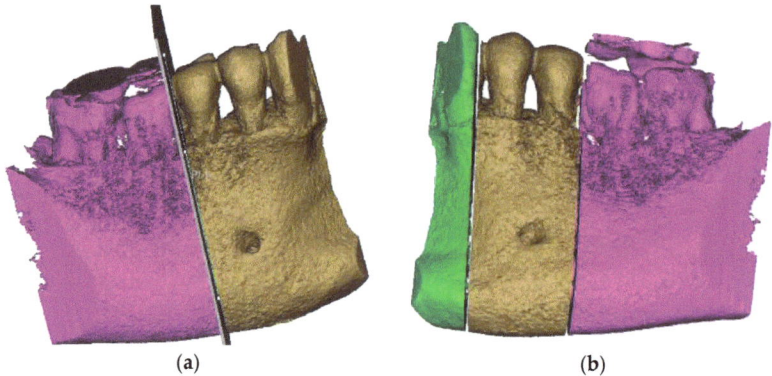

Figure 3. Sections to preserve the area of interest: (**a**) distal section; and (**b**) mesial section.

By replicating the "crop" function, we managed to isolate the area of interest, where the presence of the abfraction at the bundle level is visible on the buccal faces of the two premolars (Figure 4a). The phenomenon is similar to the compression cracking produced in the case of cold plastic deformation of metallic materials (Figure 4b). The "editing" of the premolars is a laborious operation in the case of processing images obtained from CBCT.

The Mimics program is being developed for studies based on images without artifacts. The elimination of artifacts (Figure 4c) was effectuated "pixel by pixel" on each slice of the tomography.

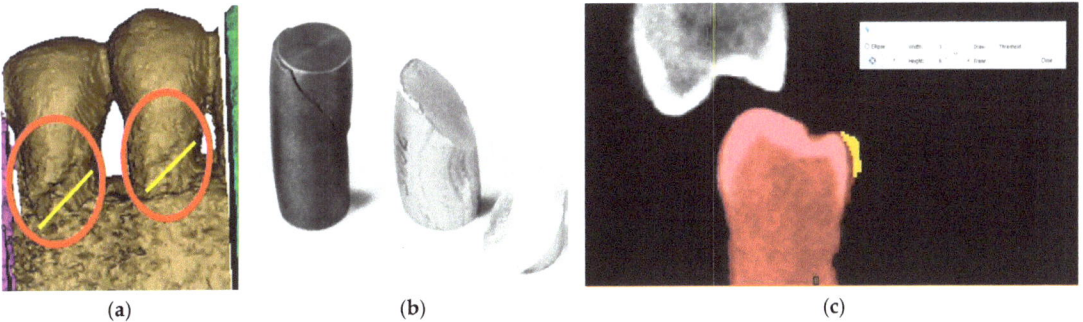

Figure 4. (**a**) Highlighting of abfraction areas; (**b**) compression fracture for cast iron and aluminum: "classic" fracture surface at 45°; and (**c**) selecting artifacts for removal.

After the complete separation of the area of interest from possible artifacts, the data obtained with Mimics was further processed in 3-matic, the second component of the suite (Figure 5a). In 3-D, the anatomical components of interest were separated step by step so that, finally, the premolars were visualized as separate 3D objects (Figure 5b). To reach this stage, for each of the three objects (mandible, first and second premolar), we need to go through several stages of "repairing" their surfaces to be able to move from an external surface to 3D objects with volumetric consistency, which allows performing complex mechanical analyses with finite elements. It can be seen that the 2nd premolar presents a more extensive area of abfraction in surface and depth, which is why all calculations were subsequently performed only on this anatomical element. To perform a relevant analysis, cementum and enamel were separated in Mimics. This was done using density filtering of the original CBCT information (Hounsfield units), and then separate 3D objects were generated (Figure 5c).

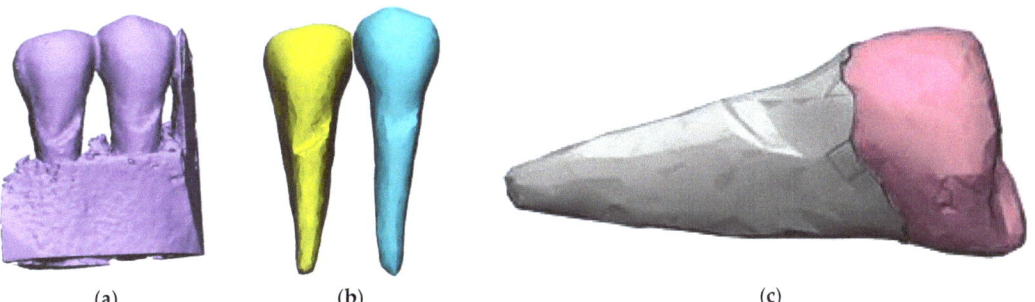

Figure 5. (**a**) Introducing data into 3-matic; (**b**) the steps for separating the anatomical components of interest in the 3-matrix; and (**c**) separation of cementum from enamel.

After the stage of obtaining an error-free 3D object, the recalculation of the triangulation mesh follows in order to move from the triangles that define the outer contour to tetrahedral elements through which the outer contour acquires an inner, volumetric "consistency". The recalculation of the triangle mesh can be conducted in several ways, and it is even possible to reduce the number of tetrahedral elements to reduce the duration of the numerical calculation procedures. Figure 6a shows the situation after recalculation with a gradient mesh (procedure called gradient remesh). If the previous steps have gone correctly, the creation of the volumetric mesh can proceed (Figure 6b), and if the volumetric meshes has been calculated successfully, the anatomical objects processed in this way can be exported to numerical analysis programs with finite elements, in this case ANSYS © ANSYS Inc. (Houston, TX, USA) (Figure 6c).

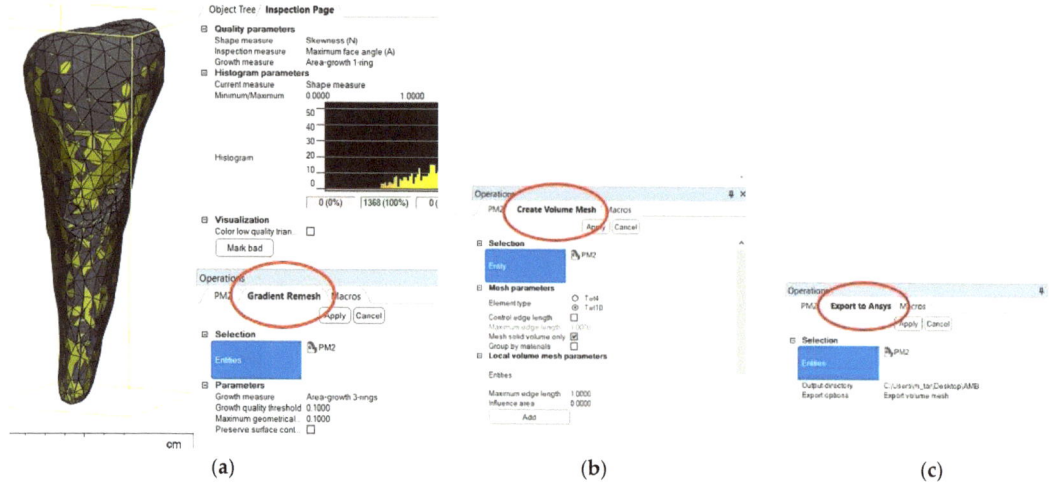

Figure 6. (**a**) Gradient remesh procedure; (**b**) creating the volumetric network; and (**c**) volumetric mesh export in ANSYS.

After importing the volumetric meshes into ANSYS, the structure of the module was selected for calculating the effects of the applied stress (Figure 7).

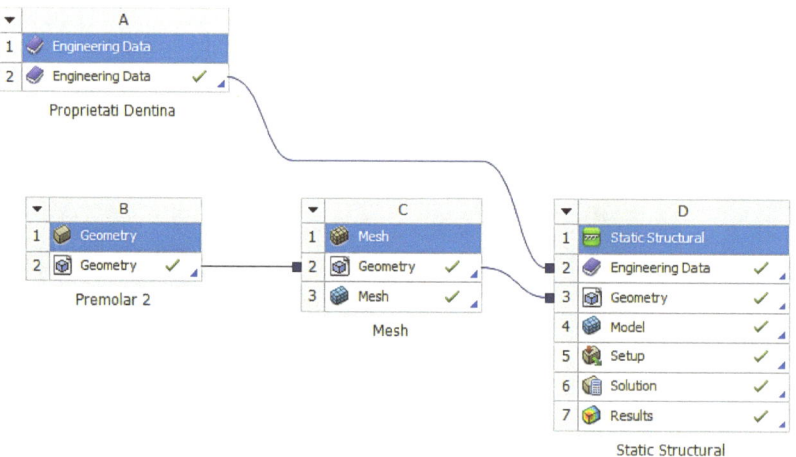

Figure 7. The structure of the module for calculating the effects of applied stress.

In the analyzed case, we selected the Static Structural calculation mode, within which the objects that, through their geometry, constitute the model and the properties of the materials involved in the calculations (Engineering Data) were defined. Next, the definition of the Support (support of the volumetric element) and the means of applying mechanical stress (Force) were determined. In the Solution section, the mechanical elements that required calculation by FEA were determined. The adjacent diagram shows the requirements. Then, the program started to find results in the Solution section. In the case of the second premolar, the support area A inside the alveolus (blue area) and the area B for applying the pressure force to the occlusal surface (red areas) were defined (Figure 8).

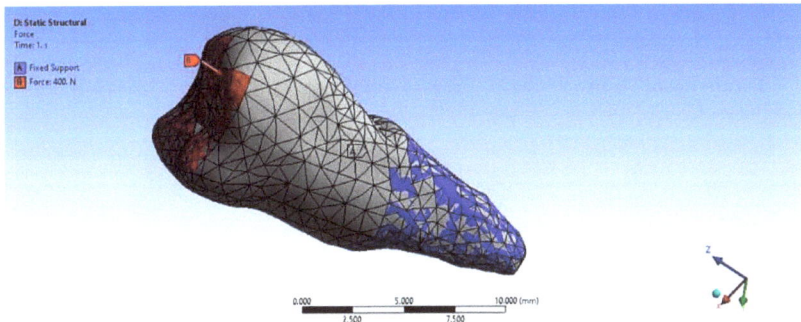

Figure 8. Definition of support area and force application areas.

In the Engineering Data (Figure 9), the material constants characterizing the tooth required for performing the analysis with finite elements were entered. A force of 400 N at 35 °C was used in two positioning variants: perpendicular to the tooth crown and inclined at 45°, to simulate mastication (the first variant) and stress due to bruxism (the second variant).

	A	B	C
1	Property	Value	Unit
2	Material Field Variables	Table	
3	Isotropic Elasticity		
4	Derive from	Young's Mod...	
5	Young's Modulus	1.961E+04	MPa
6	Poisson's Ratio	0.31	
7	Bulk Modulus	1.72E+10	Pa
8	Shear Modulus	7.486E+09	Pa
9	Tensile Ultimate Strength	90	MPa
10	Compressive Ultimate Strength	300	MPa

Figure 9. Material constants used in calculations.

The elastic properties of cementum and enamel, entered into the software to perform the numerical simulations, are presented in Table 1.

Table 1. Elastic properties of dental cement and enamel.

	Elastic Properties of Cement	Elastic Properties of Enamel
Young's modulus, MPa	18,600	84,000
Poisson's ratio	0.31	0.3
Global Modulus, MPa	16.316	70.000
Transverse Modulus, MPa	7099.2	32.308

Table 2 shows the characteristics of the two meshes (enamel and cement).

Table 2. Characteristics of dental components.

Material	Condition	Statistics	
		Nodes	Elements
Cement	Built mesh	2685	1402
Enamel		2578	1316

Figure 10 shows the enamel–cement assembly, the two layers that cover the crown and the root.

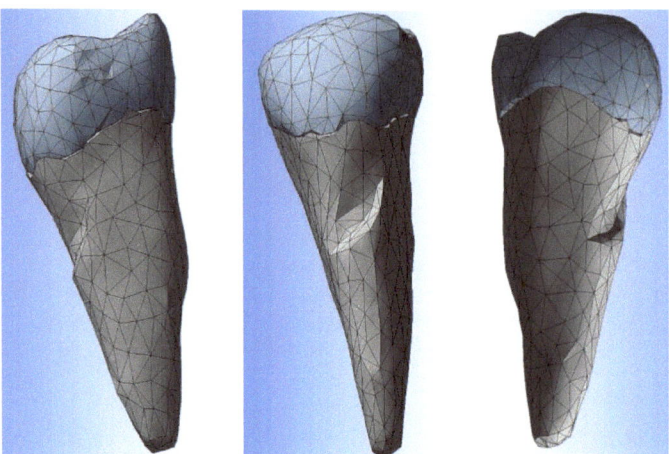

Figure 10. Enamel–cement assembly.

Figure 11 shows the application of the experimental force perpendicular to the occlusal surface. Figure 12 presents the applying of the inclined force. In both figures, the root zone where the support in the alveolus was defined is marked in blue.

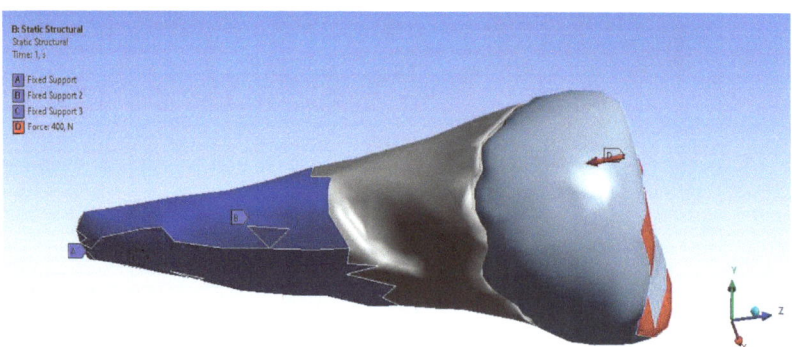

Figure 11. The force applied perpendicular to the occlusal surface and the support in the alveolus.

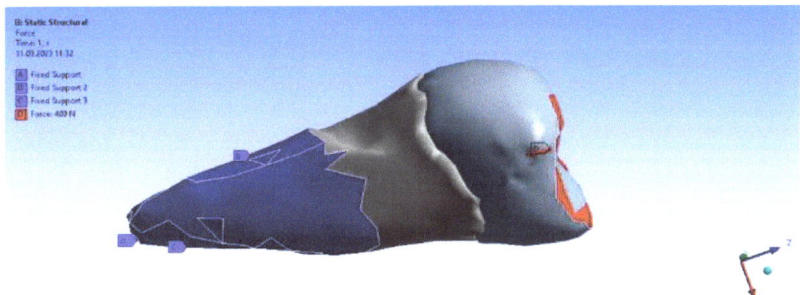

Figure 12. The force applied at an angle and the support in the alveolus.

Table 3 present the distribution of the experimental forces applied perpendicularly and inclined at 45° on the 3 axes OX, OY, and OZ.

Table 3. The distribution of the applied experimental perpendicular load and 45° load.

Experimental Load Applied Perpendicularly		Experimental Load Applied Inclined at 45°	
Type	Load	Type	Load
X component	−78 N (slope)	X component	−55 N (slope)
Y component	−78 N (slope)	Y component	−253 N (slope)
Z component	−385 N (slope)	Z component	−305 N (slope)
Resultant	400 N	Resultant	400 N

Tables 4 and 5 show the centralized maximum and minimum values of the stresses and deformations produced as a result of the experimental solicitations applied perpendicularly and at a 45° inclination to the occlusal surface of the premolar.

Table 4. Results obtained from the solicitation applied perpendicular to the occlusal surface.

	Total Deformation	Deformation in X Direction	Deformation in Y Direction	Deformation in Z Direction	Equivalent Stress	Normal Stress X	Normal Stress Y	Normal Stress Z	Maximum Main Stress	Minimum Main Stress	Tangential Stress XY	Tangential Stress YZ	Tangential Stress XZ
Minimum	0 mm	-4.24×10^{-3} mm	-2.52×10^{-2} mm	-1.56×10^{-2} mm	1.01×10^{-6} MPa	-35.6 MPa	-57.1 MPa	-104 MPa	-15.2 MPa	-152 MPa	-43.7 MPa	-39.6 MPa	-56.3 MPa
Maximum	2.77×10^{-2} mm	3.57×10^{-3} mm	6.98×10^{-4} mm	4.78×10^{-3} mm	248 MPa	61.5 MPa	177 MPa	72.2 MPa	195 MPa	21.4 MPa	44.2 MPa	117 MPa	22.2 MPa
Minim. in	Cementum	Cementum	Enamel	Enamel	Cementum	Cementum	Enamel	Enamel	Enamel	Cementum	Enamel	Enamel	Cementum
Maxim. in	Cementum	Enamel	Enamel	Enamel	Cementum	Enamel	Enamel	Enamel	Enamel	Enamel	Cementum	Cementum	Cementum

	Maximum Tangential Stress	Main Elastic Relative Deformation	Main Maximum Elastic Relative Deformation	Main Minimum Elastic Relative Deformation	Maximum Tangential Elastic Relative Deformation	Relative elastic Normal X Deformation	Relative Elastic Normal Y Deformation	Relative Elastic Normal Z Deformation	Relative Elastic Tangential XY Deformation	Relative Elastic Tangential YZ Deformation	Relative Elastic Tangential XZ Deformation
Minimum	5.4×10^{-7} MPa	6.36×10^{-11} mm/mm	-1.33×10^{-5} mm/mm	-1.05×10^{-2} mm/mm	7.6×10^{-11} mm/mm	-2.26×10^{-3} mm/mm	-1.43×10^{-3} mm/mm	-3.45×10^{-3} mm/mm	-2.81×10^{-3} mm/mm	-4.09×10^{-3} mm/mm	-7.93×10^{-3} mm/mm
Maximum	143 MPa	1.33×10^{-2} mm/mm	9.66×10^{-3} mm/mm	1.09×10^{-5} mm/mm	2.01×10^{-2} mm/mm	1.37×10^{-3} mm/mm	1.89×10^{-3} mm/mm	3.14×10^{-3} mm/mm	6.23×10^{-3} mm/mm	1.65×10^{-2} mm/mm	3.13×10^{-3} mm/mm
Minim. in	Cementum	Cementum	Enamel	Cementum	Cementum	Cementum	Cementum	Cementum	Cementum	Cementum	Cementum
Maxim. in	Cementum	Cementum	Cementum	Enamel	Cementum	Cementum	Cementum	Enamel	Cementum	Cementum	Cementum

Table 5. Results obtained from the solicitation applied at 45° to the occlusal surface.

	Total Deformation	Deformation in X Direction	Deformation in Y Direction	Deformation in Z Direction	Equivalent Stress	Normal Stress X	Normal Stress Y	Normal Stress Z	Maximum Main Stress	Minimum Main Stress	Tangential Stress XY	Tangential Stress YZ	Tangential Stress XZ
Minimum	0 mm	-6.1×10^{-3} mm	-9.02×10^{-2} mm	-3.99×10^{-2} mm	1.02×10^{-6} MPa	-112 MPa	-199 MPa	-278 MPa	-65.5 MPa	-470 MPa	-148 MPa	-176 MPa	-178 MPa
Maximum	9.28×10^{-2} mm	1.83×10^{-2} mm	1.38×10^{-3} mm	3.12×10^{-2} mm	780 MPa	61.5 MPa	649 MPa	304 MPa	704 MPa	73.8 MPa	134 MPa	370 MPa	78.6 MPa
Minim. in	Cementum	Cementum	Enamel	Enamel	Cementum	Cementum	Enamel	Enamel	Enamel	Enamel	Cementum	Enamel	Cementum
Maxim. in	Enamel	Enamel	Cementum	Enamel	Cementum	Enamel	Enamel	Enamel	Enamel	Enamel	Cementum	Cementum	Cementum

	Maximum Tangential Stress	Main Elastic Relative Deformation	Main Maximum Elastic Relative Deformation	Main Minimum Elastic Relative Deformation	Maximum Tangential Elastic Relative Deformation	Relative Elastic in Normal X Deformation	Relative Elastic in Normal Y Deformation	Relative Elastic in Normal Z Deformation	Relative Elastic Tangential XY Deformation	Relative Elastic Tangential YZ Deformation	Relative Elastic Tangential XZ Deformation
Minimum	5.45×10^{-7} MPa	6.42×10^{-11} mm/mm	-1.31×10^{-5} mm/mm	-3.26×10^{-2} mm/mm	7.68×10^{-11} mm/mm	-7.42×10^{-3} mm/mm	-5.42×10^{-3} mm/mm	-7.58×10^{-3} mm/mm	-6.29×10^{-3} mm/mm	-9.77×10^{-3} mm/mm	-2.51×10^{-2} mm/mm
Maximum	450 MPa	4.19×10^{-2} mm/mm	3.08×10^{-2} mm/mm	7.02×10^{-5} mm/mm	6.34×10^{-2} mm/mm	4.72×10^{-3} mm/mm	6.75×10^{-3} mm/mm	9.91×10^{-3} mm/mm	1.88×10^{-2} mm/mm	5.21×10^{-2} mm/mm	1.11×10^{-3} mm/mm
Minim. in	Cementum	Cementum	Enamel	Cementum	Cementum	Cementum	Cementum	Cementum	Cementum	Cementum	Cementum
Maxim. in	Cementum	Cementum	Cementum	Enamel	Cementum	Cementum	Cementum	Enamel	Cementum	Cementum	Cementum

The total deformation (Figure 13a,b) is apparently distributed similarly regardless of the direction of the experimental forces, except when the perpendicular forces are applied, when a value approximately three times than the effect produced after the inclined application of force is observed.

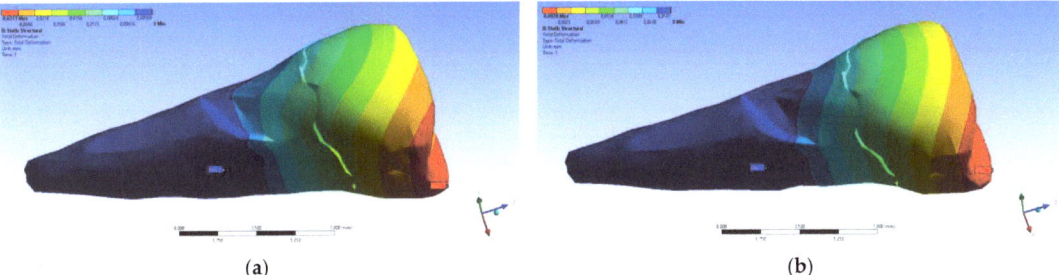

Figure 13. (**a**) The total deformation when the experimental force is applied perpendicular to the occlusal surface; and (**b**) the total deformation when the experimental force is applied at 45° on the occlusal surface.

A small contraction ($\sim -2 \times 10^{-3}$ mm) was recorded in the X direction (Figures 14 and 15) in the area bordering the abfraction. If the greatest contraction is manifested buccally at the enamel–cementum junction and lingually in the coronal region, a low elongation occurs ($\sim 3 \times 10^{-4}$ mm).

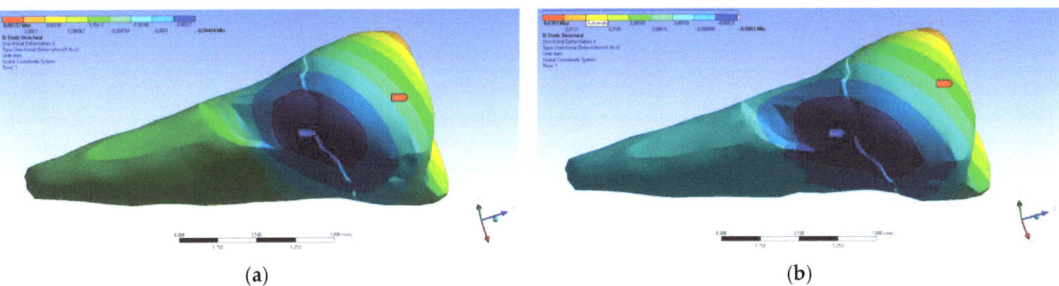

Figure 14. Deformation in the X direction when the experimental force is applied perpendicular to the occlusal surface: (**a**) mesio-buccal aspect; and (**b**) buccal aspect.

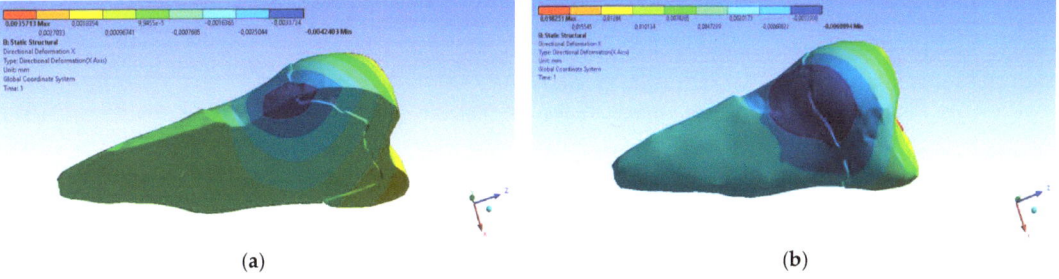

Figure 15. *Cont.*

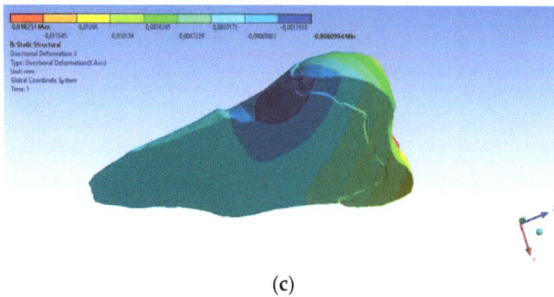

(c)

Figure 15. Deformation in the X direction when the experimental force is applied at 45° on the occlusal surface: (**a**) bucco-lingual section; (**b**) mesio-buccal aspect; and (**c**) mesio-buccal section.

As for the deformation in the Y direction, the behavior was similar (Figures 16 and 17), but it was found that the inclination of the force causes 3–4 times larger deformations.

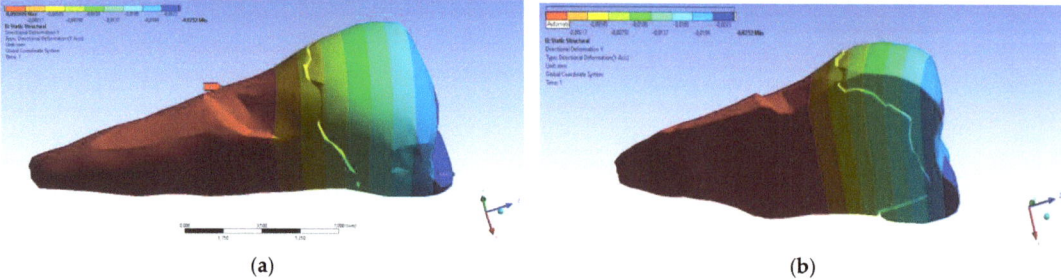

Figure 16. Deformation in the Y direction when a perpendicular experimental force is applied to the occlusal surface: (**a**) mesio-buccal aspect; and (**b**) section.

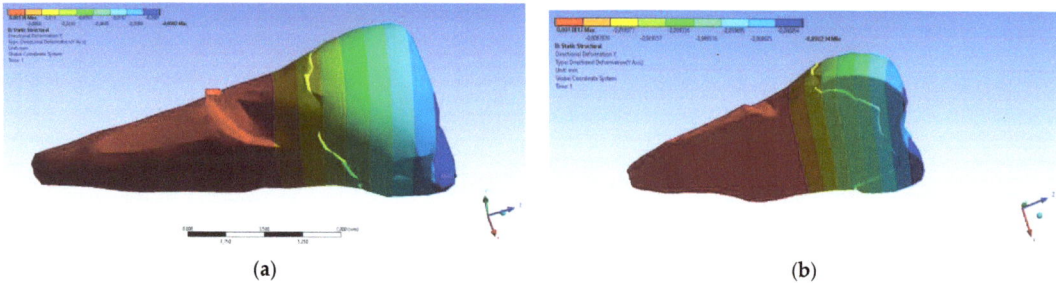

Figure 17. Deformation in the Y direction when a 45° experimental force is applied on the occlusal surface: (**a**) mesio-buccal aspect; and (**b**) section.

In the Z direction (Figures 18 and 19), the deformation was also greater in the case of a 45° angle in the experimental force direction on the occlusal surface.

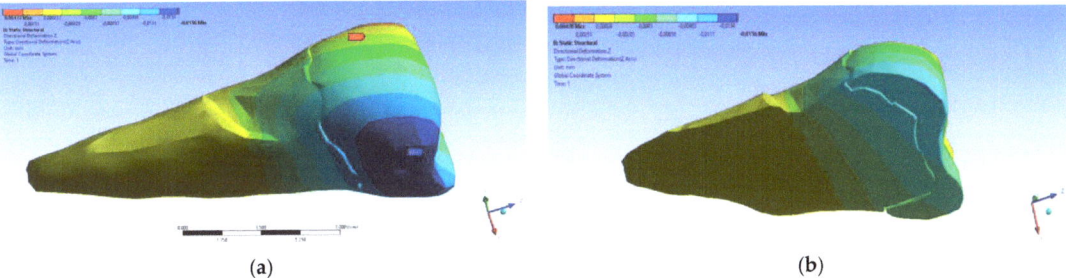

Figure 18. Deformation in the Z direction when the experimental force is applied perpendicular to the occlusal surface: (**a**) mesio-buccal aspect; and (**b**) section.

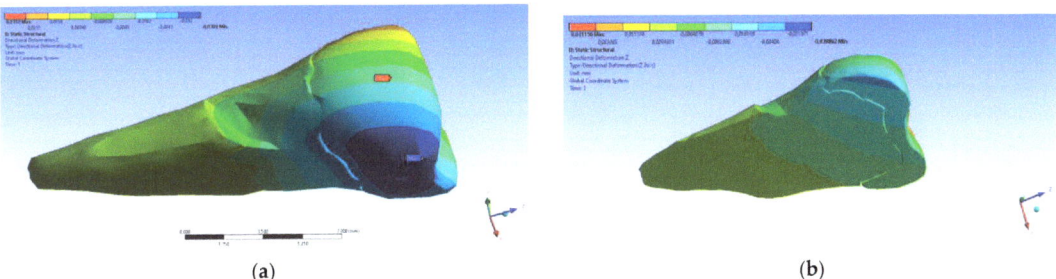

Figure 19. Deformation in the Z direction when the 45° experimental force is applied on the occlusal surface: (**a**) mesio-buccal aspect; and (**b**) section.

In the case of perpendicular force application, the affected area of the abfraction lesion manifested relatively moderate values of the equivalent stress (80 MPa) (visible in Figure 20a). Higher maximum stresses (~3 times) developed in the case of inclined force application (Figure 20b), but it can be seen that the stress transmission was only superficial.

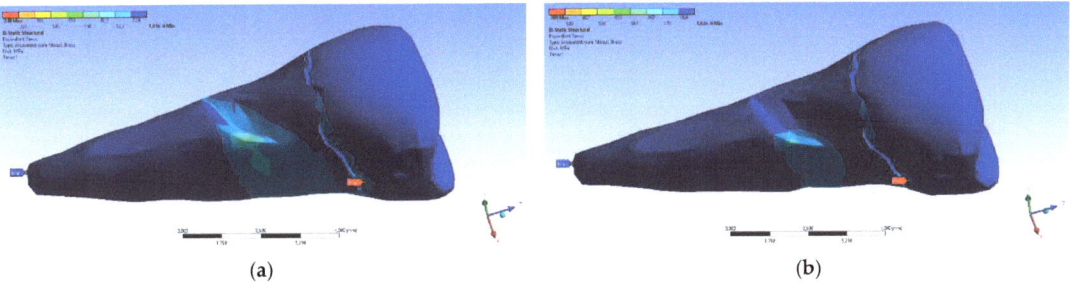

Figure 20. Equivalent stress when the experimental force is applied: (**a**) perpendicular to the occlusal surface (mesio-buccal aspect); and (**b**) at 45° on the occlusal surface (section).

On the lower flank of the abfraction area, a normal compressive stress on the X axis appears, with a value of -35.6 MPa, visible in Figure 21a,b. An almost similar situation, but with stresses that were three times higher, occurred in the case of the inclined force application (Figure 22a,b).

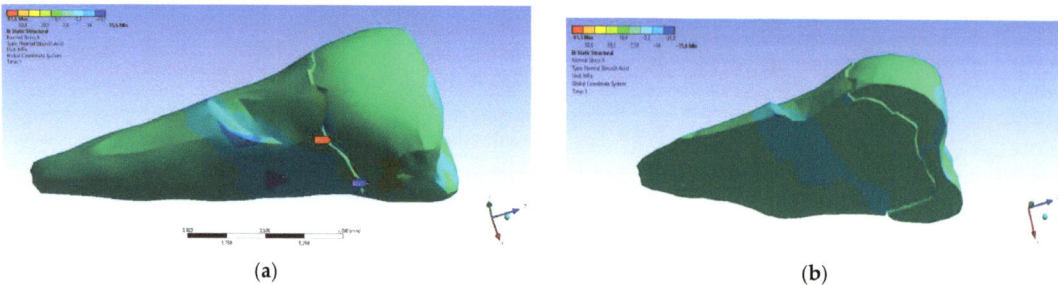

Figure 21. Localizations of normal stress X when a perpendicular experimental force is applied on the occlusal surface: (**a**) mesio-buccal aspect; and (**b**) section.

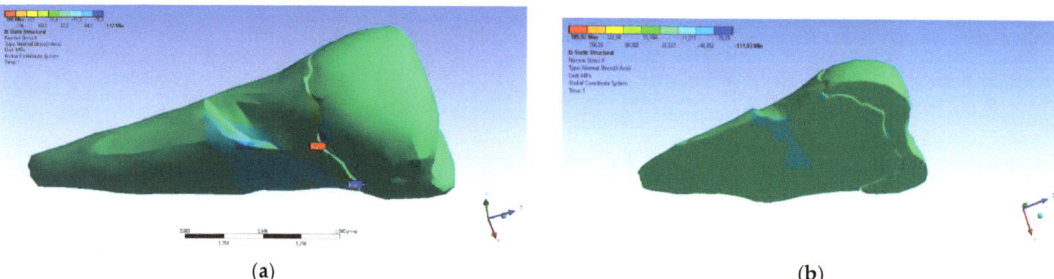

Figure 22. Localizations of normal stress X when an experimental force at 45° is applied on the occlusal surface: (**a**) mesio-buccal aspect; and (**b**) section.

In the Y direction, relatively high compressive stresses (~−20 MPa) appeared in the parcel area, which also propagated to the section of the affected area. The recorded values were 3–4 times higher when the force was applied in an inclined direction (Figures 23 and 24).

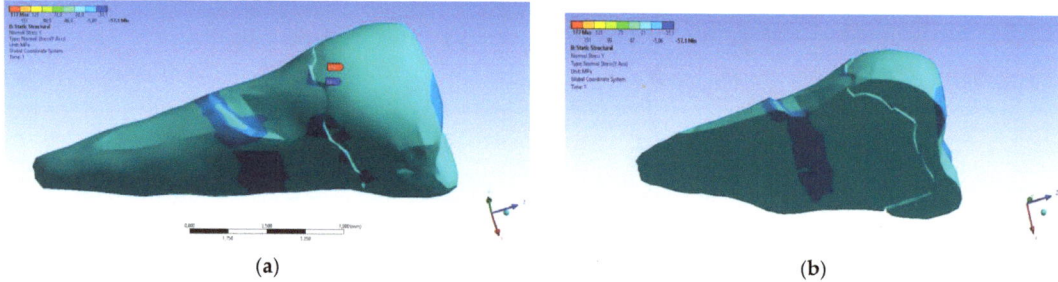

Figure 23. Localizations of normal stress Y when a perpendicular experimental force is applied on the occlusal surface: (**a**) mesio-buccal aspect; and (**b**) section.

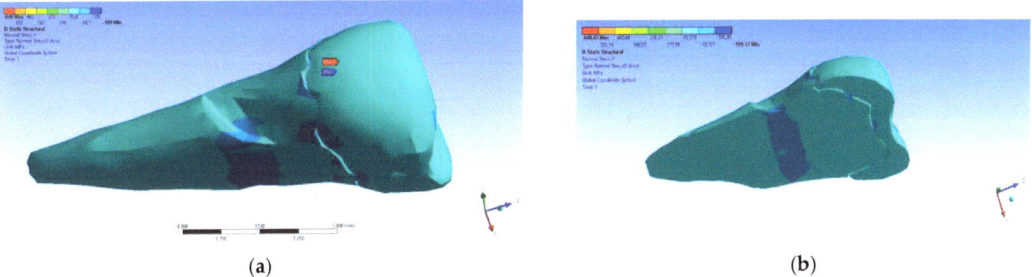

(a)   (b)

Figure 24. Localizations of normal stress Y when an experimental force is applied at 45° on the occlusal surface: (**a**) mesio-buccal aspect; and (**b**) section.

In the Z direction, the same tendency was maintained (Figure 25).

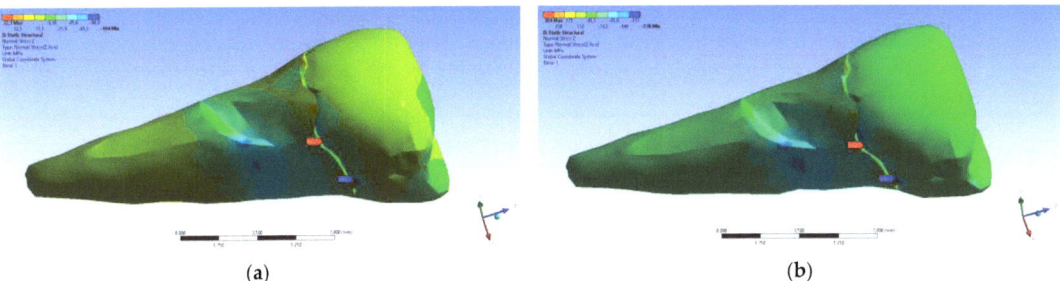

(a)   (b)

Figure 25. Localizations of normal stress Z when experimental forces are applied to the occlusal surface: (**a**) perpendicular forces (mesio-buccal aspect); and (**b**) a 45° force is applied to the occlusal surface (aspect).

The maximum principal stress registered maximum values in the package area, both when the experimental force was applied perpendicular to the occlusal surface (Figure 26a) and when it was applied at an angle of 45° (Figure 26b).

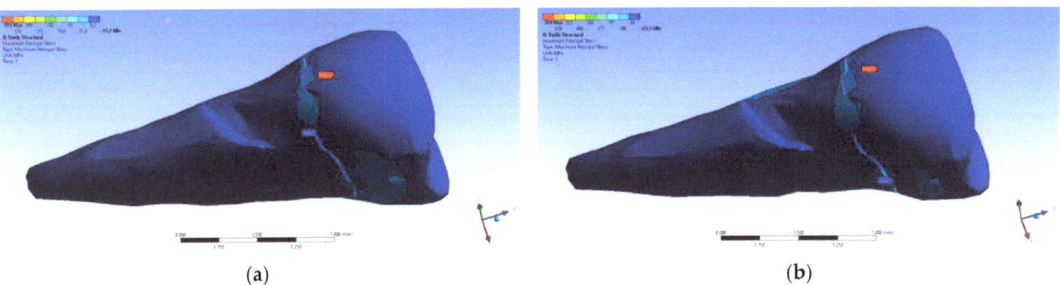

(a)   (b)

Figure 26. Mesio-buccal aspect of maximum principal stress when experimental force is applied to the occlusal surface: (**a**) perpendicularly; and (**b**) at 45°.

If, in the apical 2/3 of the root and in the coronal area of the tooth, the minimum main stresses were tensile around the abfraction zone, when the applied experimental force was perpendicular to the occlusal surface, in the cervical 1/3 of the root, these stresses changed and became compressive, as depicted in Figure 27a. In accordance with previous observations, the behavior was similar when a 45° experimental force was applied to the occlusal surface, like in Figure 27b.

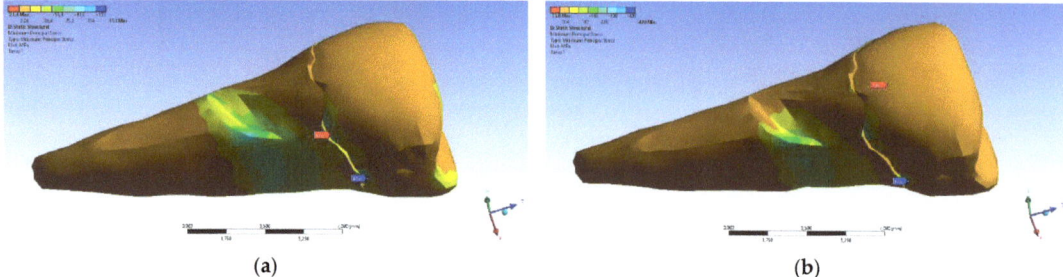

Figure 27. Maximum principal stress when experimental forces are applied to the occlusal surface: (**a**) perpendicularly; and (**b**) at 45°.

The tangential stresses in the XY, YZ, and XZ directions were manifested in the same way on the higher values, corresponding to the inclined application of the forces (Figures 28 and 29).

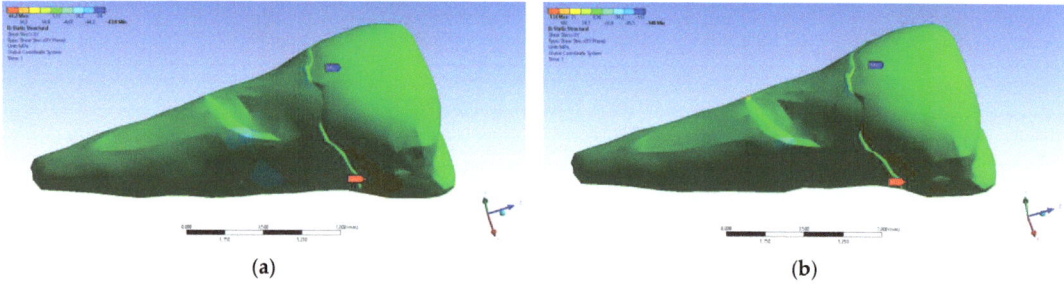

Figure 28. Mesio-buccal aspect of tangential tension XY when the experimental force is applied to the occlusal surface: (**a**) perpendicularly; and (**b**) at 45°.

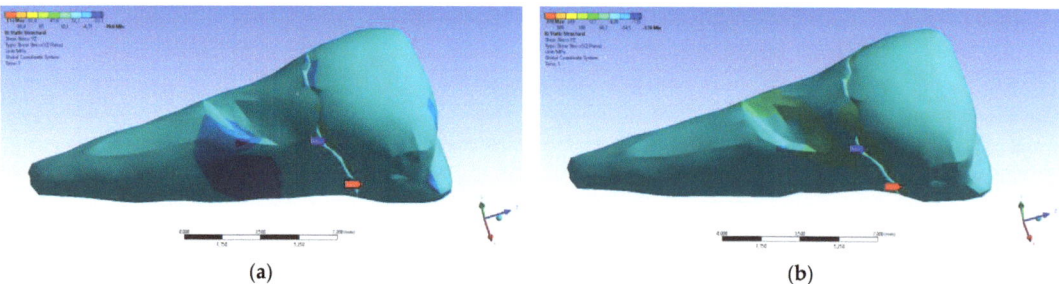

Figure 29. Mesio-buccal aspect of tangential tension YZ when the experimental force is applied to the occlusal surface: (**a**) perpendicularly; (**b**) at 45°.

The tangential stresses in the YZ plane were compressive (~−20 MPa), while the rest of the tooth was predominantly subjected to slightly higher but tensile stresses. Moderate compressive stresses were manifested in the XZ plane, but also precisely in the affected area (Figure 30).

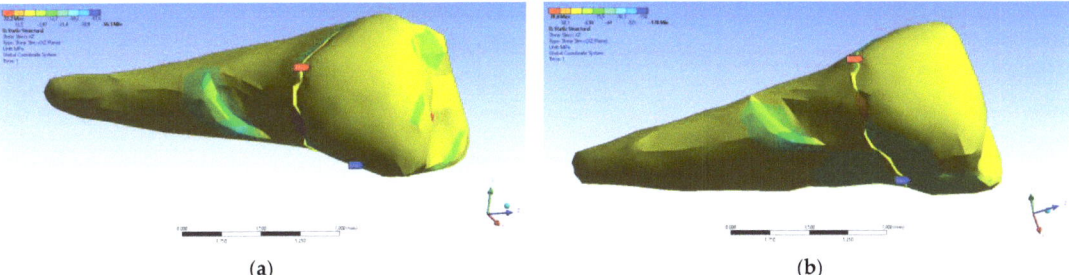

(a) (b)

Figure 30. Mesio-buccal aspect of tangential tension XZ when the experimental force is applied to the occlusal surface: (**a**) perpendicularly; and (**b**) at 45°.

Figure 31 presents the mesio-buccal aspects of the maximum tangential stress when the experimental force was applied to the occlusal surface perpendicularly (a) and at 45° (b). The developed maximum tangential stress was tensile, and in the affected area it had a moderate value.

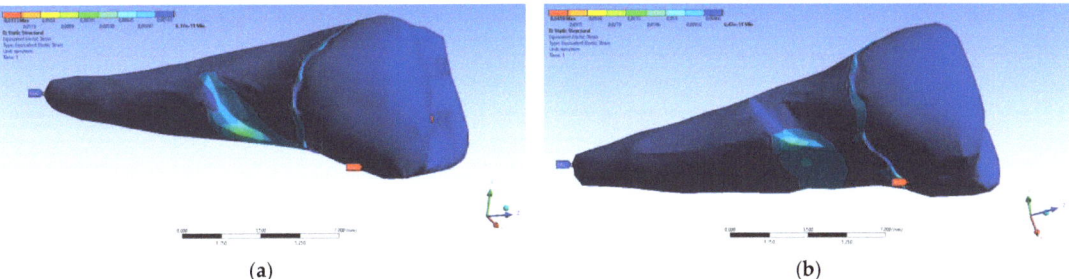

(a) (b)

Figure 31. Mesio-buccal aspects of the maximum shear elastic strain when applying the experimental force to the occlusal surface: (**a**) perpendicularly; (**b**) in 45°.

When determining elastic relative deformation (Figure 32a,b), normal elastic relative deformation X (Figure 33a,b), Y (Figure 34a,b), Z (Figure 35a,b), the relative tangential elastic deformation XY (Figure 36a,b), YZ (Figure 37a,b) and XZ (Figure 38a,b), the cervical third of the root around the abfraction area always behaves differently than the other areas of the tooth.

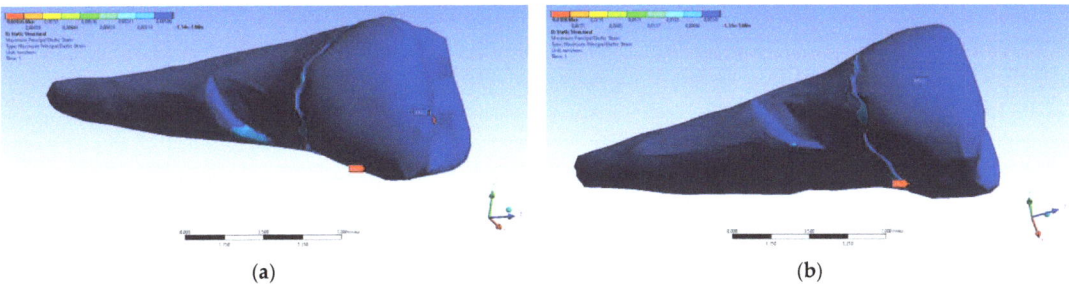

(a) (b)

Figure 32. Mesio-buccal aspects of the maximum principal elastic strain when applying the experimental force to the occlusal surface: (**a**) perpendicularly; and (**b**) at 45°.

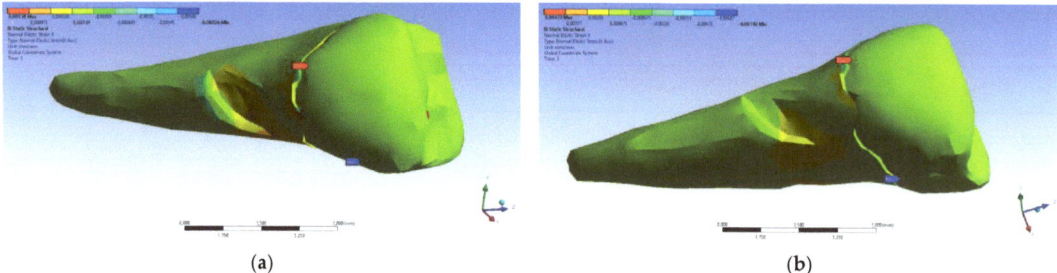

Figure 33. Mesio-buccal aspects of the normal elastic strain X when applying the experimental force to the occlusal surface: (**a**) perpendicularly; and (**b**) at 45°.

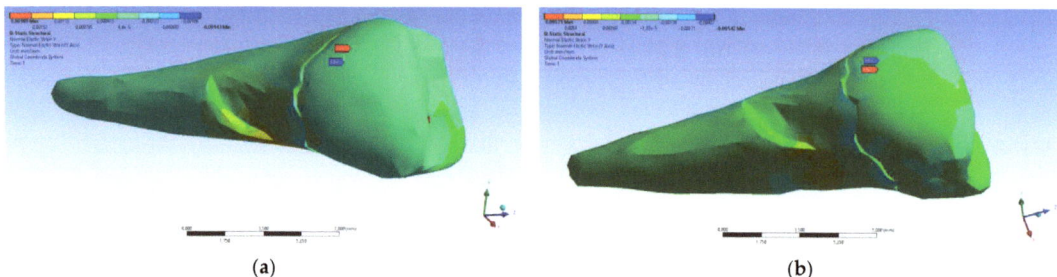

Figure 34. Mesio-buccal aspects of the normal elastic strain Y when applying the experimental force to the occlusal surface: (**a**) perpendicularly; and (**b**) at 45°.

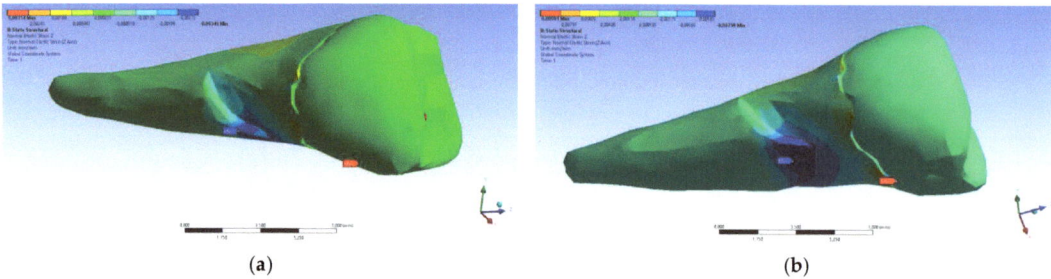

Figure 35. Mesio-buccal aspects of the normal elastic strain Z when applying the experimental force to the occlusal surface: (**a**) perpendicularly; and (**b**) at 45°.

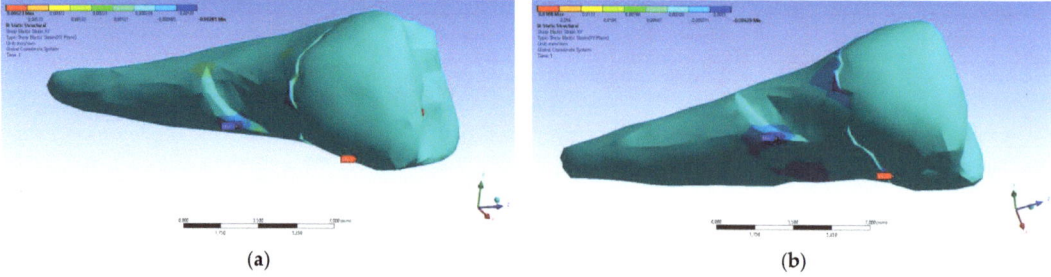

Figure 36. Mesio-buccal aspects of the shear elastic strain XY after the application of an experimental force to the occlusal surface: (**a**) perpendicularly; and (**b**) at 45°.

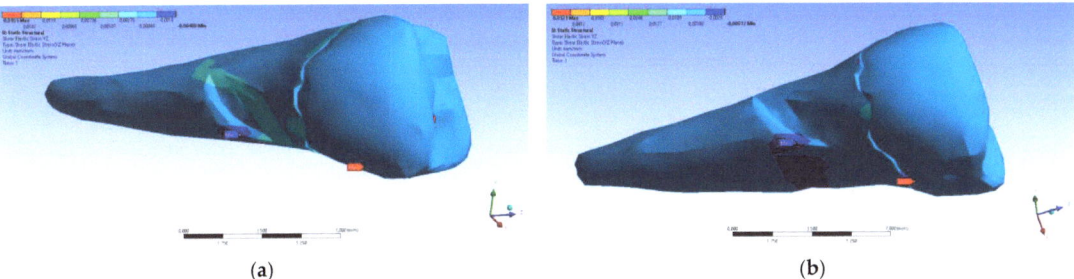

Figure 37. Mesio-buccal aspects of the shear elastic strain YZ after the application of an experimental force to the occlusal surface: (**a**) perpendicularly; and (**b**) at 45°.

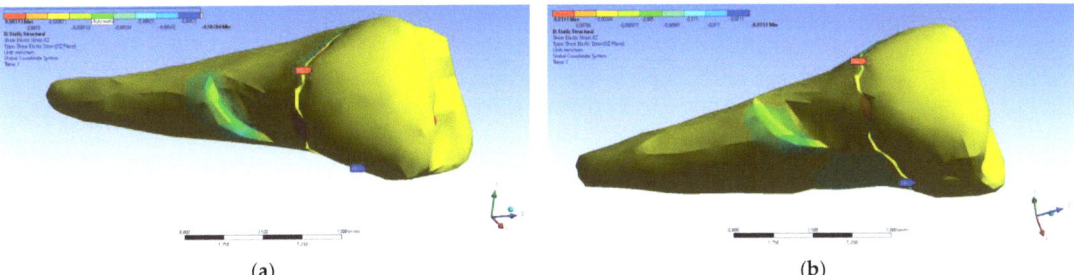

Figure 38. Mesio-buccal aspects of the shear elastic strain XZ after the application of an experimental force to the occlusal surface: (**a**) perpendicularly; and (**b**) at 45°.

As in the case of the other determinations, the inclined application of the forces will lead to the development of more important deformations than in the case of the perpendicular application of the occlusal stresses.

The experimental FEA research of the forces exerted on the lower premolars with abfraction lesions was carried out in order to demonstrate the fact that the axial overstressing forces and those applied at an angle of 45 degrees possibly induce the appearance of unwanted effects on the dental hard tissues in their cervical areas.

The patient was assessed during further dental visits every month for 3 months. She continued to complain about the signs of bruxism, but without experiencing the painful sensitivity in the lower right premolars with abfraction. For this reason, it was indicated that the patient should continue wearing the custom-made mouth guard.

After 8 months of wearing the customized thermoformed mouth guard, the patient agreed to participate in the recording of dynamic occlusal measurements using a digital T-Scan device. This device determined the levels of occlusal loads on the teeth of both dental arches, especially on the lower mandibular premolars that had abfraction lesions. In this way, the subsequent dental therapy necessary to obtain a stable occlusion of the patient's teeth could be established.

4. Literature Review

To accomplish this systematic literature review, a bibliographic survey was carried out in national and international scientific journals indexed in medical databases such as EBSCO, Medline, Google Scholar, PubMed, SciELO, Scopus, Web of Science. The keywords included "noncarious cervical lesion (NCCL)", "abfraction", "premolars", "finite element method (FEM)", and "finite element analysis (FEA)" in the title or abstract.

These searches included English-language articles published between January 2014 and December 2023, tracking original research with full access. All identified articles were chosen according to their relevance and objectivity in relation to the topic under study. Data collection involved the study's selection and data extraction. The article selection for review was undertaken separately by two reviewers towards their possible inclusion after their eligibility criteria were determined. In the first phase, 198 articles and abstracts were chosen.

The inclusion criteria were as follows: the presence of the keywords applied for searching, articles with the search terms in the title or abstract, and original articles published between the years 2014 and 2023.

The exclusion criteria were as follows: non-English language specialty literature; case reports; abstracts; editorial letters; laboratory and animal studies; studies based on questionnaires; treatment management studies; literature reviews, citations, patents, books, dissertation theses, reference books, print-ahead articles, articles that were outside the theme researched for the review, and published before 2014 or after 2023.

Thirty-four articles were eliminated as not related to the research topic. The remaining 29 articles were screened to exclude duplicates and irrelevant papers. Eighteen articles published before 2014 or after 2023 were discarded after reading and analysis according to the exclusion criteria.

In the next stage, references in the included articles were also read in order to identify additional relevant literature. Three researchers extracted the data, and the other three validated it. The eligibility of the articles included in the review was resolved by consensus, with no disagreements. After applying all the selection criteria (derived from the inclusion and exclusion criteria), only eleven articles remained in the study for this review.

A brief description of the included articles in this study is presented in Table 6, and the results and conclusions related to those articles are shown in Table 7 [24–34].

Table 6. Brief description of included articles in the study [24–34].

Author, Reference No., Year	Title of Article	Aim of Study	Methodology/Data Analyzed with FEM	Values, Location of Load
Jakupović S. et al. 2014 [24]	Analysis of the abfraction lesions formation mechanism by the FEM	The authors evaluated stress in the lower premolar under static solicitations.	The intact tooth was scanned with a µCT 1076 SkyScan scanner (Kontich, Belgium). The images were reconstructed with the Nrecon (Skyscan) program into trans-axial sections. The additional reduction of input data was implemented, and the reconstruction of the 3D model was realized. Analyses of µCT section data were performed with the CTAn program (Skyscan), by using a 3D CAD tooth model (Matlab, Creo Parametric 1.0) with the Ansys Workbench 14.0 program.	200 N Paraxial 40°
Soares P.V. et al. 2015 [25]	Loading and composite restoration assessment of different non-carious cervical lesions morphologies—3D FEA	The impacts of various occlusal loadings on premolars with NCCLs (unrestored or restored with composite resins) were studied with 3D FEA.	The intact tooth was set in a contact scanner (MDX-40, Roland Co., Osaka, Japan). The 3D models of FEA were manufactured by simulating an intact tooth model, models with NCCL morphologies, and restored models of all types of lesions. For creating the volume of external and internal shapes of hard and soft tissues of tooth, the STL files were exported to CAD (Computer Assisted Design; Rhino3D 4.0, Rhinoceros, USA) software. NCCL morphologies and their restorations were obtained through Boolean operations. The models were examined with the biomechanical analysis software ANSYS 12.0 (Ansys Workbench 12.0.1, PA, EUA), with STEP format software, for pre-processing, processing, and post-processing. After the conversion mesh test, the solid quadratic tetrahedral components with ten nodes were utilized.	100 N Vertical Paraxial 45° buccal and palatal loading

Table 6. Cont.

Author, Reference No., Year	Title of Article	Aim of Study	Methodology/Data Analyzed with FEM	Values, Location of Load
Zeola I.F. et al. 2015 [26]	Influence of non-carious cervical lesions depth, loading point application and restora-tion on stress distribution pattern in lower pre-molars: A 2D FEA	The authors investigated the biomechanical behavior of lower premolars (the NCCL depth, load type, and restoration status) using FEA.	The intact extracted lower premolar scan images were studied with two-dimensional FEM. The scan data were exported to computer-aided design software (Autodesk Mechanical Desktop 6; Autodesk Inc., San Rafael, CA, USA) to generate the external contours of tooth structure and the polyether/polystyrene cylinder. The polyline module of CAD software was used for defining the tooth shapes, points, and line associations. The generated 2D FEA models were the healthy tooth, the three sizes of NCCL (small, medium, and deep), and the restored lesions. The obtained data were exported to CAE (computer-aided engineering) software (ANSYS 12.0, ANSYS Inc., Houston, TX, USA), using the *.IGES format. In the pre-processing phase, eight-noded isopara-metric plane elements were utilized (PLANE 183). The quantitative examination of strain (MPa) was determined at the enamel surface (on its upper wall), dentin (at the bottom wall), and dentin (on the lower wall) of the NCCLs.	100 N Oblique loads on buccal cusp: on internal occlusal surface; on outer buccal cusp surface
Jakupović S. et al. 2016 [27]	Biomechanics of cervical tooth region and non-carious cervical lesions of different morphology three dimensional finite element analysis	The authors examined, through 3D FEA, the stress distribution and the biomechanical behavior of two types of occlusal charging of hard dental tissues of the lower first premolar with abfraction.	Three-dimensional models of the lower first premolar with wedge-shaped lesions and saucer-shaped lesions (U lesions) were realized. Microcomputed tomography (μCT) X-ray images were obtained. A scanner (type SkyScan 1076 Kontich, Belgium) was used. The images were rebuilt into transaxial sections by using Nrecon and CTAn program software (SkyScan). A total of 570 horizontal sections were selected for the making of the 3D models. MATLAB program packages (MathWorks, Inc., Natick, MA, USA) and Creo Parametric 1.0 CAD software were used for obtaining the volumetric 3D CAD tooth model of the lower first premolar with abfraction lesions. FEM analysis of strain under functional and nonfunctional occlusal charging was realized with CTAn program 1.10 and ANSYS Workbench version 14.0.	200 N 40°
Zeola L.F. et al 2016 [28]	Effects of non-carious cervical lesion size, occlusal loading and restoration on biomechani-cal behaviour of premolar teeth	Investigation of the influence of NCCL dimensions, of restorations, and of occlusal loading direction on biomechanical behavior, as well as load tests and fracture toughness tests in the mandibular premolars, by FEA.	The intact extracted lower premolar scan images were studied with 2D FEM. The scan data were exported to computer-aided design software (Autodesk Mechanical Desktop 6; Autodesk Inc., San Rafael, CA, USA) to generate the external contours of tooth structure and the polyether/polystyrene cylinder. The polyline module of CAD software was used for defining the tooth shapes, points, and line associations. The generated 2D FEA models were the healthy tooth, the three sizes of NCCL (small, medium, and deep), and the restored lesions. The obtained data were exported to CAE (computer-aided engineering) software (ANSYS 12.0, ANSYS Inc., Houston, USA), using the *.IGES format. In the pre-processing phase PLANE 183 program was utilized. The quantitative examination of strain (MPa) was determined at the enamel surface (on its upper wall), dentine (at the bottom wall), and dentine of the NCCLs (on the lower wall).	100 N Loads on outer and inner slopes of buccal cusp
Costa L.S.V. et al 2017 [29]	Influence of the occlusal contacts in formation of abfraction lesions in the upper premolar	The authors used FEA to observe the repartition of the stress over the upper premolar, applying centric contact, working contact, and balancing contact occlusal loading, to realize a biomechanical comparison of these contacts with increased potential to induce NCCLs.	In the 3D model, a first maxillary premolar was used, along with their specific oral tissues (enamel, dentin, a periodontal ligament), and the fixation cylinder. The file was acquired with CAD software (Rhinoceros 5.0 McNeel, North America, OH, USA) in STL format. The anatomic contours were designed using the Biocad method. Analysis software ANSYS 15.0, ANSYS Inc., Houston, TX, USA, was used. The meshes were generated by applying the tetrahedral elements and the convergence test. The mechanical properties were taken from the specialty literature and then inserted into the software for the static structural analysis. Axial and paraxial loads (40°) were reproduced for central occlusion, laterality on the occlusal slope of the oral working cusp, and interference contact to balance movement on the occlusal slope of the facial cusp. The shapes of dental elements were examined through the colorimetric scale for the determination of qualitative similarity in the simulated occlusions. The stress distribution over the course of the loadings was displayed by colorimetric graphs.	Axial loads Paraxial 40° loads on oral and buccal cusp

Table 6. Cont.

Author, Reference No., Year	Title of Article	Aim of Study	Methodology/Data Analyzed with FEM	Values, Location of Load
Machado, A.C. et al. 2017 [30]	Stress-strain analysis of premolars with non-carious cervical lesions: influence of restorative material, loading direction and mechanical fatigue.	The purpose of the study was to evaluate the stress and strain dispersion in upper pre-molars affected by NCCLs in accordance with factors such as restorative technique, direction of occlusal loads, and mechanical fatigue.	A 3D finite element analysis linear elastic investigation was conducted using the anatomical shape of the hard periodontal tissues of the tooth (pulp, dentin, enamel, periodontal ligament, and cortical and medullar bones). The 14 models were generated by Rhinoceros 3D software (Rhinoceros, Miami, FL, USA) and simulated the sound tooth, unrestored buccal saucer-shaped NCCLs, and restored NCCLs with different types of dental materials (resin-modified glass ionomer, flowable composite resin, conventional nanofilled composite resin, lithium disilicate glass ceramic, and conventional nanofilled composite resin core associated with a 0.5-mm lithium disilicate glass ceramic laminate). With the processing analysis software (ANSYS 12.0, Ansys Workbench 12.0.1, Canonsburg, PA, USA) and the Standard for the Exchange of Product Data (STEP) format, the preprocessing, processing, and postprocessing analyses were performed. A strain gauge was connected to the buccal surface of the analyzed tooth for the registration of tooth strains before and after cyclic loading (200,000 cycles, 50 N).	150 N Axial loads on both cusps Paraxial loads at a 45° angle on palatine cusp
Stănuși, A. et al. 2019 [31]	Effects of occlusal loads in the genesis of non-carious cervical lesions—a finite element study	The size and repartition of stress in a maxillary first premolar of a 14-year-old patient suspected of having normal and heavy occlusal loads was studied.	A 3D model of the upper first premolar was realized through the CT images. Eight scenarios for the vertical loads and eight scenarios for the horizontal loads were used. To obtain the 3D model, the scanned images were converted by the MIMICS program and then processed in Abaqus/CAE so that they could be studied with FEA. The 3D virtual model contained the upper right first premolar tooth (enamel, dentine, and pulp) and their alveolar bone. The tooth was not presented rigidly in the bone, and between them existed the periodontal ligament with a 0.069 GPa elastic modulus. The FEA model presented tetrahedral elements (47,548 elements and 68,504 nodes). MIMICS Program and Abaqus/CAE were used. The 3D virtual model represented by the maxillary right first premolar and their alveoli were considered a parallelepiped.	180 N and 532 N Horizontal loads Vertical loads
Vuković, A.A. et al. 2019 [32]	Occlusal Stress Distribution on the Mandibular First Premolar—FEM Analysis.	The purpose of this paper was to realize an FEM investigation of the dispensation of stress and of the deformation in a lower first premolar by applying two types of loads.	Microcomputed tomography (μCT) and a scanner (SkyScan 1076 Kontich, Belgium) were used on an intact premolar tooth under two types of loading. So a volumetric 3D CAD tooth model was obtained by the utilization of MATLAB (MathWorks, Inc., Natíck, MA, USA) program packages and Creo Parametric 1.0 CAD software. On the tooth model, a wedge-shaped abfraction lesion was formed, and then the models were transferred to the FEA software ANSYS Workbench (14.0). A FE-mesh of models was implemented. The properties of the tooth tissues were utilized. The model was fixed to simulate the periodontal ligament movement under 300μm loads and the contact points with neighboring teeth.	200 N Axial load Paraxial load
Stănuși, A. et al. 2020 [33]	Analysis of stress generated in the enamel of an upper first premolar: a finite element study	The aim of this article was to present the distribution and dimension of stress that appeared in the enamel of a maxillary first bicuspid tooth after exerting normal and excessive occlusal loadings.	A virtual model of the maxillary first premolar without any lesion was utilized to realize five models with distinct degrees of dental occlusal abrasion. The CT images of the maxillary premolar were transformed into 3D data by the MIMICS program (Materialise NV, Leuven, Belgium, 1992), and FEA was applied to study the resulting stresses. The scenarios obtained for occlusal loading of the 3D virtual model (14 in number) were investigated using the Abaqus/CAE program (ABAQUS Software, S.A.R.L., Versailles, France, 1994). The loads were exerted in the vertical and horizontal directions. The 3D models were tetrahedral elements with an average size of around 0.5 mm per surface.	180 N and 532 N Horizontal load Vertical load

Table 6. Cont.

Author, Reference No., Year	Title of Article	Aim of Study	Methodology/Data Analyzed with FEM	Values, Location of Load
Peres, T.S. et al. 2022 [34]	Influence of non-carious cervical lesions, bone attachment level, and occlusal load on the stress distribution pattern in maxillary premolars: finite element analysis.	The purpose of the study was to analyze the stress distribution design by using 3D FEA in upper premolars with and without NCCL prior to and after rehabilitation with composite resin. The impact of different occlusal loads on various bone attachment levels and tooth structure was also evaluated.	Nine CAD models were obtained after the intact models, through Rhinoceros 3D software (Rhinoceros, Miami, FL, USA). The design of the cervical area varied (intact tooth, wedge-shaped NCCL, restored NCCL with composite resin, but also normal level of bone, or with vertical and horizontal bone loss). For each model, vertical, buccal, and palatal loads were simulated. The analysis software ANSYS 12.0 (Ansys Workbench 12.0.1, Canonsburg, PA, USA). The Standard for the Exchange of Product Data (STEP) format was used, with preprocessing, processing/data calculation, and post-processing/analysis of stress dispersation. Stress values were collected after processing the models (maximum principal stress and minimum principal stress).	100 N Vertical load Buccal load Palatal load

Table 7. Description of included articles in the study (results and conclusion) [24–34].

No.	Author, Reference No., Year of Publishing	Main Results and Conclusions
1	Jakupović S. et al. [24] 2014	The action of occlusal loads (especially paraxial one) induces considerable stress in the cervical sub-superficial stratum of enamel. The stress values of the cervical area due to the paraxial loads are about five times higher in comparison with the superficial enamel layer.
2	Soares P.V. et al. [25] 2015	The morphology of NCCLs presented reduced consequences for the stress distribution design. The loading type and existence of composite resin restorations affected the biomechanical comportment of the maxillary premolars.
3	Zeola I.F. et al. [26] 2015	The depth of NCCLs is related to the intensification of the magnitude and the expansion of strain concentration. The application of loads on the external slope of the buccal cusps in mandibular premolars created a higher possibility of fracture in comparison with the application on the internal slope. Resin composite restoration of lesions augments the structural integrity and the biomechanics of roundabout NCCLs close to the healthy teeth.
4	Jakupović S. et al. [27] 2016	The exposure to occlusal loadings induces the progression of abfraction lesions. The type of action of these loadings impacts the stress intensity in the cervical area of teeth. The shape of abfraction lesions represents a major factor in the dispersal of internal stress. Underneath occlusal loads, V-shaped abfraction lesions presented notably higher stress accumulation in comparison with U-shaped abfraction lesions.
5	Zeola L.F. et al [28] 2016	The exposure to occlusal loadings induces the progression of abfraction lesions. The type of action of these loadings determines the stress intensity in the cervical area of teeth. The eccentric occlusal loads induced excessive calculated stress values in all hard tissues of the tested tooth models. The shape of the abfraction lesions also impacts the partition of internal stress in the hard tissues of the tooth.
6	Costa L.S.V. et al [29] 2017	For the quantitative comparison, the results appear in a table. The maximum values, which represent the concentrations of higher stress, are located in the enamel rather than the dentine. Eccentric contacts also present a higher possibility of progressing the abfraction lesions in the cervical area of the teeth and thus developing the size of tensile and shear stresses.
7	Machado, A.C. et al. [30] 2017	The presence of NCCLs associated with paraxial loads determined a higher stress concentration in the cervical area of the tooth. The paraxial load represented the major factor that impacted the biomechanical behavior of teeth affected by NCCLs. The restored NCCLs with composite resin alone or with ceramic laminates appears to be the optimum manner of direct rehabilitation since their biomechanical behaviors were almost identical with those of the sound teeth.

Table 7. Cont.

No.	Author, Reference No., Year of Publishing	Main Results and Conclusions
8	Stănuși, A. et al. [31] 2019	The highest values of stress were situated in the oral cervical area, but may appear in other tooth regions too, where NCCLs are not commonly found. This fact implies that the genesis of cervical noncarious lesions is multifactorial.
9	Vuković, A.A. et al [32] 2019	Under the action of occlusal paraxial loads, the strain values were greater and more notable in the cervical area. In an abfraction lesion, under a paraxial load, the measured stress values were extremely high. Exposure to the stress of V abfraction lesions will determine their deepening. The deformation of the tooth below the paraxial load was approximately 10 times greater than below the axial load.
10	Stănuși, A. et al. [33] 2020	Compressive stress predominated in the simulations of premolar models with horizontal occlusal abrasion. Both compressive and tensile stresses appeared in the simulations of the affected tooth models with oblique occlusal abrasions. The exceeding vertical and horizontal loads were prejudicial, regardless of their magnitude.
11	Peres, T.S. et al. [34] 2022	The presence of NCCL intensified the tensile stress concentration in the cervical third of the buccal surface. The tensile stress concentrations were the same in healthy and restored models. The stress level at the periodontal bone level was not affected by the presence or absence of NCCL, but it was associated with the occlusal load. The existence of NCCL contributed to the apparition of an excessive stress concentration in the tooth model cervical area, particularly when the oblique occlusal loads acted.

5. Discussion

Dental enamel, the densest calcified tissue in the body, contains, by weight, 96% inorganic material (represented by hydroxyapatite, HA), 1–2% organic material (proteins), and water. [35–37]. HA crystal orientation confers the notable mechanical properties of enamel [38]. The cement–enamel junction (CEJ) is a very sensitive zone in the cervical area of teeth, and the physiologic biomechanics of enamel and CEJ functions are difficult to study [39,40]. In the lateral areas of dental arches with interferences, the existence of parafunctional forces can influence the normal morphology of the CEJ. The amount of the organic phase at the interface influences the deformation of dental hard tissues at the enamel–dentine junction. The repeated parafunctional forces can generate excessive compressive or shearing pressure, which induces the apparition of microcracks in the HA crystals. The crack propagation in the enamel is less due to its rigid structure, and most cracks appear near the external coat of the enamel. In time, the microcracks can extend until the enamel and dentin are degraded and determine the deformation of that area [41–43]. The deformation differs at the enamel–dentine (EDJ) and cement–dentine (CDJ) junctions. The propagation of cracks is due to the rigid structure of the external layer of enamel, where the majority of microcracks are located [43,44]. The ability to maintain, through fluid percolation, the crystalline integrity in the hydroxyapatite of enamel and dentin under occlusal loads is limited [37,43]. Exposure to repetitive mechanical loads results in cumulative fatigue damage. The dysfunctional and excessive action of masticatory forces applied non-axially to malpositioned or bruxing teeth causes flexion of the teeth's crystalline structure, which induces destruction of the prismatic architecture of HA and the apparition of the specific shape of abfraction lesions due to the low packing density of the Hunter–Schreger band (HSB) in the cervical area [8,10,11]. The highest occurrence of abfractions is found in the mandibular premolars, followed by the maxillary premolars, and then by the molars, canines, and incisor teeth. This fact is probably induced by the presence of the furcation in the area adjacent to the cervical coronal area, the cervical constriction of the crown, and its small volume [7,8,10]. Chewing cycle loads can cause significant bending and flexural loads on the cusps of posterior teeth in the time of functional and parafunctional occlusal movements [45,46]. These occlusal loads can theoretically cause the occurrence of the horizontal force component too, which can determine the accumulation of tensile stress and further, the apparition of cracks in the inter-crystalline space [46,47].

The knowledge of the etiological factors in abfraction lesions and in all types of NCCLs is of major significance in order to conduct a proper diagnosis and, therefore, to realize accurate therapeutic management of NCCLs. The utilization of virtual investigations, like finite element analysis (FEA), represents an actual tendency in dentistry. Through FEA, it is possible to examine the stresses and strains of intricate systems like the orofacial system. This involves the mathematical conversion and analysis of the mechanical parameters of an object [19,21,22,35]. FEA allows for the simulation of possible clinical situations that may be encountered in practice in order to estimate the behavior of some dental structures under conditions of maximum stress [21,33,48].

Abfraction lesions represent a demineralization of the human body and can occur in association with pathological wear of the tooth due to the interaction of chemical, biological, and behavioral factors [36]. The biomechanics of abfraction lesions can also be indirectly evaluated by using the FEA method [10,19]. In our FEA study, 400 N extrinsic forces were applied perpendicularly and tilted at 45° on three axes, XY, OY, and OZ, which were high enough to induce the breakdown of cement and dentine HA crystals.

Tanaka et al. [49] realized an analysis of stress on a maxillary central incisor and mandibular first molar by using the two-dimensional finite element method (FEM) and applying the elasto–plastic deformation theory. They observed that the oblique loading spreads on the enamel surface near the CEJ and provokes plastic distortions, which in time can lead to the apparition of NCCLs. Stănuși et al. [31] observed that the values and distribution of strain were not favorable in the application of excessive horizontal loads on the studied undamaged tooth. They also pointed out that the tooth that was undamaged was the most affected by stress, regardless of the force used. In another FEA study with occlusal loads in a maxillary first premolar, the zones with an excessive concentration of forces were highlighted. The authors observed that in all models (with horizontal or oblique wear on intact tooth), stress was situated especially in the cervical area of the buccal surface of the tooth, and that the most harmful effects were caused by the excessive intensity of applied forces [33]. In conformity with the results of our FEA study, the inclined application induced stresses and deformations that were three to four times higher than in the case of the perpendicular application of experimental forces.

The dental cracks can be understood as predecessors to the formation of NCCLs, and many researchers have reported an interrelationship between occlusal loads and stress and the development of NCCLs [12,30,33,48,50–52]. Research by Donovan et al. [53] indicated that excessive vertical occlusal loads are associated with the progression of all types of NCCLs. The results of our study are in accordance with their findings, and the investigations also showed that the inclined application of the forces will lead to the development of more important deformations than in the case of a perpendicular application of occlusal stresses. Our study revealed, also, that there is a correlation between perpendicular and 45°-inclined occlusal loads and the occurrence of stress in the buccal-cervical area of the tooth.

After the research conducted by Poiate et al. [54], FEA has become appropriate for quantitative stress analysis and provides important results related to stress and displacement that are fundamental to planning preventive and restorative approaches in abfractions. Vuković A. et al. [32] used the FEA method to evaluate the distribution of stress and deformation on the lower first premolar by applying 200 N axial and non-axial loads. The stress values situated in the cervical area of the intact tooth were higher in the region of the EDJ, and the deformation values of the tooth under para-axial loads were approximately 10 times higher than the value of the deformation under an axial load.

The FEA study performed by Yang et al. [55] indicated that the developed stress appeared in axial and non-axial occlusal charges according to the level of periodontal bone support, which was induced by the hard and soft tissues of a mandibular premolar. The applied stress of 90 N was on the same buccal cusp occlusal slope, both axially and non-axially (at 45°). The stress in both the radicular dentine and the periodontal bone ridge was unevenly distributed due to the non-axial forces that were used. There was a significant increase in cases of severe bone reduction (≥50%). The authors also found that the decrease in periodontal bone support can induce the apical expansion of the tooth defect. Our analysis reported that the occlusal stresses' perpendicular solicitations lead to less significant deformations than in the case of the inclined application of the forces.

Excessive loads exerted on teeth can induce the development of periodontal disorders. In their research, Luchian et al. studied, through FEM, the occurrence of periodontal damage to mandibular incisors under the action of different degrees of orthodontic forces and the potential risks for the development of periodontal diseases, although these effects were still not clinically recognized. They concluded that the anatomical particularities should be taken into consideration in the application of orthodontic forces to incisors with damaged periodontal tissues [56].

Many authors consider that, although time-consuming, FEA analysis helps us to explain the occurrence of a series of unwanted phenomena at the level of some teeth, implants, direct or indirect restorations, and the dental materials used, and can indicate the vulnerable areas where maximum stresses and deformations are developed [57–62]. Jakupović A. et al. [63] found that the type of tooth loading has the greatest influence on the intensity of stress. The values of the obtained stresses in the restorative material and dental tissues differ due to the different mechanical properties of the materials. Restoration of NCCLs significantly reduces extremely high stress values at their bottom. Dam Van et al. [64] underlined that FEA is an important tool in implant dentistry to study the stress distribution on the adjoining bone, the biomechanics of dental implants and bone, the implant and bone interface, and their fatigue behaviors. Other authors concluded that since the experimental capabilities in implant dentistry are greatly limited by the ethical aspects of research on human subjects, FEAs are useful procedures for understanding the micro-displacements of dental implants and the mode of transmission of stresses, strains, and deformations at the bone level, with direct implications for the involved tissues [19,65–70].

Finite element analysis is appropriate for quantitative static stress analysis and provides important results for both stress and displacement. These are fundamental to planning preventive and restorative approaches in NCCLs [69–71]. Although this FEA study has useful results for establishing correlations with clinical data, it still has limitations, which should be considered.

The controversial etiology and questionable diagnosis of NCCLs have often led to an erroneous approach to their therapeutic management. Through FEA results, the stress distribution values of dental hard tissues, which are appreciably impacted by their properties, like the elastic modulus and surface properties, can be highlighted [72]. FEA also enables the evaluation of the fracture risk of a tooth or dental implant in accordance with the distribution and orientation of stress [62,64].

Our study is limited in that it examined a single case. Longitudinal studies in enlarged samples will make it possible to assess the development of abfraction lesions due to occlusal loads and interferences and test the efficiency of dental materials and restorative treatments. Another limitation of the study is that FEA is a computerized investigation realized after patient data were input from CBCT, which means that the clinical conditions may not have been totally reproduced. FEA studies should always be completed with a personalized clinical evaluation. The exactitude and the material properties of the data utilized in the model influence the FEA predictions [19]. Currently, the involvement of occlusal forces in the formation of structural defects in abfractions is beyond question.

The detection of non-carious abfraction lesions in the cervical area of the dental hard tissues by the clinician (especially at the level of the upper canines and the maxillary and mandibular premolars) indicate that the patient will require occlusal balancing therapy in the future. Various ulterior occlusion analysis systems can be used to record detailed data regarding the existence of excessive occlusal forces (including the T-Scan digital device), but these types of analyses can only be performed in the presence of the patient.

This study recognized the relationship between the morphology of the studied teeth and the effect of axial and inclined forces on the apparition and advancement of NCCLs.

The clinical relevance of the study is that it reinforces the use of FEA to realize scientific validation of the biomechanical features regarding hard dental structures, their supporting tissues, and the dental biomaterials used in direct and indirect oral rehabilitation.

The results of this study may not be postulated to the general population because the cause of abfraction lesions is multifactorial and, at the same time, each patient presents individual characteristics that conventionally cannot be generalized.

The implications of this study for current dental practice should be emphasized. When examining a patient for the first time, the presence of abfraction lesions located in the cervical area of the teeth can indicate, to the clinician, possible overloading of the occlusal forces, which is why the clinician must perform a detailed history of the disease, a thorough anamnesis, and a complete examination of the patient. Future applications should focus on strategies for decreasing or eliminating paraxial loads in the optimization of temporomandibular joint models, teeth, dental implants, dentures, orthodontic appliances, etc., for proper dental therapeutic management.

The diagnosis and correction of occlusal imbalances are easier to achieve with interdisciplinary collaboration. In this manner, the choice of treatment should be realized in accordance with other clinical and complementary examinations in order to increase the patient's quality of life, because oral health is a major critical factor for general health and wellbeing.

6. Conclusions

The realized FEA demonstrated that the most vulnerable areas, where shears, stresses, and maximum deformations occurred, were in the cervical areas of the abfraction lesions.

The stresses occurred regardless of the ways in which the force was applied (perpendicular or inclined at $45°$). In all cases, the inclined application led to a three-fourths higher development of stresses and deformations than in the case of the perpendicular application of the experimental forces.

Using computer simulations in imaging analysis and mechanical efforts through FEA can provide valuable information and offer solutions for a better understanding of the mechanisms involved in the masticatory stresses and strains on teeth.

Author Contributions: Conceptualization, A.B. (Alexandru Burcea), B.C.C. and E.S.B.; data curation, A.B. (Alexandru Burcea) and A.B. (Anamaria Bechir); formal analysis, A.B. (Alexandru Burcea), L.L.M. and M.T.; investigation, A.B. (Anamaria Bechir) and L.L.M.; methodology, A.B. (Alexandru Burcea), B.C.C., E.S.B. and L.L.M.; project administration, B.C.C. and L.L.M.; resources, B.C.C., A.B. (Alexandru Burcea) and E.S.B.; software, E.S.B. and M.T.; supervision, A.B. (Anamaria Bechir), E.S.B., L.L.M. and M.T.; validation, A.B. (Anamaria Bechir) and M.T.; visualization, A.B. (Alexandru Burcea), B.C.C. and L.L.M.; writing—original draft preparation, A.B. (Anamaria Bechir), B.C.C. and M.T.; writing—review and editing, A.B. (Anamaria Bechir), M.T. and E.S.B. M.T., A.B. (Alexandru Burcea) and L.L.M. contributed equally to this work. All authors have read and agreed to the published version of the manuscript.

Funding: This research received no external funding.

Institutional Review Board Statement: The study was accomplished by the implementation of the ethical principles of the Declaration of Helsinki and of the good clinical practice. The protocol was authorized by the Ethics Committee of Dental Medicine Faculty, Titu Maiorescu University of Bucharest (No. 7 of 14 January 2019).

Informed Consent Statement: Informed consent was obtained from the subject involved in the study. Written informed consent has been obtained from the patients to publish this paper.

Data Availability Statement: Data supporting the reported results are contained within the article.

Conflicts of Interest: The authors declare no conflicts of interest.

References

1. Tsuchida, S.; Nakayama, T. Recent Clinical Treatment and Basic Research on the Alveolar Bone. *Biomedicines* **2023**, *11*, 843. [CrossRef] [PubMed]
2. Foster, B.L.; Ao, M.; Salmon, C.R.; Chavez, M.B.; Kolli, T.N.; Tran, A.B.; Chu, E.Y.; Kantovitz, K.R.; Yadav, M.; Narisawa, S.; et al. Osteopontin regulates dentin and alveolar bone development and mineralization. *Bone* **2018**, *107*, 196–207. [CrossRef] [PubMed]
3. Jiang, N.; Guo, W.; Chen, M.; Zheng, Y.; Zhou, J.; Kim, S.G.; Embree, M.C.; Songhee Song, K.; Marao, H.F.; Mao, J.J. Periodontal Ligament and Alveolar Bone in Health and Adaptation: Tooth Movement. *Front. Oral Biol.* **2016**, *18*, 1–8. [CrossRef] [PubMed]
4. Bănuț Oneț, D.; Barbu Tudoran, L.; Delean, A.G.; Șurlin, P.; Ciurea, A.; Roman, A.; Bolboacă, S.D.; Gasparik, C.; Muntean, A.; Soancă, A. Adhesion of Flowable Resin Composites in Simulated Wedge-Shaped Cervical Lesions: An In Vitro Pilot Study. *Appl. Sci.* **2021**, *11*, 3173. [CrossRef]
5. Zabolotna, I. Study of the morphological structure of enamel and correlation of its chemical composition with dentin in intact teeth and with a cervical pathology. *J. Stomatol.* **2021**, *74*, 9–15. [CrossRef]
6. Goldberg, M. Non-carious cervical lesions (NCCL). *J. Dent. Health Oral Disord. Ther.* **2021**, *12*, 67–72. [CrossRef]
7. Nascimento, M.M.; Dilbone, D.A.; Pereira, P.N.; Duarte, W.R.; Geraldeli, S.; Delgado, A.J. Abfraction lesions: Etiology, diagnosis, and treatment options. *Clin. Cosmet. Investig. Dent.* **2016**, *3*, 79–87. [CrossRef] [PubMed]
8. Badavannavar, A.N.; Ajari, S.; Nayak, K.U.; Khijmatgar, S. Abfraction: Etiopathogenesis, clinical aspect, and diagnostic-treatment modalities: A review. *Indian J. Dent. Res.* **2020**, *31*, 305–311. [CrossRef] [PubMed]
9. Konagala, R.K.; Mandava, J.; Anupreeta, A.; Mohan, R.B.; Murali, K.S.; Lakshman, V.U. AbfractionParadox—A Literature Review on Biomechanics, Diagnosis And Management. *Int. J. Sci. Res.* **2018**, *7*, 46–49.
10. Rusu Olaru, A.; Popescu, M.R.; Dragomir, L.P.; Rauten, A.M. Clinical Study on Abfraction Lesions in Occlusal Dysfunction. *Curr. Health Sci. J.* **2019**, *45*, 390–397. [CrossRef]
11. David, M.C.; Almeida, C.P.; Almeida, M.P.; Araújo, T.S.B.; Vanzella, A.C.B.; Filho, I.J.Z.; Bernardes, V.L. Prevalence of Non-Carious Cervical Lesions and Their Relation to Para-functional Habits: Original Study. *Health Sci. J.* **2018**, *12*, 557. [CrossRef]
12. Zuza, A.; Racic, M.; Ivkovic, N.; Krunic, J.; Stojanovic, N.; Bozovic, D.; Bankovic-Lazarevic, D.; Vujaskovic, M. Prevalence of non-carious cervical lesions among the general population of the Republic of Srpska, Bosnia and Herzegovina. *Int. Dent. J.* **2019**, *69*, 281–288. [CrossRef] [PubMed]
13. Peumans, M.; Politano, G.; Van Meerbeek, B. Treatment of noncarious cervical lesions: When, why, and how. *Int. J. Esthet. Dent.* **2020**, *15*, 16–42. [PubMed]
14. Cruz, S.E.T.; Gadelha, V.R.; Gadelha, V.M. Non-carious cervical injuries: Etiological, clinical and therapeutic considerations. *Rev. Cubana Estomatol.* **2019**, *56*, 1–17.
15. Plevris, V.; Tsiatas, G.C. Computational Structural Engineering: Past Achievements and Future Challenges. *Front. Built Environ.* **2018**, *4*, 21. [CrossRef]
16. Liu, Y.; Wu, R.; Yang, A. Research on Medical Problems Based on Mathematical Models. *Mathematics* **2023**, *11*, 2842. [CrossRef]
17. Agarwal, S.K.; Mittal, R.; Singhal, R.; Hasan, S.; Chaukiyal, K. Stress evaluation of maxillary central incisor restored with different post materials: A finite element analysis. *J. Clin. Adv. Dent.* **2020**, *4*, 22–27. [CrossRef]
18. Liu, W.K.; Li, S.; Park, H.S. Eighty Years of the Finite Element Method: Birth, Evolution, and Future. *Arch. Comput. Methods Eng.* **2022**, *29*, 4431–4453. [CrossRef]
19. Bandela, V.; Kanaparthi, S. *Finite Element Analysis and Its Applications in Dentistry*; IntechOpen: London, UK, 2021; Available online: https://www.intechopen.com/chapters/74006 (accessed on 6 October 2022). [CrossRef]
20. Cipollina, A.; Ceddia, M.; Di Pietro, N.; Inchingolo, F.; Tumedei, M.; Romasco, T.; Piattelli, A.; Specchiulli, A.; Trentadue, B. Finite Element Analysis (FEA) of a Premaxillary Device: A New Type of Subperiosteal Implant to Treat Severe Atrophy of the Maxilla. *Biomimetics* **2023**, *8*, 336. [CrossRef]
21. Lisiak-Myszke, M.; Marciniak, D.; Bieliński, M.; Sobczak, H.; Garbacewicz, Ł.; Drogoszewska, B. Application of Finite Element Analysis in Oral and Maxillofacial Surgery-A Literature Review. *Materials* **2020**, *13*, 3063. [CrossRef]
22. Shruti, S.; Shrishail, K.V.; Priyanka, T. Applications of finite element analysis in dentistry: A review. *J. Int. Oral Health* **2021**, *13*, 415–422.
23. Ornelas, D.A.T.; Vela, M.O.R.; García Palencia, P. Abfraction: Etiopathogenesis, clinical aspect, diagnosis and treatment, a review literature. *Int. J. Appl. Dent. Sci. (IJADS)* **2022**, *8*, 97–100. [CrossRef]
24. Jakupovic, S.; Cerjakovic, E.; Topcic, A.; Ajanovic, M.; Konjhodzic-Prcic, A.; Vukovic, A. Analysis of the Abfraction Lesions Formation Mechanism by the Finite Element Method. *Acta Inform. Medica* **2014**, *22*, 241–245. [CrossRef]
25. Soares, P.V.; Machado, A.C.; Zeola, L.F.; Souza, P.G.; Galvão, A.M.; Montes, T.C.; Pereira, A.G.; Reis, B.R.; Coleman, T.A.; Grippo, J.O. Loading and composite restoration assessment of various non-carious cervical lesions morphologies—3D finite element analysis. *Aust. Dent. J.* **2015**, *60*, 309–316. [CrossRef] [PubMed]
26. Zeola, L.F.; Pereira, F.A.; Galvão, A.; Da, M.; Montes, T.C.; De Sousa, S.C.; Teixeira, D.N.R.; Reis, B.R.; Soares, P.V. Influence of noncarious cervical lesions depth, loading point application and restoration on stress distribution pattern in lower premolars: A 2D finite element analysis. *Biosci. J.* **2015**, *31*, 648–656. [CrossRef]
27. Jakupović, S.; Anic, I.; Ajanovic, M.; Korac, S.; Konjhodzic, A.; Dzankovic, A.; Vuković, A. Biomechanics of cervical tooth region and noncarious cervical lesions of different morphology; three dimensional finite element analysis. *Eur. J. Dent.* **2016**, *10*, 413–418. [CrossRef]

28. Zeola, L.F.; Pereira, F.A.; Machado, A.C.; Reis, B.R.; Kaidonis, J.; Xie, Z.; Townsend, G.C.; Ranjitkar, S.; Soares, P.V. Effects of non-carious cervical lesion size, occlusal loading and restoration on biomechanical behaviour of premolar teeth. *Aust. Dent. J.* **2016**, *61*, 408–417. [CrossRef] [PubMed]
29. Costa, L.S.V.; Tribst, J.P.M.; Borges, A.L.S. Influence of the occlusal contacts in formation of Abfraction Lesions in the upper premolar. *Braz. Dent. Sci.* **2017**, *20*, 115–123. [CrossRef]
30. Machado, A.C.; Soares, C.J.; Reis, B.R.; Bicalho, A.A.; Raposo, L.; Soares, P.V. Stress-strain analysis of premolars with non-carious cervical lesions: Influence of restorative material, loading direction and mechanical fatigue. *Oper. Dent.* **2017**, *42*, 253–265. [CrossRef]
31. Stănuși, A.; Mercuț, V.; Scrieciu, M.; Popescu, M.S.; Crăițoiu Iacob, M.M.; Dăguci, L.; Castravete, S.; Vintilă, D.D.; Vătu, M. Effects of occlusal loads in the genesis of non-carious cervical lesions—A finite element study. *Rom. J. Oral Rehabil.* **2019**, *11*, 73–81.
32. Vuković, A.; Jakupović, S.; Zukić, S.; Bajsman, A.; Gavranović Glamoč, A.; Šečić, S. Occlusal Stress Distribution on the Mandibular First Premolar—FEM Analysis. *Acta Med. Acad.* **2019**, *48*, 255–261. [CrossRef] [PubMed]
33. Stănuși, A.; Mercuț, V.; Scrieciu, M.; Popescu, S.M.; Iacov Crăițoiu, M.M.; Dăguci, L.; Castravete, Ș.; Amărăscu, M.O. Analysis of stress generated in the enamel of an upper first premolar: A finite element study. *Stoma Edu J.* **2020**, *7*, 28–34. [CrossRef]
34. Peres, T.S.; Teixeira, D.N.R.; Soares, P.V.; Zeola, L.F.; Machado, A.C. Influence of non-carious cervical lesions, bone attachment level, and occlusal load on the stress distribution pattern in maxillary premolars: Finite element analysis. *Biosci. J.* **2022**, *38*, e38072. [CrossRef]
35. Shaik, I.; Dasari, B.; Shaik, A.; Doos, M.; Kolli, H.; Rana, D.; Tiwari, R.V.C. Functional Role of Inorganic Trace Elements on Enamel and Dentin Formation: A Review. *J. Pharm. Bioallied Sci.* **2021**, *13* (Suppl. 2), S952–S956. [CrossRef] [PubMed]
36. Lee, E.-S.; Wadhwa, P.; Kim, M.-K.; Bo Jiang, H.; Um, I.-W.; Kim, Y.-M. Organic Matrix of Enamel and Dentin and Developmental Defects. In *Human Tooth and Developmental Dental Defects—Compositional and Genetic Implications*; IntechOpen: London, UK, 2022; Available online: https://www.intechopen.com/chapters/77993 (accessed on 21 April 2023). [CrossRef]
37. Roberts, W.E.; Mangum, J.E.; Schneider, P.M. Pathophysiology of Demineralization, Part I: Attrition, Erosion, Abfraction, and Noncarious Cervical Lesions. *Curr. Osteoporos. Rep.* **2022**, *20*, 90–105. [CrossRef]
38. Stifler, C.A.; Jakes, J.E.; North, J.D.; Green, D.R.; Weaver, J.C.; Pupa, G. Crystal misorientation correlates with hardness in tooth enamels. *Acta Biomater.* **2021**, *120*, 124–134. [CrossRef]
39. Koju, S.; Maharjan, N.; Yadav, D.K.; Bajracharya, D.; Baral, R.; Ojha, B. Morphological analysis of cementoenamel junction in permanent dentition based on gender and arches. *J. Kantipur Dent. Coll.* **2021**, *2*, 24–28.
40. Nguyen, K.-C.T.; Yan, Y.; Kaipatur, N.R.; Major, P.W.; Lou, E.H.; Punithakumar, K.; Le, L.H. Computer-Assisted Detection of Cemento-Enamel Junction in Intraoral Ultrasonographs. *Appl. Sci.* **2021**, *11*, 5850. [CrossRef]
41. Yap, R.C.; Alghanem, M.; Martin, N. A narrative review of cracks in teeth: Aetiology, microstructure and diagnostic challenges. *J. Dent.* **2023**, *138*, 104683. [CrossRef]
42. Stănuși, A.; Ionescu, M.; Cerbulescu, C.; Popescu, S.M.; Osiac, E.; Mercuț, R.; Scrieciu, M.; Pascu, R.M.; Stănuși, A.Ș.; Mercuț, V. Modifications of the Dental Hard Tissues in the Cervical Area of Occlusally Overloaded Teeth Identified Using Optical Coherence Tomography. *Medicina* **2022**, *58*, 702. [CrossRef]
43. Shen, L.; Barbosa de Sousa, F.; Tay, N.; Lang, T.S.; Kaixin, V.L.; Han, J.; Kilpatrick-Liverman, L.; Wang, W.; Lavender, S.; Pilch, S.; et al. Deformation behavior of normal human enamel: A study by nanoindentation. *J. Mech. Behav. Biomed. Mater.* **2020**, *108*, 103799. [CrossRef] [PubMed]
44. Bhanderi, S. Facts about cracks in teeth. *Prim. Dent. J.* **2021**, *10*, 20–27. [CrossRef]
45. Wan, B.; Shahmoradi, M.; Zhang, Z.; Shibata, Y.; Sarrafpour, B.; Swain, M.; Li, Q. Modelling of stress distribution and fracture in dental occlusal fissures. *Sci. Rep.* **2019**, *9*, 4682. [CrossRef] [PubMed]
46. Morimoto, S.; Lia, W.K.C.; Gonçalves, F.; Nagase, D.Y.; Gimenez, T.; Raggio, D.P.; Özcan, M. Risk Factors Associated with Cusp Fractures in Posterior Permanent Teeth—A Cross-Sectional Study. *Appl. Sci.* **2021**, *11*, 9299. [CrossRef]
47. Wilmers, J.; Bargmann, S. Nature's design solutions in dental enamel: Uniting high strength and extreme damage resistance. *Acta Biomater.* **2020**, *107*, 1–24. [CrossRef] [PubMed]
48. Goodacre, C.J.; Roberts, W.E.; Munoz, C.A. Noncarious cervical lesions: Morphology and progression, prevalence, etiology, pathophysiology, and clinical guidelines for restoration. *J. Prosthodont.* **2023**, *32*, e1–e18. [CrossRef] [PubMed]
49. Tanaka, M.; Naito, T.; Yokota, M.; Kohno, M. Finite element analysis of the possible mechanism of cervical lesion formation by occlusal force. *J. Oral Rehabil.* **2003**, *30*, 60–67. [CrossRef] [PubMed]
50. Maayan, E.; Ariel, P.; Waseem, H.; Andrey, G.; Daniel, R.; Rachel, S. Investigating the etiology of non-carious cervical lesions: Novel μCT analysis. *J. Dent.* **2023**, *136*, 104615. [CrossRef] [PubMed]
51. Teixeira, D.N.R.; Zeola, L.F.; Machado, A.C.; Gomes, R.R.; Souza, P.G.; Mendes, D.C.; Soares, P.V. Relationship between noncarious cervical lesions, cervical dentin hypersensitivity, gingival recession, and associated risk factors: A cross-sectional study. *J. Dent.* **2018**, *76*, 93–97. [CrossRef]
52. Lim, G.E.; Son, S.A.; Hur, B.; Park, J.K. Evaluation of the relationship between non-caries cervical lesions and the tooth and periodontal tissue: An ex-vivo study using micro-computed tomography. *PLoS ONE* **2020**, *15*, e0240979. [CrossRef]
53. Donovan, T.E.; Marzola, R.; Murphy, K.R.; Cagna, D.R.; Eichmiller, F.; McKee, J.R.; Metz, J.E.; Albouy, J.P.; Troeltzsch, M. Annual Review of Selected Scientific Literature: Report of the Committee on Scientific Investigation of the American Academy of Resto-rative Dentistry. *J. Prosthet. Dent.* **2017**, *118*, 281–346. [CrossRef] [PubMed]

54. Poiate, I.; Muramatsu, M.; Mori, M.; Campos, T.; Matsuda, K.; Lopez, M.; Poiate, E., Jr. Abfraction lesion in central incisor tooth: Displacement and stress evaluation by laser speckle and finite element analysis. *Med. Res. Arch.* **2023**, *11*, 1–20. [CrossRef]
55. Yang, S.; Chung, H. Three-dimentional finite element analysis of a mandibular premolar with reduced periodontal support under a non-axial load. *Oral Biol. Res.* **2019**, *43*, 313–326. [CrossRef]
56. Luchian, I.; Martu, M.A.; Tatarciuc, M.; Scutariu, M.M.; Ioanid, N.; Pasarin, L.; Kappenberg-Nitescu, D.C.; Sioustis, I.A.; Solomon, S.M. Using fem to assess the effect of orthodontic forces on affected periodontium. *Appl. Sci.* **2021**, *11*, 7183. [CrossRef]
57. Alemayehu, D.B.; Jeng, Y.R. Three-Dimensional Finite Element Investigation into Effects of Implant Thread Design and Loading Rate on Stress Distribution in Dental Implants and Anisotropic Bone. *Materials* **2021**, *14*, 6974. [CrossRef] [PubMed]
58. Germán-Sandoval, R.; Ortiz-Magdaleno, M.; Sánchez-Robles, P.; Zavala-Alonso, N.; Fernando Romo-Ramírez, G. Analysis of the Mechanical Behavior and Effect of Cyclic Fatigue on the Implant-Abutment Interface. *Odovtos Int. J. Dent. Sci.* **2021**, *23*, 104–114. [CrossRef]
59. Nie, H.; Tang, Y.; Yang, Y.; Wu, W.; Zhou, W.; Liu, Z. Influence of a new abutment design concept on the biomechanics of peri-implant bone, implant components, and microgap formation: A finite element analysis. *BMC Oral Health* **2023**, *23*, 277. [CrossRef] [PubMed]
60. Comaneanu, R.M.; Mihali, T.; Gioga, C.; Pangica, A.-M.; Perlea, P.; Coman, C.; Hancu, V.; Botoaca, O.; Voiculeanu, M.; Tarcolea, M. FEA on the biomechanical behavior of immediately loaded implants with different sizes. *Rom. J. Stomatol.* **2023**, *69*, 116–122. [CrossRef]
61. Gönder, H.Y.; Mohammadi, R.; Harmankaya, A.; Yüksel, İ.B.; Fidancıoğlu, Y.D.; Karabekiroğlu, S. Teeth Restored with Bulk–Fill Composites and Conventional Resin Composites; Investigation of Stress Distribution and Fracture Lifespan on Enamel, Dentin, and Restorative Materials via Three-Dimensional Finite Element Analysis. *Polymers* **2023**, *15*, 1637. [CrossRef]
62. Schmid, A.; Strasser, T.; Rosentritt, M. Finite Element Analysis of Occlusal Interferences in Dental Prosthetics Caused by Occlusal Adjustment. *Int. J. Prosthodont.* **2023**, *36*, 436–442. [CrossRef]
63. Jakupović, S.; Šehić, A.; Julardžija, F.; Gavranović-Glamoč, A.; Sofić, A.; Bajsman, A.; Kazazić, L. The Influence of Different Occlusal Loading on Six Restorative Materials for Restoration of Abfraction Lesions—Finite Element Analysis. *Eur. J. Dent.* **2022**, *16*, 886–894. [CrossRef] [PubMed]
64. Dam Van, V.; Trinh Hai, A.; Dung Dao, T.; Hai Trinh, D. Applications of Finite Element in Implant Dentistry and Oral Rehabilitation. *Open Dent. J.* **2021**, *15*, 392–397. [CrossRef]
65. Reddy, M.S.; Sundram, R.; Eid Abdemagyd, H.A. Application of Finite Element Model in Implant Dentistry: A Systematic Review. *J. Pharm. Bioallied Sci.* **2019**, *11* (Suppl. 2), S85–S91. [CrossRef] [PubMed]
66. Rathod, D.K.; Chakravarthy, C.; Suryadevara, S.S.; Patil, R.S.; Wagdargi, S.S. Stress Distribution of the Zygomatic Implants in Post-mucormycosis Case: A Finite Element Analysis. *J. Maxillofac. Oral Surg.* **2023**, *22*, 695–701. [CrossRef] [PubMed]
67. Lee, C.-H.; Mukundan, A.; Chang, S.-C.; Wang, Y.-L.; Lu, S.-H.; Huang, Y.-C.; Wang, H.-C. Comparative Analysis of Stress and Deformation between One-Fenced and Three-Fenced Dental Implants Using Finite Element Analysis. *J. Clin. Med.* **2021**, *10*, 3986. [CrossRef] [PubMed]
68. Zupancic Cepic, L.; Frank, M.; Reisinger, A.; Pahr, D.; Zechner, W.; Schedle, A. Biomechanical finite element analysis of short-implant-supported, 3-unit, fixed CAD/CAM prostheses in the posterior mandible. *Int. J. Implant Dent.* **2022**, *8*, 8. [CrossRef] [PubMed]
69. Ma, D.; Qian, J. Three-dimensional finite element stress analysis of surface-mounted inlays in repairing pulp-penetrating non-carious cervical lesion of maxillary first premolar. *Hua Xi Kou Qiang Yi Xue Za Zhi* **2023**, *41*, 541–553, (In English and Chinese). [CrossRef] [PubMed]
70. Kamenskikh, A.A.; Sakhabutdinova, L.; Astashina, N.; Petrachev, A.; Nosov, Y. Numerical Modeling of a New Type of Prosthetic Restoration for Non-Carious Cervical Lesions. *Materials* **2022**, *15*, 5102. [CrossRef] [PubMed]
71. Sender, R.S.; Strait, D.S. The biomechanics of tooth strength: Testing the utility of simple models for predicting fracture in geometrically complex teeth. *J. R. Soc. Inteface* **2023**, *20*, 20230195. [CrossRef]
72. Pala, E.; Ozdemir, I.; Grund, T.; Lampke, T. The Influence of Design on Stress Concentration Reduction in Dental Implant Systems Using the Finite Element Method. *Crystals* **2024**, *14*, 20. [CrossRef]

Disclaimer/Publisher's Note: The statements, opinions and data contained in all publications are solely those of the individual author(s) and contributor(s) and not of MDPI and/or the editor(s). MDPI and/or the editor(s) disclaim responsibility for any injury to people or property resulting from any ideas, methods, instructions or products referred to in the content.

MDPI AG
Grosspeteranlage 5
4052 Basel
Switzerland
Tel.: +41 61 683 77 34

Diagnostics Editorial Office
E-mail: diagnostics@mdpi.com
www.mdpi.com/journal/diagnostics

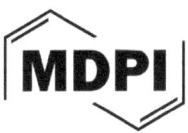

Disclaimer/Publisher's Note: The title and front matter of this reprint are at the discretion of the Guest Editors. The publisher is not responsible for their content or any associated concerns. The statements, opinions and data contained in all individual articles are solely those of the individual Editors and contributors and not of MDPI. MDPI disclaims responsibility for any injury to people or property resulting from any ideas, methods, instructions or products referred to in the content.